Psychopharmacology
An Introduction

Fourth Edition

René Spiegel
Clinical Development & Medical Affairs, Neuroscience
Novartis Pharma AG
CH-4002 Basel, Switzerland
and
Faculty of Psychology
University of Basel, Switzerland

With contributions by S. Hossein Fatemi, Conrad Gentsch,
Ferenc Martenyi, Mark Schmidt and Ed Snyder

WILEY

Other Wiley Editorial Offices

John Wiley & Sons Inc., 111 River Street, Hoboken, NJ 07030, USA

Jossey-Bass, 989 Market Street, San Francisco, CA 94103-1741, USA

Wiley-VCH Verlag GmbH, Boschstr. 12, D-69469 Weinheim, Germany

John Wiley & Sons Australia Ltd, 33 Park Road, Milton, Queensland 4064, Australia

John Wiley & Sons (Asia) Pte Ltd, 2 Clementi Loop #02-01, Jin Xing Distripark, Singapore
129809

John Wiley & Sons Canada Ltd, 22 Worcester Road, Etobicoke, Ontario, Canada
M9W 1L1

Wiley also publishes its books in a variety of electronic formats. Some content that
appears in print may not be available in electronic books.

Library of Congress Cataloging-in-Publication Data

Spiegel, René
  [Einführung in die Psychopharmakologie. English]
  Psychopharmacology an introduction / René Spiegel; with contributions
  by S. Hossein Fatemi ... [et al.].-- 4th ed.
    p. ; cm.
  Includes bibliographical references and index.
  ISBN 0 471 56039 1 (cloth : alk. paper) -- ISBN 0 470 84691 7 (pbk. : alk. paper)
    1. Psychopharmacology. I. Fatemi, S. Hossein. II. Title.
  [DNLM: 1. Psychopharmacology--methods. 2. Mental Disorders--drug therapy.
  3. Psychotropic Drugs--therapeutic use. QV 77 S755p 2003a]
  RM315.S6513 2003
  615'.78--dc21   2003049746

British Library Cataloguing in Publication Data

A catalogue record for this book is available from the British Library

ISBN: 0 471 56039 1 (cloth)
ISBN: 0 470 84691 7 (paper)

Typeset by Dobbie Typesetting Ltd, Tavistock, Devon
Printed and bound in Great Britain by TJ International, Padstow, Cornwall
This book is printed on acid-free paper responsibly manufactured from sustainable forestry
in which at least two trees are planted for each one used for paper production.

Psychopharmacology

Contents

Preface

The prototypes of modern psychopharmaceuticals were discovered between 1952 and 1958. Since that time the effective treatment of schizophrenic psychoses, depressions, anxiety syndromes and other mental disorders has become possible and a new, multidisciplinary science – biological psychiatry – has developed. Clinical psychiatry has changed dramatically in the past 50 years: fewer patients are hospitalized long term, psychiatric care and treatment have largely shifted to outpatient departments and private practices, and new models of combined pharmacological and non-drug-based prophylactic and therapeutic interventions have been developed.

When the first edition of this book was published, more than 20 years ago, the first wave of modern psychopharmacology – triggered by the partly accidental discovery of neuroleptic, antidepressant and anxiolytic drugs – was essentially over. What some consider a second wave – the period characterized by the advent of so-called atypical antipsychotic and more specifically acting antidepressant drugs – had not yet begun; use of drugs other than benzodiazepines in anxiety disorders was unusual, mood stabilizers other than lithium were not generally recognized and pharmacological treatment of Alzheimer's disease was probably not even thought of. Nevertheless, much of the basic knowledge necessary for these more recent developments was already available at that time, and many of the clinical research concepts and instruments were identical or very similar to those used today.

This fourth edition of *Psychopharmacology: an Introduction* contains some important changes from the previous ones. Most importantly, several chapters were either thoroughly revised or completely rewritten by very competent professional colleagues. This shared authorship is a direct consequence of the enormous growth of psychopharmacology that has occurred in the past few decades and the impossibility for a single person to oversee more than a few areas of this multidisciplinary science. Readers of our book should know that, with one exception, all contributors and the main author are working in the pharmaceutical industry, all for the same drug company (Novartis Pharma).

Although this could be seen as a serious source of scientific bias, all of us have made an honest effort to minimize bias, to write as scientists without attempting to support, openly or covertly, the drugs marketed by our company. Nevertheless, it was perhaps inevitable that some of the examples and studies discussed in the text originated from our own preclinical and clinical work, and that we tend to see many issues typical of our science from a rather specific standpoint.

My thanks for help go to Drs Paul Glue and Keith Wesnes, who were kind enough to review and comment on parts of the manuscript and to suggest additional references. I am grateful to many generations of mostly psychology students at the Universities of Basel and Fribourg (Switzerland) for their attention to detail and the many critical questions that have helped to shape this book. I also thank my son Simon Spiegel for his diligent help with the list of references.

Basel, March 2003

Preface to Third Edition

Almost 14 years have passed since the first edition of this 'Introduction' was published by Kohlhammer-Verlag, and the second edition was published 7 years ago by Hans Huber. The English version of this book was first published by John Wiley & Sons in 1983, who also brought out the second edition in 1989 and have now produced this third English edition.

This third edition essentially retains the structure of the second edition but its contents have been revised, with considerable changes in some parts. Thus, account is taken of the fact that a new generation of antidepressants has been available for some years, that concepts of the mechanisms of neuroleptic action have altered several times and have led to products with new mechanisms of action, and that therapeutic advances have even been recorded in a field that was only recently considered to be hopeless, namely Alzheimer's disease. New methodological developments, especially in the use of imaging techniques in psychiatry, and changes in opinions on the best possible use of psychopharmaceuticals and their duration of use in schizophrenia and depression have been suitably taken into account.

This book is aimed at doctors, psychologists and members of other professions dealing with patients and clients receiving short-term or continuous treatment with psychopharmaceuticals. It presents the desired actions and adverse effects of modern psychopharmaceuticals, their therapeutic uses and limitations, the history of psychopharmacology and research into potential new psychopharmaceuticals. The emphasis lies on the clinical and psychological aspects of psychopharmacology and psychopharmacotherapy, with only a basic consideration of the neurophysiological, molecular biological and neuroendocrinological aspects.

As in the previous editions, it was my aim to write a compact, interesting and easily readable book, and to avoid specialist jargon and technical details as far as possible, but without losing sight of my own interests. I hope that the reader will profit from this effort. I thank Mrs A. R. Knecht, who, in addition to her other duties, advanced the production of this new edition through her great personal endeavors. My thanks also go to the management at Sandoz Pharma AG, who have consistently encouraged my activities as a lecturer and author, and the Clinical Psychology students of the Universities of Basel and Fribourg, whose questions, comments and thoughts have contributed in many ways to the production of this book.

Please note that when referring to doctors, patients, students, etc. I have used the pronoun 'he' as an abbreviation of the more politically correct form 'he/she'.

Basel, July 1995

Preface to Second Edition

This introduction to psychopharmacology is a thorough revision of *Psychopharmacology*, written in conjunction with Mr H.-J Aebi and published for the first time in 1981 by Kohlhammer, Stuttgart and in 1983 by John Wiley, Chichester. Mr Aebi has for some years now been active in another field and declined co-authorship of the new edition.

This book is aimed at psychologists, psychiatrists and members of other professions dealing with patients and clients who (need to) take psychopharmaceuticals. The book presents the desired and adverse actions of modern psychopharmaceuticals, the therapeutic uses and limitations of these medicaments, the history of psychopharmacology and research into potential new psychopharmaceuticals. The emphasis lies on the clinical and psychological aspects of psychopharmacology and somewhat less on neurobiological and pharmacological topics.

It was my aim to write a compact, interesting and easily readable book, and to avoid specialist jargon and technical details as far as possible, but without losing sight of my own interests. I am sensitive to the echoes of readers and ask them not to hesitate in voicing criticisms and suggestions with a view to any new edition that may be produced.

I thank Mrs L. Brünger, who advanced the production of this book with her speedy and reliable work. My thanks also go to the superiors and colleagues at Sandoz, whose moral and material support was always welcome. My particular appreciation goes to my family for their constant consideration.

Basel, December 1988

Foreword

The fourth edition of René Spiegel's *Psychopharmacology: an Introduction* is very welcome. First, it comes after nearly a decade of exceptional growth in knowledge in the areas covered by this book: the drugs which are used to treat the major mental illnesses, the mechanism of action of these drugs, the methods used to identify and develop novel compounds, their effects in normals, and societal attitudes about cost-effectiveness of these agents, which strongly influences the extent of utilization of new drugs, which are now much more costly relative to other areas of the economy than previously. Many drugs barely discussed in the previous edition are now standard treatments in many parts of the world, e.g. the atypical antipsychotic drugs, mood stabilizers, and cholinesterase inhibitors, receive deserved detailed attention in the Fourth Edition.

Because the progress in multiple areas covered by this classic text has been so profound in recent years, René Spiegel, a psychologist and psychopharmacologist who had written nearly all of the three preceding editions himself, recruited a number of experts in specific fields of knowledge to assist in this new edition. Though most of these co-authors are from the pharmaceutical industry, I could detect no bias that this introduced into the presentation of the material that relates to their particular employers or the perspective that a disinterested academic might bring to the topic, with the welcome exception that a considerable amount of attention is given to information that concerns drug discovery and development. These are important topics which drive progress in the field and are, in fact, almost the exclusive provence of industry, as academic and government groups have delegated this function to the private sector.

However, topics such as mechanism of action and clinical applications of psychotropic drugs are given the most detailed coverage. The organization of the Third Edition has been largely retained because of its effectiveness, but with addition of two new chapters, one on Psychopharmacology and Health Economics, the other on the use of neuroimaging techniques, and broadening of the focus of the chapter on Psychopharmacology and Memory to other domains of cognition. The advantages of a single authored text have been preserved despite the expanded scope and number of authors, due, no doubt, to good communication among the various authors and skillful final editing. The final product is an exceptionally readable and informative volume which should meet the varied needs of readers at many levels of sophistication. While fulfilling the promise of the title as an Introduction to Psychopharmacology, one of the outstanding features of this book is the depth of information it provides in a number of key areas, particularly those that are clinically relevant.

This book will be of particular value to the broad range of clinicians who now have the privilege and responsibility to prescribe psychotropic drugs to clients and patients.

Chapter 1, Modern Psychopharmaceuticals, written by Dr Hossein Fatemi, and *Chapter 8*, Psychopharmaceuticals and the Treatment of Mental Disorders, provide succinct, up to date, and well-referenced information on how to use the major classes of psychotropic drugs. The latter chapter discusses in a frank and balanced manner the ambivalence towards the use of pharmacologic agents in mental disorders felt by some, and the limitations on the achievements of current drugs as ideal therapies for schizophrenia, bipolar disorder and major depression in particular. Clearly, much has been accomplished, but many needs, especially for prevention of relapse, removal of specific types of symptoms, and restoraton of work and social function, remain to be accomplished by drug and psychosocial therapies.

Chapter 2, the History of Psychopharmacology, provides one of the best short essays on this fascinating topic to be found anywhere. Although psychopharmaceuticals in today's sense have been available only for about 50 years, doctors, priests, medicine men, herbalists and others – witches! – have at all times owned knowledge of various ingredients, mainly from plants, for the relief or cure of mental suffering. Time and again the history of psychiatry shows swings between 'soft' methods of treatment (soothing, protecting, relieving, understanding the patient) and dramatically violent procedures (discipline, drill, intimidation, punishment) which, surprisingly, reached their high point in the Europe of the so-called Enlightenment. Many will also find the description of the prescribing habits of Emil Kraepelin and Eugen Bleuler, the historically most important figures in the history of schizophrenia, of great interest.

Chapter 3, Effect of Psychotropic Medications on Healthy Subjects, is rarely dealt with in texts of psychopharmacology, and is superbly treated here. As the use of psychotropic drugs spreads beyond the major diagnostic categories for which they were developed and approved, understanding the effects of psychotropic drugs on those with normal physiology has become of greater importance. Novel methods are required to assess these effects and the techniques of current interest are well described here. The study of the effects of these agents in normals has yielded considerable information that clarifies their mechanism of action in clinical conditions.

Chapter 4, Mechanisms and Action in Man and Animals, written by Dr Conrad Gentsch, provides a concise introduction to neurobiology at the cellular through systems level which facilitates understanding the range of theories about the mechanism of action of the current generation of psychotropic drugs. Where there is no consensus about mechanism of action, the most widely held views are described. The chapter is very readable and will enable beginning students to understand the major theories of mechanism of action of psychotropic drugs. It is particularly strong in the description of behavioral animal models that are used for discovery and preclinical characterization of potential new psychopharmaceuticals.

Chapter 5, Clinical Research in Psychopharmacology, written by Dr Ferenc Martenyi, offers a good description of how drugs are developed in man. It is written from the perspective of someone in the pharmaceutical industry who has first-hand knowledge of the myriad issues that lead to the enormous attrition in compounds that appear to have merit from test tube and animal studies, and then fail somewhere along the way to meet the rigid criteria for efficacy and safety, as well as tolerability, that are required of a successful addition to the list of approved drugs. Pharmacokinetics and clinical trial design, including the most important rating instruments for assessment of efficacy are discussed in considerable detail.

Chapter 6, Neuroimaging Studies in Psychopharmacology, by Dr Mark Schmidt, describes studies with modern techniques that allow direct "on-line" observations of biological processes occurring in intact and fully functional animals and human brains, and how these processes are altered by centrally acting drugs. The chapter covers the most important aspects of techniques known as SPECT (Single Photon Emission Computer Tomography), PET (Positron Emission Tomography) and fMRI (functional Magnetic Resonance Imaging), and it describes the types of scientific questions pursued with these methods as well as some limitations of the different approaches.

Chapter 7, Psychotropic Drugs and Cognitive Function, covers an area of psychopharmacology that has attracted much interest in recent years: the impact of psychopharmaceuticals on human cognitive functioning. Separate sections describe cognitive deficiencies often or regularly observed in patients with schizophrenia, depression, bipolar disorder, anxiety syndromes etc., and how these deficits are affected by antipsychotic, antidepressant, mood stabilizing, and anxiolytic etc. drugs. The current, albeit limited range of drugs useful for palliative purposes to treat Alzheimer disease and to limit its progression is also discussed.

Chapter 8, which was updated by Dr Hossein Fatemi, an experienced clinician, as mentioned above, provides expert guidance on the use of psychotropic drugs for the major mental disorders. This is the section of the book, along with Chapter 1, that clinicians in training as well as those in practice, will find most useful. It is organized by disorder and provides the necessary information to select and utilize drug treatment, with realistic guidelines about expected efficacy and side effect profiles.

Chapter 9, Psychopharmacology and Health Economics, authored by Dr Ed Snyder, explains the principles of pharmacoeconomics and its applications in psychopharmacology. Readers will find a clear statement of the methodology employed in this still developing field which is of immense importance to day. Major decisions which affect the availability of psychotropic drugs and clinical decisions by individual practitioners are often based on poorly informed concepts of cost-benefit analysis. This chapter will greatly increase the sophistication of many readers on this topic.

The *Epilogue* contains some thoughts as to how psychopharmacology has influenced modern psychiatry and psychology in practice and theory. This brief chapter also contains an account of the controversy about extending prescription authority to non-medical psychotherapists.

In summary, the new edition of Spiegel's *Psychopharmacology: an Introduction* should finds its way to the desks and bookshelves of many individuals who are seeking an up to date, thorough, practical, readable, concise summary of the best and newest knowledge in this dynamic field of knowledge which has few peers for importance to the quality of life of the general population.

Herbert Y. Meltzer, MD
Bixler Professor of Psychiatry and Professor of Pharmacology
Vanderbilt University School of Medicine

April 2003

1

Modern Psychopharmaceuticals

Revision by
HOSSEIN FATEMI

1.1 DEFINITION AND CLASSIFICATION

Psychopharmaceuticals are medications that can affect the behavior and subjective state of man and are used therapeutically on account of these 'psychotropic' effects. Apart from psychopharmaceuticals, there are many other substances with psychotropic action, such as alcohol, nicotine, cocaine and heroin, which are characterized as social or addictive products and have no generally recognized therapeutic applications in Western medicine. Analgesics and members of other drug classes also have direct or indirect actions on subjective state and behavior but are not considered to be psychopharmaceuticals because they are not used primarily for their psychotropic effects.

Like other medications also, psychopharmaceuticals can be classified according to various principles: the chemist characterizes them by their chemical structure, the pharmacologist by their actions in representative biological test systems and the doctor by their therapeutic uses or indications. The classification according to *clinical criteria* today covers the following classes of psychopharmaceuticals:

- Antipsychotics for the symptomatic treatment of schizophrenia and states of agitation occurring in other psychiatric syndromes; these medicines are also occasionally called neuroleptics or major tranquillizers.

Psychopharmacology, Fourth Edition. By R. Spiegel
© 2003 John Wiley & Sons, Ltd: ISBN 0 471 56039 1: 0 470 84691 7 (PB)

Table 1.1 Classification of psychotropic substances

Position of recognized psychotropic effect	Medications having a therapeutic action	Substances having no recognized therapeutic action
Psychotropic effect is the main effect, with the desired action	*Psychopharmaceuticals* Antipsychotics Antidepressants Mood stabilizers Anxiolytics, hypnotics Psychostimulants Nootropics, antidementia drugs	*'Social drugs', 'drugs'* Alcohol Nicotine Cocaine, heroin, etc.
Psychotropic effect is a side effect, with undesired action	Analgesics Narcotics Antihistamines Antihypertensives Appetite suppressants	

- Antidepressants for the treatment of depression; other names are thymoleptics (i.e. mood stabilizers) or thymeretics (i.e. mood activators) for a more stimulant group of antidepressants.
- Mood stabilizers for the treatment of mania or hypomania, mixed states of mania and depression or rapid cycling between mania and depression.
- Anxiolytics for the treatment of states of anxiety and tension of varied origins; they are also called minor tranquillizers. The sleep-inducing agents (hypnotics) most used today are chemically and pharmacologically closely related to tranquillizers.
- Psychostimulants are medications that can increase drive and performance. Their most frequent use is in attention deficit hyperactivity disorder (ADHD) and in narcolepsy. They are also called stimulants or, less commonly today, analeptics.
- Nootropics are substances that, especially in the elderly, may have a beneficial effect on cognitive functions without inducing general stimulation. They are being superseded by a new class of compound, the so-called antidementia drugs.

Apart from psychopharmaceuticals, there are many other substances that also affect subjective state and behavior: *'social drugs'* such as alcohol and caffeine have little or no therapeutic applications in Western medicine but undoubtedly affect subjective state and behavior, whereas the use of *'drugs'* such as marijuana, LSD, cocaine and heroin involves risks that, according to today's opinion, outweigh the possible benefits.

Other medications, which will not be discussed in the following chapters, have psychotropic actions that are considered to be side effects or adverse effects. Thus, some antihistamines (i.e. products used to counteract allergic reactions) induce fatigue and drowsiness, and the same applies to some myorelaxants. Older antihypertensives (i.e. agents reducing blood pressure) such as alpha-methyldopa (Aldomet®) or clonidine (Catapres®) can cause fatigue and depression.

Many medications have indirect psychotropic effects in that they relieve pain and other complaints and so improve well-being. Analgesics, antipyretics and anti-inflammatory products are the best-known examples. They are not considered to be psychotropic substances because they have no direct action on behavior and subjective state when given in therapeutic doses.

The following sections of this chapter concentrate on psychopharmaceuticals in the sense of Table 1.1, i.e. antipsychotics, antidepressants, mood stabilizers, anxiolytics and psychostimulants; attention also will be paid to hypnotics and antidementia drugs.

1.2 ANTIPSYCHOTICS

1.2.1 CLINICAL ACTIONS AND USES

Antipsychotics are calming medications used to counteract marked inner unrest, psychomotor agitation and severe insomnia. These states can arise within the following contexts:

- Schizophrenic psychoses, especially catatonic and paranoid forms (ICD F20.0 and F20.2, also F20.9, 23.1, 23.2, etc.).
- Mania (ICD F30.1–30.9, F31.1 and 31.2).
- Psychotic syndromes as sequelae of organic brain disorders (e.g. old age paranoia, ICD F22.0).
- Depressions, especially those with anxious, agitated symptoms (ICD F23.2 and F33.3).

Patients treated with antipsychotics find that these drugs have a pronounced calming effect that differs from that of other sedative medications (anxiolytics and hypnotics) in two major respects. Firstly, in contrast to most anxiolytics, most antipsychotics are not myorelaxant and, unlike sleep inducers, are not narcotic even in high doses. Secondly, apart from their calming action they also act on some psychotic symptoms (hence the expression 'antipsychotics'). The antipsychotic effects of these drugs generally develop only after several days or weeks of treatment. Delusions and ideas of persecution recede and partially or entirely lose their frightening character, and threatening and demanding voices become quieter or are totally silenced. The patient gives the impression of being able to cope with his surroundings in a more meaningful and comprehensible manner; his subjective state and behavior are less 'psychotic'.

The therapeutic effect of antipsychotics consists of a "calming action on psychomotor agitation, aggressive behaviour, affective tensions, psychotic illusions, psychotic delusions, catatonic behavioural disturbances, and schizophrenic ego-disturbances" (Benkert and Hippius, 1980, p. 86). This descriptive list also expresses the fact that neuroleptics have a primarily sedative action at the start of a treatment. Delay and Deniker (1953), the discoverers of the first antipsychotic, chlorpromazine (see Chapter 2), described the gradual waning of the general calming effect and the appearance of the antipsychotic action during therapy as follows: "Following a transient, somnolent phase, the patients seem calm, indifferent and distant (in French 'lointains'), their bearing is affectively and emotionally neutral and passive, although the intellectual faculties do not appear to be impaired" (Delay and Deniker, 1953, p. 350).

On the basis of studies with healthy subjects and observations in psychotic patients, Degkwitz (1967, p. 108) distinguished between three phases of action of antipsychotic drugs:

- First phase (duration about one week): the patient tends to doze and sleep, even during daytime, and his drive is clearly reduced; he has no initiative and appears lethargic and indifferent to his environment; there is a certain detachment from worries and anxieties, also from those psychotic in nature, i.e. delusions, ideas of reference and paranoid–hallucinatory experiences become less frequent.
- Second phase (duration about one week): the sedative effect recedes while the 'antipsychotic' effect is retained; during this phase, despite a pronounced reduction in emotional tension, there is still a danger of unexpected emotional outbreaks and over-reactions.
- Third phase: the general loss of drive is only minor whereas emotional responsiveness is still reduced; the patient seems to be indifferent and shows little spontaneity; the antipsychotic drug effect is retained and, in many cases, the patient's insight into his illness (and hence also the possibility for psycho- and sociotherapeutic measures) increases.

Some 20 years later, Keck et al. (1989) noted that the course of action of neuroleptics, particularly the onset of their specific antipsychotic action, has still not been studied accurately enough. According to these authors there have been hardly any controlled studies in which clear distinction was made between the non-specific calming action and the antipsychotic effects of neuroleptics.

1.2.2 THE BEST-KNOWN PRODUCTS

More than 30 antipsychotics are currently marketed in many European countries (and a few less in the USA and other English-speaking areas), the

Table 1.2 A selection of widely used antipsychotics

Trade name	Generic name	Customary oral daily doses (mg)
Ciatyl®, Sordinol®	Clopenthixol	20–300
Dapotum®, Lyogen®, Omca®, Prolixin®	Fluphenazine	2–20
Dipiperon®	Floropipamide	80–360
Dogmatil®	Sulpiride	100–600
Fluanxol®	Flupenthixol	1–10
Haldol®	Haloperidol	5–20
Largactil®, Megaphen®, Thorazine®	Chlorpromazine	200–800
Leponex®, Clozaril®	Clozapine	100–900
Loxitane®	Loxapine	40–100
Mellaril®	Thioridazine	150–800
Moban®	Molindone	50–225
Navane®	Thiothixene	5–30
Neuleptil®, Aolept®	Periciazine	20–150
Neurocil®, Nozinan®	Levomepromazine	50–600
Orap®	Pimozide	2–6
Prazine®, Protactyl®	Promazine	50–1000
Risperdal®	Risperidone	2–6
Sedalande®	Fluanison	5–80
Serentil®	Mesoridazine	75–300
Seroquel®	Quetiapine	150–750
Stelazine®	Trifluoperazine	5–20
Tindal®	Acetophenazine	40–120
Trilafon®	Perphenazine	8–32
Truxal®, Taractan®	Chlorprothixene	50–600
Zeldox®	Ziprasidone	40–160
Zyprexa®	Olanzapine	7.5–30

best known of which are presented in Table 1.2. The following explanations apply to this table and to the others in this chapter:

- *Trade names* (first column): they are chosen by the manufacturers and are protected as trade marks. They can vary from one country to another for the same compound. Medications are mostly designated by their trade names in everyday clinical use.
- *Non-proprietary or generic names* (second column): these give, in abbreviated form, an indication of the chemical structure of a medication and, because they are the same in all countries, promote better international understanding (in publications, congresses, etc.) than trade names.
- *Customary oral daily doses* (third column): the smallest and largest recommended daily doses of the same medication may differ by a factor of 3–20. These wide dosage ranges are due to the fact that antipsychotics are used for various indications and that their efficacy and tolerability vary

from patient to patient. Thus, elderly patients are given the smallest possible doses, whereas large doses may be required in young, acutely psychotic patients.

1.2.3 DIFFERENCES BETWEEN DIFFERENT PRODUCTS

In view of the extent of Table 1.2 and the aforementioned number of 30 or more commercially available compounds, the obvious question is whether so many antipsychotics are actually needed or in what ways the various products differ in clinical use.

Two different aspects have to be considered in the answer: economic and scientific. An economic interest to have a variety of products in the market exists on the part of those pharmaceutical companies that have developed and marketed or are developing antipsychotics. Consequently, their advertising places the emphasis on the special features and advantages of individual medications, even though the differences between many products are not always very relevant clinically. Nevertheless, the differences that actually exist between products with regard to their pharmacokinetic and pharmacodynamic properties are of scientific interest, especially those related to the effects of atypical versus typical antipsychotics:

- *Pharmacokinetics* (i.e. study of the movements of a medication): antipsychotics and other medications show differences in absorption, distribution, metabolism and excretion as a result of their different chemical structures and pharmaceutical preparations (capsule, tablet, injectable) and in relation to the conditions within the body (see Chapter 5). The transfer of a medication from the blood into the brain tissue across the so-called blood–brain barrier, its binding to specific brain structures and thus its actions depend on the physicochemical properties of the molecule. The interplay of these and other factors explains why antipsychotics of different chemical structures are not equally effective milligram for milligram (Table 1.2: column 3) and why they differ with regard to onset and duration of action.
- *Pharmacodynamics*: antipsychotics also differ in their pharmacodynamics, i.e. their pharmacological and clinical profiles of action. A rough distinction is made between highly sedative, hypnotic antipsychotics (e.g. clopenthixol, levomepromazine) and other products with weaker initial sedative action (e.g. fluphenazine and haloperidol). Sedative antipsychotics are prescribed for states of major unrest, often combined with insomnia, whereas the less sedative antipsychotics are preferred for patients suffering from delusions and hallucinations but in whom heavy sedation during daytime is undesirable.

The availability of the more recent, so-called atypical antipsychotics (clozapine, olanzapine, quetiapine, risperidone; see Table 1.2) makes it prudent that these agents be used as first-line therapeutic drugs in the treatment of all patients who are deemed psychotic/schizophrenic. This is mostly due to the safer profile of these medications versus the old typical antipsychotics (e.g. haloperidol). However, there are exceptional cases when, in emergencies and in the case of disturbed and agitated patients representing a danger to themselves and to others, the doctor may choose a medication having a pronounced sedative and initially sleep-inducing effect. Despite the very varied supply, most doctors restrict themselves to using just a few antipsychotics with which they have become familiar during their training and clinical activities.

1.2.4 SIDE EFFECTS ('ADVERSE EFFECTS') OF ANTIPSYCHOTICS

The clinical choice of an antipsychotic is not only determined by the diagnosed illness and the prevailing symptoms but also on the basis of what side effects the treating doctor regards as being acceptable in each individual case. Antipsychotics are not only strong-acting with respect to their desired effects but also with respect to their undesirable actions, known as side effects. Table 1.3 provides a summary of the commonest side effects of antipsychotics.

In general, the sedating, initially sleep-promoting antipsychotics, especially in larger doses, often induce vegetative side effects such as orthostatic hypotension, mostly accompanied by acceleration of pulse rate, modifications of myocardial activity that are revealed in the electrocardiogram (ECG), sweating, dry mouth and sometimes impaired sexual function, especially in men. In contrast, agents having a pronounced antipsychotic action often lead to extrapyramidal motor symptoms, namely dyskinesias (disturbed movements), iatrogenic (treatment-induced) Parkinsonian states and, after prolonged use, tardive dyskinesias (see Section 1.2.5). The 'atypical' antipsychotic clozapine and, to a lesser extent, olanzapine and quetiapine are exceptions to this rule because they exhibit marked antipsychotic activity associated with a spectrum of side effects more typical of a sedating, weakly antipsychotic agent. Irrespective of the type of action, antipsychotics may also trigger adverse hormonal shifts (elevation of prolactin levels) and often, as a result, amenorrhea and (transient) sterility, breast enlargement (gynecomastia) and lactation.

In view of the large number of potential adverse effects, the benefits and risks of antipsychotic treatment have to be weighed carefully against each other in each individual patient: the unrestricted prescription of these medications is just as unwarranted as total abstinence from medications.

1.2.5 NEUROLEPTICS AND TARDIVE DYSKINESIAS: UNANSWERED QUESTIONS

Tardive dyskinesias are motor disturbances that sometimes arise following long-term treatment with neuroleptics. The first symptoms to appear are

Table 1.3 Side effects of antipsychotics

Vegetative disorders[a] (particularly with sedative–hypnotic antipsychotics)
- Decrease in blood pressure, especially on standing up (i.e. orthostatic hypotension)
- Acceleration of pulse rate
- Modification of myocardial activity (ECG changes)
- Sweating, dry mouth, constipation
- Impotence, ejaculation disorders, anorgasmia

Extrapyramidal motor disorders (particularly with antipsychotics having a pronounced antipsychotic action)

Early dyskinesia and dystonias (uncontrolled movements and postures that may arise at the start of therapy)
- Spasms of the tongue, visual spasms, pharyngospasms
- Grimacing, stiff neck, trismus
- Gyratory and rotatory movements of the upper extremities

Parkinsonism
- Restriction of motor movement (akinesia)
- Loss of facial expression (hypomimia), festinating gait
- Increased muscle tension (rigor), trembling (tremor)

Akathisia
- Restlessness, inability to remain seated
- Urge to move continuously

Tardive dyskinesia
- Involuntary chewing, smacking of lips, swallowing and rolling movements of the tongue
- Gyratory and flailing movements of the extremities

---

[a]The *neuroleptic malignant syndrome* (NMS; see Shalev and Munitz, 1986), a rare but very hazardous complication of neuroleptic treatment, is counted among the vegetative disorders but may occur also after the use of neuroleptics with pronounced antipsychotic action. This syndrome is characterized by immobility, rigidity, tremor, greatly elevated body temperature (i.e. hyperthermia), accelerated pulse, bouts of sweating and white blood count shifts. Figures for the incidence of NMS vary from 0.4% to 1.4% of all patients treated with neuroleptics (Pope *et al.*, 1986); young men are affected relatively more frequently (Kellam, 1990).

generally rolling and gyratory movements of the tongue. These are followed by sucking and smacking movements of the lips and, finally, the trunk and extremities may be affected. The dyskinesias disappear entirely during sleep and subside during wakefulness when the parts of the body involved are moved intentionally, e.g. during talking, eating or writing.

Opinions vary as to the incidence and causes of tardive dyskinesias and their precise connection with the use of neuroleptics. Estimates of their incidence extend from 0.5% to 56% of all chronically hospitalized psychiatric patients – a discrepancy that is attributed primarily to the differences in criteria governing the selection of patients for various investigations and to heterogeneous assessment criteria (Kane and Smith, 1982; Meltzer and Fatemi, 2001). Tardive dyskinesias may arise during treatment with neuroleptics but are also observed months or years after the medication has been discontinued. Tardive dyskinesias are more commonly seen in older patients, although motor disturbances in varying forms are, in any event, more frequent in advanced age (Varga *et al.*, 1982). Moreover, older patients being treated with neuroleptics generally have a longer history of illness and drug therapy than do younger patients. Some authors take the view that the cumulative neuroleptic dose over a period of time (and not the duration of treatment) represents the decisive risk factor for the appearance of tardive dyskinesias. However, this view has been contradicted on the basis of empirical studies (Bergen *et al.*, 1992).

1.3 ANTIDEPRESSANTS

1.3.1 CLINICAL ACTIONS AND USES

Antidepressants are medications used to treat depression, i.e. states of severe dejection lasting for weeks or months. The term 'depression' does not designate a single disease but a syndrome that needs to be characterized more precisely on the basis of the prevailing symptoms present and taking the patient's prior history into account. On the basis of the patient's clinical status, differentiation is made between inhibited and agitated forms of depression; states of depression that are almost exclusively expressed in the form of physical complaints and symptoms are also termed somatized or masked depressions.

Antidepressants are primarily prescribed for their mood-elevating action, which develops after several days of treatment and often only after some weeks. The expressions 'thymoleptic' (i.e. mood-stabilizing medicament) and 'thymeretic' (i.e. mood-activating medicament) designate two antidepressant groups that differ partially in their pharmacological and clinical actions. Neither thymoleptics nor thymeretics act to improve mood or produce euphoria in healthy, non-depressed subjects, so in this respect their mood-lightening effect can be considered disease-specific.

A major indication for antidepressants is endogenous depression, which, by definition, has its origin neither in a physical cause nor in a psychologically traceable development or cause. In the case of so-called psychogenic depression or depression mostly due to situational factors, on the other hand, antidepressants are of only secondary importance; in such cases therapy should begin with psychotherapeutic procedures and then, if not responsive, be extended to medications.

Combined pharmacotherapeutic and psychotherapeutic approaches are also successful in psychogenic depression (see Chapter 8). In the case of somatogenic depression, which by definition is based on a physical illness, causal therapy is, wherever possible, directed at the underlying physical ailment, antidepressants possibly being used to provide an additional symptomatic relief.

Thymoleptics and thymeretics are not 'happy pills', nor are they euphorics. In the case of endogenous depression there is a balancing out of pathological low mood, an effect that is normally obtained in two to three weeks or even longer in many cases. The first effect to become apparent in most cases of depression is the calming one, with the result that anxiousness, unrest and sleep disturbances can be reduced quickly and hence the patient's confidence in the treatment increases. Drugs that may be stimulating or cause euphoria in healthy volunteers, such as amphetamine, alcohol or cocaine, are not suitable for use as antidepressants.

If an antidepressant is discontinued too early, rapid and serious relapse may result. This indicates that, whereas antidepressants may shorten or curb a depressive episode, they cannot definitely end – and hence cure – it. The attenuation of depressive symptoms is thus not a sufficient criterion for withdrawing drug therapy (Chapter 8). The decision as to when an antidepressant may be discontinued is often difficult – and also dependent on the chronicity of the patient's depression and the number of episodes of depression experienced.

1.3.2 THE BEST-KNOWN PRODUCTS

There are about 30 antidepressants marketed at present in most European countries (fewer in the USA), differing in their pharmacokinetic and pharmacodynamic properties. The best-known products are listed in Table 1.4. In clinical terms, distinction is made between initially-sedative, drive-neutral and activating antidepressants. Initially-sedative antidepressants, such as amitriptyline and doxepine, are prescribed primarily for depressions with anxious–agitated symptoms and act initially to calm the patient and promote sleep; their mood-lightening effect develops later. Weakly sedative and activating antidepressants (e.g. nortriptyline, desipramine, fluoxetine) are prescribed when sedation of the patient is not indicated or is undesirable (Fig. 1.1). Products that have been introduced in the last 10 years are generally characterized by better tolerability and greater safety.

1.3.3 HOW EFFECTIVE ARE ANTIDEPRESSANTS?

It is not always easy to assess the success of antidepressant treatment accurately because depression often tends to spontaneous healing or remission. Cyclic and periodic forms of endogenous depression follow a phasic pattern: the depressive episode lasting weeks or months can, in the bipolar form, shift into mania or there is a gradual lightening of the depression, as may be

Table 1.4 A selection of well-known antidepressants

Trade name (UK and US)	Generic name	Customary oral daily doses (mg)
Agedal[®][a]	Noxiptiline	75–450
Anafranil[®]	Clomipramine	130–250
Aventyl[®]	Nortriptyline	50–150
Effexor[®][b]	Venlafaxine	37.5–450
Insidon[®]	Opipramol	150–300
Lexapro[®][c]	Escitalopram oxalate	10–20
Ludiomil[®]	Maprotiline	150–230
Luvox[®][d]	Fluvoxamine	50–300
Manerix[®], Aurorix[®][e]	Moclobemide	150–600
Molipaxin[®][f] (UK) Desyrel[®] (US)	Trazodone	50–400
Noveril[®][a]	Dibenzepine	120–720
Pertofran[®]	Desipramine	150–300
Prozac[®][d]	Fluoxetine	20–80
Remeron[®][f]	Mirtazapine	15–45
Seropram[®], Celexa[®][d]	Citalopram	20–60
Seroxat[®], Paxil[®][d]	Paroxetine	20–60
Serzone[®][f]	Nefazodone	150–600
Sinequan[®]	Doxepin	150–300
Surmontil[®]	Trimipramine	150–300
Tofranil[®]	Imipramine	150–300
Tolvon[®]	Mianserin	10–60
Tryptizol[®], Amyline[®] (UK) Elaril[®], Endep[®], Elavil[®] (US)	Amitryptiline	150–300
Vivalan[®][a]	Viloxazine	150–200
Vestra[®][b]	Reboxetine	4–10
Wellbutrin[®], Zyban[®][f]	Bupropion	100–450
Zoloft[®][d]	Sertraline	50–200

[a]Not currently marketed in the USA.
[b]Serotonin norepinephrine reuptake inhibitor (SNRI).
[c]S-Enantiomer of citalopram.
[d]Selective serotonin reuptake inhibitor (SSRI).
[e]Reversible inhibitor of monoamine oxidase activity (RIMA).
[f]Atypical agent.

observed in the unipolar forms. The depressions of middle and old age (involutional and late depressions) are also subject to spontaneous remission or healing, even though the tendency to chronicity is intensified and the risk of recurrence of depression is greater (review by Jablensky, 1987). Psychogenic depression often subsides when the exterior (social, familial) circumstances or inner (psychodynamic) conditions of the patient change, whereas somatic depression is generally also relieved when the physical cause is eliminated. In the individual case it is consequently often difficult to distinguish between a

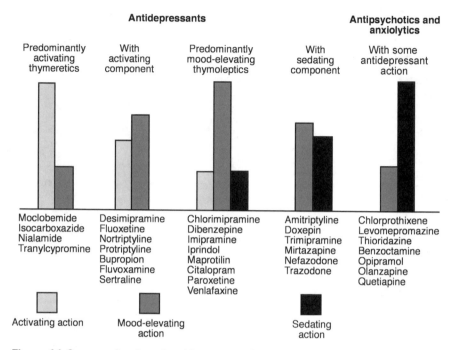

Figure 1.1 Spectra of action of antidepressants. The diagram (modified after Pöldinger, 1975, reproduced by permission of Editiones 'Roche', Basel) shows some typical medication used to treat depression. The activating drugs on the left with little or no sedative action are mainly used in inhibited forms of depression. The antipsychotics and anxiolytics with some antidepressant properties on the right are used in patients with more agitated forms of depression. In the middle are the typical antidepressants with, relatively speaking, the most pronounced mood-elevating effect

cure *post hoc* or *propter hoc*: has the antidepressant agent contributed to the shortening of the depressive phase, or would it have subsided spontaneously?

The difficulties associated with a reliable assessment of the success of treatment in each individual case are also reflected to some extent in the published results of controlled clinical studies with antidepressants in larger groups of patients. Controlled trials, i.e. comparisons between an active product such as an antidepressant and placebo (a medicament containing no active ingredient), do not always produce the expected results (Table 1.5). According to an early review by Morris and Beck (1974), placebo was therapeutically equal to the studied antidepressant in 31 of 88 published comparative trials, i.e. in 35% of all studies. With these figures it also has to be considered that trials with a 'negative' outcome (i.e. no significant difference between active product and placebo) have a much smaller chance of being

Table 1.5 Efficacy of first-generation antidepressants (controlled studies against placebo: results of 88 comparative trials, modified from Morris and Beck, 1974)

	Hospitalized		Outpatients		Mixed groups		Total	
	Better than placebo	Not better	Better than placebo	Not better	Better than placebo	Not better	Better than placebo	Not better
Imipramine	23	15	6	4	1	1	30	20
Desipramine	3	2	1	0	0	0	4	2
Amitriptyline	7	4	7	2	0	0	14	6
Nortriptyline	4	3	1	0	0	0	5	3
Protriptyline	1	0	2	0	0	0	3	0
Doxepin	1	0	0	0	0	0	1	0
Total	39	24	17	6	1	1	57	31

The figures correspond to the number of comparative, placebo-controlled clinical studies in which the superiority of the antidepressant in question over placebo was demonstrated or could not be demonstrated.

published than studies with a 'positive' outcome, suggesting that the percentage of negative trials is even higher in reality.

It is thus understandable why some earlier authors previously doubted the efficacy of antidepressants in general (Welner *et al.*, 1980) or the advantages of newer antidepressants compared with 'classical' products (Song *et al.*, 1993). However, the great majority of doctors and scientific authors consider that the efficacy of first-generation antidepressants (imipramine, amitriptyline, nortriptyline) has been proved beyond any reasonable doubt, and that efficacy also has been demonstrated for newer products such as trazodone, the selective serotonin reuptake inhibitors (SSRIs) and serotonin norepinephrine reuptake

Table 1.6 The most common side effects of first-generation antidepressants

Mental symptoms
- Tiredness, pronounced daytime sleepiness, sleep disturbances
- Delirium (following overdosage, particularly in elderly patients)

Somatic symptoms
- Dry mouth, bad taste in the mouth, constipation
- Urinary retention, impotence
- Accommodation disorders (difficulty in near–far focusing of the eyes)
- Orthostatic hypotension, collapse (in elderly patients)
- Dizziness, headaches, palpitations
- Increased sweating

Complications
- Switch from depression to mania (in bipolar disorder)
- Attempted suicide (particularly with activating antidepressants)

Table 1.7 The most common side effects of SSRIs, SNRIs and other newer antidepressants (Sadock and Sadock, 2001)

SSRIs	
In general	Sexual inhibition (inhibited orgasm, decreased libido), nausea, anorexia, weight gain, headaches, insomnia, somnolence, vivid dreams, tremor, seizure, akathisia, hyponatremia, serotonin syndrome
Fluoxetine	Headaches, anxiety, insomnia, neutropenia
Paroxetine	Weight gain, constipation, dry mouth, somnolence, neutropenia
Sertraline	Gastrointestinal disturbance, diarrhea, insomnia, somnolence
Fluvoxamine	Insomnia, somnolence
Citalopram	Gastrointestinal disturbance, somnolence
Escitalopram	Nausea, insomnia, ejaculation disorder, somnolence, increased sweating, fatigue
SNRIs	
Venlafaxine	Nausea, somnolence, dry mouth, dizziness, anxiety, blurred vision, increase in blood pressure (>300 mg/day)
Reboxetine	Urinary hesitancy, headache, constipation, nasal congestion, perspiration, dizziness, dry mouth, decreased libido, insomnia
Atypicals	
Bupropion	Headache, insomnia, nausea, restlessness, agitation, psychosis, seizure with >400 mg/day
Trazodone	Sedation, orthostatic hypotension, dizziness, headache, nausea, gastric irritation, priapism
Nefazodone	Headache, dry mouth, somnolence, nausea, dizziness, constipation, elevation in liver enzymes
Mirtazapine	Somnolence, dry mouth, increased appetite, constipation, weight gain, dizziness
RIMA	
Moclobemide	Insomnia, headache, dry mouth, dizziness, fatigue, nausea, diarrhea

RIMA, reversible inhibitor of monoamine oxidase activity.

inhibitors (SNRIs). Nevertheless, about one third of all depressed patients are considered refractory to therapy, i.e. do not respond to adequate doses of antidepressants within four to six weeks (Möller, 1991).

Methodological questions regarding the proof of efficacy of psychopharmaceuticals will be discussed in more detail in Chapter 5.

1.3.4 SIDE EFFECTS OF ANTIDEPRESSANTS

The most common side effects of the older antidepressants, especially those of the sedative type, are vegetative and mostly due to the anticholinergic action of these products: dry mouth, difficulties of visual accommodation, constipation, impotence in men, dizziness, increased sweating and palpitations. Of medical significance, especially in older patients, are decreases in blood pressure going as far as orthostatic collapse, delirium (state of confusion with disorientation in time and space) after overdosage and heart function disorders (Table 1.6).

The side effects of antidepressants, sometimes very unpleasant, often lead patients to interrupt their treatment or to reduce the drug dose, which involves a great risk in view of the high relapse rate and danger of suicide in depression. The newer antidepressants, such as trazodone, fluoxetine and other SSRIs and moclobemide, are characterized by better tolerability and lower toxicity and are therefore preferred in the treatment of outpatients and elderly patients (Rudorfer and Potter, 1989). A detailed list of general and specific common side effects associated with the newer generation of antidepressants is seen in Table 1.7.

1.4 MOOD STABILIZERS

1.4.1 CLINICAL ACTIONS AND USES

Mood stabilizers are a variable group of medications that stabilize the mood in a manic or hypomanic patient. This class of medications is mainly used for acute and maintenance treatment of patients who suffer from bipolar disorder or manic–depressive illness or those suffering from schizoaffective illness. Bipolar disorder is a debilitating mood disorder characterized by episodes of mania or hypomania alternating with depression. The manic symptoms may consist of an expansive, elated or irritable mood, pressured speech, flight of ideas, decreased need for sleep, distractibility and excessive participation in activities that have a potential for painful consequences (APA, 1994). The symptoms may last for one week and cause marked impairment in social and occupational function or lead to hospitalization. In general, a manic phase may lead into either a euthymic or depressed period. Depressive periods are extremely severe and prompt the patient to seek psychiatric help. The suicide rate is quite high and is estimated at 10–25%.

DSM-IV (APA, 1994) criteria recognize two types of bipolar disorder. In type I bipolar disorder, a patient exhibits mania and depression. In type II disorder, mania is replaced by hypomania (a less severe form) and alternates with depression. Several course modifiers are recognized in the evaluation of subjects with bipolar disorder, e.g. mixed states, rapid cycling and dysphoric mania. A mixed manic state is characterized by the simultaneous presence of both depressive and manic symptoms. Dysphoric mania is characterized by complaints of depression, anxiety and anger while experiencing mania (Janicak et al., 2001). Rapid cycling characterizes a group of treatment-resistant bipolar patients who experience a minimum of four episodes (hypomania, mania, depression, mixed mania) during a period of 1 year (Dunner et al., 1977; APA, 1994; Janicak et al., 2001).

The treatment of bipolar disorder is contingent on correct diagnosis because initiation of a mood-stabilizing agent may significantly alter the course of disease. Classically, lithium has been the main agent, which not only treats the manic/hypomanic symptoms but also treats the depressive symptoms. In contrast to the antidepressants described so far in this book, lithium is not a complex synthetic compound but a metal found in nature in the form of a number of salts. Lithium has a prophylactic action against manic and depressive episodes occurring in the context of bipolar disorder. Under lithium medication, the intervals between the individual episodes gradually become longer and the protection against relapse becomes all the more pronounced the longer lithium is regularly taken (Baldessarini, 1985). Recently, a number of other agents have been used in the treatment of bipolar disorder that may, in certain patients, be more effective or better tolerated. This issue is important because not all patients respond to lithium, and from those who do respond well to lithium a proportion cannot tolerate the varied side effects:

- Valproic acid (Depakote®) is an anticonvulsant with good antimanic action that is especially suited for patients with rapid cycling and mixed episodes (Bowden *et al.*, 1994). However, it is a poor antidepressant, necessitating the use of a low-dose SSRI in the treatment of depression that may occur in the course of bipolar disease.
- Lamotrigine, another anticonvulsant, has been shown to be a potentially good mood stabilizer with both antidepressant and antimanic efficacy (Fatemi *et al.*, 1997; Calabrese *et al.*, 1999).
- Other agents with anticonvulsant properties that may be of use in the treatment of bipolar disorder include topiramate, gabapentin, tiagabine and carbamazepine (Janicak *et al.*, 2001).

The antiepileptic agent carbamazepine (Tegretol®) has been discussed for many years as an alternative to lithium because it also has an antimanic effect and prophylactic activity against depression, with possibly better tolerability. However, carbamazepine has not yet been proven to be superior to lithium,

Table 1.8 A selection of well-known and potential mood stabilizers (Janicak *et al.*, 2001, reprinted with permission)

Trade name	Generic name	Customary oral daily dose (mg)
Depakote®, Depakene®	Valproic acid[a]	250–1500
Eskalith®, Lithonate®, Lithobid®	Lithium[a]	300–1800
Lamictal®	Lamotrigine	12.5–200
Neurontin®	Gabapentin	600–3600
Tegretol®	Carbamazepine	200–1200
Topamax®	Topiramate	300–600
Zyprexa®	Olanzapine[a]	10–20

[a]Approved by the US Food and Drug Administration for the treatment of acute mania.

Table 1.9 The most common side effects of mood stabilizers (Sadock and Sadock, 2001). Reproduced by permission of Lippincott Williams & Wilkins

Lithium	Neurological: tremor, ataxia, seizures Endocrine: hypothyroidism Cardiovascular: T wave changes, sinus node dysfunction Renal: polyuria, nephrogenic diabetic insipidus Dermatological: hair loss, acne, psoriasis, rash Gastrointestinal: nausea, diarrhea Miscellaneous: fluid retention, weight gain, weakness
Valproic acid	Common: gastrointestinal irritation, nausea, sedation, tremor, weight gain, hair loss Uncommon: vomiting, diarrhea, ataxia, dysarthria
Carbamazepine	Dose-related: double vision, vertigo, gastrointestinal disturbance Idiosyncratic: agranulocytosis, Stevens–Johnson syndrome, aplastic anemia
Lamotrigine	Rash (approximately 10%)

and its precise indications have not been adequately defined (Prien and Gelenberg, 1989), so it is mostly reserved for those patients who do not tolerate lithium or do not respond to it.

Several other agents of different chemical classes have been found to be of help in the acute treatment of bipolar disease, such as clozapine, olanzapine and nimodipine (Janicak *et al.*, 2001) (Table 1.8).

1.4.2 SIDE EFFECTS OF MOOD STABILIZERS

By far the most untoward side effects belong to lithium (Table 1.9). A fine tremor often becomes apparent at the beginning of and during therapy. In addition, some patients complain of nausea, bloating and other gastrointestinal disorders. Thirst, polyuria (increased excretion of urine) and muscular weakness are not unusual and although disturbances of thyroid and possibly kidney function are not common they call for regular check-ups for the patient receiving lithium. Weight gain is another side effect of lithium; about 20% of all long-term patients gain 10 kg or more in weight. Because lithium has a narrow therapeutic range (i.e. the range between the therapeutically effective and the toxic dose), the concentration in the patient's blood has to be monitored regularly.

1.5 ANXIOLYTICS AND HYPNOTICS

1.5.1 CLINICAL ACTIONS AND USES

Anxiolytics are medications with a calming action that are used in states of unrest, anxiety and tension of many types. The anxiolytics used today almost all belong to the *benzodiazepine* group and have the advantage of lower toxicity and generally better tolerability than other sedative drugs.

Another group of anxiolytic compounds, the so-called beta-receptor blockers (Gastpar and Rimpel, 1993), which are not psychopharmaceuticals in the conventional sense, will be dealt with briefly in Chapter 8.

Whereas antipsychotics and antidepressants are used mainly in 'major psychiatry', i.e. in the treatment of schizophrenia and depression, anxiolytics are also used in general medicine for the treatment of neurotic, vegetative, psychosomatic and even purely physical conditions. This multiple usage is promoted by the fact that anxiolytics of the benzodiazepine type have an almost exclusively central action so that vegetative effects (dry mouth, sweating, visual disturbances, urine retention, constipation, fall in blood pressure), which can be unpleasant for patients or even hazardous, are practically absent.

Many of the *hypnotics* used today are also benzodiazepines or closely related to them. Hypnotics differ from anxiolytics mainly with regard to the timing of their action: they generally have a fast onset of action, but fading after a few hours so that there is no hangover in the form of tiredness or lack of alertness on the following morning. Compared with barbiturates, often used previously as sleeping pills, the modern hypnotics are characterized by greater safety; successful suicide attempts are rare with benzodiazepine derivatives and related drugs.

1.5.2 THE BEST-KNOWN PRODUCTS

Some 25 anxiolytics and hypnotics are marketed at present; the best known of these are listed in Table 1.10. Here, again, there are striking differences between the doses of these products, which can be explained in the same way as for antipsychotics. The benzodiazepine derivatives and related compounds show few qualitative differences; nevertheless, the time–effect features, i.e. the timing of onset of action and peak action as well as duration of action, mean that it is sensible to use different products for different purposes.

1.5.3 ANXIOLYTICS OR PSYCHOTHERAPY?

What are the accepted indications for anxiolytics? Generally speaking, these medications are given nowadays when a patient suffers from anxiety states or symptoms to such an extent that his daily routine is considerably disrupted. It is quite clear from this formulation that the indications for anxiolytics are less sharply defined than those of the antipsychotics and antidepressants: when do anxiety symptoms impair daily routine to an extent that one can speak of considerable disruption? And who is to determine whether a disruption is considerable or trivial: the patient, the doctor, the relatives?

Table 1.10 A selection of well-known anxiolytics and hypnotics

Trade name (UK and US)	Generic name	Dose (mg)	Use
Adumbran®, Seresta® (UK), Serax® (US)	Oxazepam	20–150	Anxiolytic, sedative
Ambien®	Zolpidem	5/10	Insomnia
Ativan®	Lorazepam	2–10	Anxiolytic
Buspar®	Buspirone	15–30	Anxiolytic
Centrax®	Prazepam	20–60	Hypnotic
Dalmane®	Flurazepam	15–30	Hypnotic
Doral®	Quazepam	7.5/15	Hypnotic
Euhynos®, Normison®, Tenox®	Temazepam	10–60	Hypnotic
Frisium®	Clobazam	20–60	Anxiolytic
Halcion®	Triazolam	0.25–1.0	Hypnotic
Klonopin®	Clonazepam	1–6	Panic disorder, anticonvulsant, alcohol withdrawal, social phobia, acute mania
Lexotan®	Bromazepam	3–24	Anxiolytic
Librium® (UK), Limbitrol® (US)	Chlordiazepoxide	5–150	Anxiolytic
Nitrados®, Somnite® (UK), Mogadon® (US)	Nitrazepam	5–15	Hypnotic
Noctamid®	Lormetazepam	0.5–2.0	Hypnotic
Paxipam®	Halazepam	60–160	Hypnotic
Prosom®	Estazolam	1/2	Hypnotic
Restoril®	Temazepam	15–30	Hypnotic
Rohypnol®	Flunitrazepam	2–6	Hypnotic
Sonata®	Zaleplon	10	Insomnia
Tranxene®	Clorazepate Dipotassium	10–60	Anxiolytic
Valium®	Diazepam	5–60	Anxiolytic
Versed®	Midazolam	5/50 i.v.	Anesthetic
Xanax®	Alprazolam	0.5–4	Anxiolytic

Like almost all relevant authors, Lader and Petursson (1983) also advise against the long-term use of anxiolytics and they emphasize that most anxiety states and phases of insomnia generally last for only a limited period of time; either the acute stress fades or the patient becomes used to the situation (or copes with it successfully), or a spontaneous remission occurs. In many cases the patient can be managed with advice and reassurance, and thus without medicaments.

Many patients with symptoms of anxiety and tension reject psychotherapy out of hand, often using extraneous and rather irrelevant grounds as a pretext.

In addition, states of anxiety, tension and other forms of ego pain are frequently somatized, i.e. they manifest themselves in the form of physical complaints. Muscle tension, headaches, gastrointestinal disorders, sleep disturbances and other symptoms are often the somatic equivalents of states of psychic tension, and the worries and anxieties of patients are then directed at the physical symptoms, with the result that the original cause recedes into the background and is emotionally relieved. It thus becomes clear why there are broad and major fields of application for anxiolytics outside psychiatry, mainly in internal medicine, rheumatology, gynecology and pediatrics. Anxiolytics are often referred to as panaceas, i.e. a cure for everything and everyone – a criticism that is only partly justified in the opinion of many doctors: should counseling or psychotherapeutic measures be ruled out in a patient for extraneous or pertinent inner reasons, then it would not be seen as 'medically ethical' to refrain on reasons of principle from trying to treat the patient with an anxiolytic drug.

1.5.4 SIDE EFFECTS OF ANXIOLYTICS

The generally excellent tolerability of these preparations has contributed greatly to the widespread use of anxiolytics. The commonest side effects (Table 1.11) are tiredness and muscle relaxation and these usually can be avoided or attenuated by reducing the dose. Ataxia and paradoxical reactions such as irritability and increased agitation occasionally arise in the elderly but are rare in younger patients. Much attention has been focused on the negative effects of benzodiazepines on memory and other cognitive functions (see Chapter 7).

1.5.5 DEPENDENCY ON BENZODIAZEPINES

With their low toxicity, their action limited almost exclusively to the central nervous system and their other practical advantages (few pharmacokinetic interactions with other medicaments), anxiolytics and hypnotics of the benzodiazepine group apparently represent almost ideal medications. However, it is precisely the good tolerability and lack of subjectively unpleasant side effects that can lead to problems: whereas hardly a single patient wants to take antipsychotics or antidepressants without a clinical need, there is a great risk of anxiolytic drug abuse. These medications have a relaxing and calming action, the world seems friendlier and more harmonious and real personal problems become less pressing. On the other hand, unrest, anxiety and distress reappear quickly and are often intensified after withdrawal of these medications, so it is difficult to give up anxiolytics once the use of them has become a habit.

The problems of withdrawal of anxiolytics and hypnotics have been described in innumerable publications (reviews by Owen and Tyrer, 1983; Griffiths and Sannerud, 1987). Schöpf (1985) produced a compilation of the

Table 1.11 Side effects of anxiolytics (somewhat similar to the after-effects of benzodiazepine hypnotics)

- Sedation: feeling of fatigue, drowsiness, inattention
- Deterioration of performance: decreased concentration and decreased physical capacity; anterograde amnesia (see Chapter 7)
- Muscle relaxation, disturbed coordination, ataxia
- States of disorientation: mostly in elderly patients
- Paradoxical reactions: excitement, agitation, irritability, aggressiveness
- Euphoria, withdrawal symptoms, risk of dependency
- So-called alcohol potentiation: the sedative action of tranquillizers is potentiated by alcohol. Relevant impairments are possible after a combined intake of tranquillizer doses and amounts of alcohol that when taken alone would produce no detectable actions (Mattila, 1984)

most common symptoms found after discontinuation of long-term benzodiazepine medication. According to him, the following symptoms arise 'frequently to regularly': dysphoria (ill humor), anxiety, insomnia, muscle pain and twitches, tremor, restlessness, nausea, loss of appetite and weight, headaches, sweating and blurred vision, i.e. to a large extent those symptoms against which the benzodiazepines were prescribed in the first place.

More striking are withdrawal phenomena having no connection with the original symptoms, namely disturbances of perception and sense of reality. These include hypersensitivity to noise, light and other sensory stimuli, as well as distorted perception in the visual, kinesthetic and acoustic spheres. Disturbances affecting the sense of reality include transient depersonalization and derealization phenomena. Although these disturbances do not arise regularly (but according to Schöpf in about 50% of cases), they are unpleasant for those affected, often causing anxiety and low spirits, especially as few doctors are aware of these symptoms and therefore cannot suitably prepare their patients for withdrawal of anxiolytics.

Many regimens intended to prevent the appearance of benzodiazepine dependency or to make the unavoidable withdrawal symptoms more tolerable have been devised and published (Marks, 1988; Sartory and Maurer, 1991). Controlled trials have also been performed to compare abrupt and gradual withdrawal regimens and to assess the appearance of withdrawal symptoms after discontinuing benzodiazepines with long and short half-lives (Busto et al., 1986; Rickels et al., 1990; Schweizer et al., 1990). The results of these trials can be summarized as follows:

(1) Withdrawal symptoms are common after the discontinuation of benzodiazepines following prolonged use, and arise both with abrupt and gradual withdrawal and with products having short and long half-lives.

(2) After abrupt discontinuation, the withdrawal symptoms described by Schöpf (1985) and others are particularly severe and frequent during the first few days but then fade; with gradual discontinuation, the withdrawal symptoms are less frequent but show slower decrease with the passage of time.

(3) The subjectively perceived severity of withdrawal symptoms and the readiness to withstand them without recourse to rescue medication vary greatly from one person to another.

(4) The discontinuation of benzodiazepines with a short half-life is particularly difficult and there is a great tendency to use rescue medication after both abrupt and gradual withdrawal.

Many authors (Allgulander 1986; Uhlenhuth *et al.*, 1988; Chen and Lader, 1990) have debated the question of whether the use of benzodiazepines forms an epidemic that should be countered by more specific legislation. On the basis of a representative survey in more than 3000 adult Americans, Mellinger *et al.* (1984) concluded that only a small percentage of the population (1.6%) can be considered 'long-term consumers' of these medicaments and that these patients are characterized by the following features: greater age, more women, more mental symptoms and more health problems. Because most long-term consumers were found to maintain regular contact with their doctor and take their medicine as prescribed, Mellinger *et al.* saw no grounds for alarm or for restrictive measures against benzodiazepines. However, this is a view not shared by all authors.

1.5.6 ALTERNATIVES TO BENZODIAZEPINES

In principle, all drugs with damping action on the central nervous system could be used as anxiolytics or hypnotics, but the pharmacological and/or pharmacokinetic properties of most compounds are not appropriate for their therapeutic use:

- As a substance known in almost all cultures, alcohol has only a non-specific sedating action, it quickly creates dependency and is quite toxic.
- Opiates and the other natural products discussed in Chapter 2 are toxic and/ or quickly create dependency.
- Barbiturates create dependency, have an unsuitable therapeutic safety margin and exhibit adverse interactions with other medicaments.
- Antihistamines, which penetrate into the central nervous system, have a non-specific sedative action, i.e. they can induce subjectively unpleasant side effects.

Because there is a great demand for anxiolytic and hypnotic substances and because the use of benzodiazepines should, in the opinion of many, be restricted, there is still great interest in obtaining effective, safe and non-habituating anxiolytics and hypnotics. The use of low doses of antipsychotics and (sedating) antidepressants has therefore been proposed in cases where a rapid onset of dependency is to be feared with benzodiazepines or where these products are contraindicated for other reasons, as in elderly patients at risk of stumbling and falling. According to the information summarized by Möller (1993), the clinical results with some low-dose neuroleptics used as anxiolytics are very good, although the potential tardive sequelae of this type of treatment are still poorly known. Positive results have also been obtained with the sedating antidepressant trimipramine, which is used in low doses as a sleeping agent primarily in elderly patients (Dietmaier and Laux, 1993), as well as with trazodone.

The product buspirone represents another alternative, being an anxiolytic with a novel mechanism of action and, unlike benzodiazepines, no anti-convulsant or myorelaxant activities. Although buspirone has anxiolytic activity, it does not induce a spontaneous feeling of relaxation or of well-being and, insofar as the available clinical experience available allows, has less potential to produce dependency than benzodiazepines. Buspirone also differs from benzodiazepines with regard to side effects: sedation, amnesia and ataxia practically do not occur, but the substance can lead to nausea, diarrhea and occasionally headache. The disadvantages of buspirone are its low bioavail-ability (less than 10%), which can make dosage difficult, and the fact that its anxiolytic action develops only after several days of regular administration. Buspirone is therefore not indicated if rapid anxiolysis is required. On the other hand, it is particularly suitable when therapy is expected to last for a long time. Finally, several new-generation antidepressants have been approved by health authorities in the treatment of anxiety disorders, e.g. paroxetine (for social phobia, obsessive–compulsive disorder, panic disorder), fluvoxamine (for obsessive–compulsive disorder), venlafaxine (for generalized anxiety disorder), sertraline (for panic disorder, post-traumatic stress disorder, obsessive–compulsive disorder) and fluoxetine (for obsessive–compulsive disorder). These drugs are suitable for longer-term treatment of anxiety disorders at similar doses as those used in depressive disorders.

1.6 PSYCHOSTIMULANTS

1.6.1 ACTIONS AND USES OF PSYCHOSTIMULANTS

Psychostimulants are psychically stimulating pharmaceuticals; synonyms are psychotonics, psychoanaleptics, psychic energizers. Using psychostimulants it is possible to prevent or suppress states of exhaustion and feelings of tiredness that appear after great exertion, during long and monotonous activity and following sleep deprivation. Alertness, concentration and enterprise are boosted through the use of psychostimulants and there may be pronounced well-being or even a state of euphoria, particularly after higher doses. The feeling of increased concentration and alertness is not merely subjective in nature; greater performance and improved consistency of performance also may be established objectively.

Despite these desirable effects, psychostimulants do not enjoy a good reputation and are very restrictively prescribed nowadays. The main reason for this is the potential for abuse of these medicaments in sport (doping) and among drug addicts (intravenously administered amphetamine products, 'speed', etc.). The uncontrolled use of stimulants in large doses can also lead to 'amphetamine psychoses', i.e. states of intense unrest and anxiety associated with delusions and (generally visual) hallucinations. Because of these risks, psychostimulants of the amphetamine type are available strictly on pre-scription only in almost all countries. Another drawback of known psychostimulants is tachyphylaxis: when used repeatedly, the products quickly lose their effect, so that long-term users are forced to increase the dose and, depending on the duration of use and dose, will go through a very unpleasant withdrawal syndrome in the form of insuperable drowsiness, lethargy or even depression if they want to stop the product temporarily or definitely.

Psychostimulants are used therapeutically in children and adolescents suffering from attention deficit hyperactivity disorder (ADHD) and in narcolepsy. Patients with ADHD are characterized by particular inattentive-ness, motor unrest, learning disorders, impulsivity and affect incontinence. The prevalence of ADHD is reported as 3–5% of all school-age children (in the USA); depending on the author, the syndrome is two to nine times more common in boys than in girls (Biedermann, 1991). Interestingly, stimulants do not cause a further increase in unrest in these children and adolescents but lead to improved attentiveness, longer times spent on the same activity, increased self-control and thus improved adjustment to school and home life (Chapter 7). This seemingly paradoxical effect of stimulants is explained by their action in regulating or stabilizing vigilance, and the success rates amount to about 70% of all treated children (Wilens and Biedermann, 1992). In patients with ADHD, psychostimulants do not lose their efficacy even after prolonged use. Use of stimulant drugs in ADHD has increased dramatically in the last 15 years in the USA, but even more so in some European countries; as a consequence, concern was raised as to whether these drugs with their known addictive potential are not heavily overprescribed (Llana and Crismon, 1999).

Narcolepsy (ICD G47.4) and other types of hypersomnia are severe disturbances of vigilance expressed as a sudden and irresistible requirement for sleep during the day, so-called sleep attacks (Aldrich, 1990). Apart from sleep attacks, the classical tetrad of narcolepsy includes cataplexy (sudden loss of muscular tone), sleep paralysis (waking from sleep with the feeling of not being able to move) and hypnagogic hallucinations (images or sequences of

Table 1.12 A selection of well-known psychostimulants (Sadock and Sadock, 2001). Reproduced by permission of Lippincott Williams & Wilkins

Trade name	Generic name	Dose (mg)	Use
Adderall®	Amphetamine-dextroamphetamine	5–30	ADHD
		5–60	Narcolepsy
Concerta®	Methylphenidate	18–54	ADHD
Cylert®	Pemoline	56.25–112.5	ADHD
Desoxyn®, Pervitin®	Methamphetamine	20–45	ADHD
Dexedrine®, Dextrostat®	Dextroamphetamine	5–30	ADHD
Provigil®	Modafinil	100–400	Narcolepsy
Ritalin®, Methidate®,	Methylphenidate	5–60	ADHD
Methylin®, Attenade®		20–30	Narcolepsy

images of great apparent reality when falling asleep). Depending on the severity of the illness, the patient drops off to sleep every few minutes or hours, even when engaged in activities in which he had interest and joy. Narcoleptic syndromes are nowadays treated symptomatically with certain antidepressants and stimulants, often in combination.

1.6.2 THE BEST-KNOWN PSYCHOSTIMULANTS

The best-known products come from the amphetamine group (see Table 1.12): Dexedrine® (generic name d-amphetamine) and Pervitin® (methamphetamine) were particularly used in the 1950s and 1960s as stimulants and also as appetite suppressants, but today play hardly any role in medical practice. Ritalin® (methylphenidate) has some relevance: its psychostimulant action is said to be weaker than that of amphetamines and it is apparently less abused than the latter. Because methylphenidate also possesses mild antidepressant activity, in some countries it is used to combat not only narcolepsy and ADHD but also mild depressions without suicide risk (Satel and Nelson, 1989).

Some of the adverse effects associated with the use of psychostimulants include: anorexia, nausea, weight loss, insomnia, nightmares, dizziness, irritability, dysphoria, agitation, tachycardia, cardiac arrhythmias, increase in tics and dyskinesias (Sadock and Sadock, 2001). Use of psychostimulants in children with ADHD may cause transient retardation of body growth.

1.7 NOOTROPICS AND ANTIDEMENTIA DRUGS

According to a definition by Coper and Kanowski (1983, p. 409), nootropics are "centrally acting drugs intended to improve higher integrative noetic brain functions such as memory and the ability to learn, perceive, think and concentrate, but for which a specific, uniform mechanism of action is not known". The expression 'nootropic' was not adopted everywhere; some authors used terms such as 'brain metabolism enhancers' for this class of compounds. Nootropics were found to have beneficial effects on mild cognitive and affective symptoms of incipient senile dementia (Orgogozo and Spiegel, 1987). The actions of these substances were considered to be of some medical significance insofar as they contributed to keeping elderly patients independent for longer so that they could continue to live in their own homes. Well-known nootropic drugs are Hydergine® (co-dergocrine mesylate) and Nootropil® (piracetam); however, owing to their limited efficacy, the use of nootropic drugs has declined in most countries in latter years.

Recently, a number of compounds with cholinesterase inhibitory action have been introduced for the treatment of mild to moderate cognitive deficits and other symptoms of Alzheimer-type dementia. These compounds increase cholinergic neurotransmission and lead to the improvement of memory and other cognitive functions compared with patients treated with placebo. Activities of daily life (ADLs) are stabilized and demented patients with behavioral symptoms may show some improvement. Examples include donepezil (Aricept®), rivastigmine (Exelon®), tacrine (Cognex®) and galantamine (Reminyl®). A more detailed account on these agents is provided in Chapter 7.

1.8 CONCLUDING COMMENT

The foregoing sections apply a classification of psychopharmaceuticals based on the major therapeutic uses of these drugs. However, it should be emphasized that the boundaries between the substance classes are not as clear-cut as the terms used might suggest. Thus, low-dose antipsychotics are sometimes used as anxiolytics or for the calming of agitated patients with depression, and some sedative antidepressants can be useful in patients with chronic insomnia. Antidepressants, in particular SSRIs and SNRIs, are increasingly being prescribed for a variety of anxiety disorders, and benzodiazepine anxiolytics in large doses or in combination with antipsychotics are sometimes applied in patients with acute schizophrenia. These overlapping clinical uses of psychopharmaceuticals also reflect the fact that schizophrenia and depression are regularly accompanied by episodes of disturbed sleep, agitation and anxiety, and that anxiety disorders and depressive syndromes may share a number of clinical features. Pharmacotherapy in psychiatry is often symptom- or syndrome- rather than disease-orientated.

2

The History of Psychopharmacology

2.1 INTRODUCTION

When was psychopharmacology born? Is it, in fact, possible to pinpoint the date of its birth? Historical accounts yield a variety of replies: Hordern (1968) begins his history of psychopharmacology with Emil Kraepelin who, in 1882, embarked on a series of trials with various psychoactive substances in the laboratory of Wilhelm Wundt in Leipzig, and who is looked upon as the founder of pharmacopsychology (see Chapter 3). Caldwell (1978) dates the birth of psychopharmacology as being 1951, with "the utilization of drugs in restoring or maintaining mental health and for exploring the mind". This year saw the discovery of the effect of chlorpromazine. In the opinion of Sack and De Fraites (1977) the modern era of psychopharmacology begins with the observation by J. Cade of the antimanic effect of lithium at the end of the 1940s.

We do not know when, and in what context, the term 'psychopharmaceutical' (psychopharmakon) was first used. In 1548, i.e. in the transitional period between the Middle Ages and modern times, a collection of prayers of consolation and prayers for the dead was published under the title *Psycho-pharmakon, hoc est: medicina animae*. The booklet was written by Reinhardus Lorichius of Hadamar, a member of the landed gentry of the German 'Land' of Hesse. Here the term 'psychopharmakon' relates to a spiritual medicine, which is to be used in miserable and hopeless situations of life.

Apart from psychopharmaceuticals in the spiritual sense, at all times and in most cultures psychotropic plant drugs have played a role in religious practices, magic rituals and healing. The substances best known in Europe and the Mediterranean area are *opium*, *hashish* and *hellebore*; in the medicine of India and other southeast Asian countries, *rauwolfia* traditionally has been of great significance (Wittern, 1983).

Psychopharmacology, Fourth Edition. By R. Spiegel
© 2003 John Wiley & Sons, Ltd: ISBN 0 471 56039 1: 0 470 84691 7 (PB)

2.2 PSYCHOPHARMACOLOGY IN THE ANCIENT WORLD AND MIDDLE AGES

2.2.1 THE MOST IMPORTANT SUBSTANCES

Opium is the solidified juice of the opium poppy (*Papaver somniferum*), which was cultivated even in prehistoric times: poppy residues have been found in Stone Age lake dwellings in northern Italy and Switzerland. The Sumerians living in the Tigris–Euphrates area 3000 years BC planted poppies and obtained its juice, which they called 'lucky' or 'happy', an indication that they well knew the mood-lightening, euphoriant action of opium. Finds from the second millennium BC in Asia Minor, Cyprus, Mycenae and Egypt show opium as a smoking material and healing agent; depending on the context, the opium poppy also stands as a symbol of fertility, sleep, death or immortality.

The sleep-inducing and analgesic actions of opium are described in the best-known medical writings from ancient times, the *Corpus Hippocraticum* and Galen's *Opus*. There is no mention of the risk of addiction, although Galen warns against overdosage and advises that the action of opium be attenuated by the addition of other substances; opium (under the name of *laudanum*) was almost always contained in the many variants of *theriak*, a compounded panacea known best in the Middle Ages.

Paracelsus, renowned physician and medical writer in the first half of the sixteenth century, called opium the philosopher's stone of immortality. In European medicine of the sixteenth and seventeenth centuries opium found wide use as an analgesic and sedative, although its abuse had become known from journeys of discovery to the Near and Far East. In the early nineteenth century a German pharmacist, Friedrich Sertürner, isolated the particularly active morphine from natural opium and this became widely used in military medicine as an analgesic and anesthetic in the latter half of that century.

The resin of hemp (*Cannabis sativa*) is known as *hashish*; the term marihuana designates the dried flowers, bracts and upper leaves of the female hemp plant. The intoxicating action of hashish was known to some peoples of ancient times but, except for its use against ear diseases, cannabis was never used in medicine. Hashish was very widely consumed in the Islamic world of the Middle Ages and even in Europe this intoxicant repeatedly appeared, although sporadically and often as a modish fad. However, hashish never played a recognized role in medicine and thus does not count as a psychopharmaceutical agent.

Hellebore root has been the psychopharmaceutical agent *par excellence* at various times. It is a plant of the Ranunculaceae family, the roots of which, as we now know, contain several glycosides, some of them rather toxic. White hellebore was traditionally used as an emetic (Vomitivum) and black hellebore as a laxative (Purgativum); in both cases the guiding principle was that a mental illness has a physical cause that can be treated by physical effects, preferably by the removal of pathogenic substances from the body. Hellebore was so well known that it was mentioned in classical comedies: Aristophanes (*Wasps*, 1489) uses "go drink hellebore" to mean "you're crazy", and Plautus (*Pseudolus*, 1185) also means much the same when he says that some people should drink hellebore, i.e. should see a psychiatrist.

Hellebore found a very wide range of uses: mania, melancholy, inflammation of the brain and mental retardation were included among the indications just as much as epilepsy, hydrophobia, violent temper and crazy ideas (Wittern, 1983, p. 14). White and black hellebore could be combined and there is no difficulty in believing the ancient authors when they state that the simultaneous emetic and laxative treatment has a good calming effect! The use of hellebore declined in the nineteenth century because the product is difficult to dose and can induce seizures in higher doses.

Decoctions of *Rauwolfia serpentina* (snakeroot) roots traditionally were used by Indians as a remedy for snake bites and also as a calming agent in some mental illnesses. The plant and its properties were known in Europe in the sixteenth and seventeenth centuries, when rauwolfia made a successful career as a remedy for almost everything but without finding a preferential position in psychiatry. Only in the early 1950s, after the active constituents of rauwolfia were discovered and produced in pure form, did the highly sedative and hypotensive alkaloid reserpine find transient use as an agent to control schizophrenic psychoses (Frankenburg, 1994).

2.2.2 PSYCHOPHARMACEUTICALS AND THE HISTORY OF PSYCHIATRY

The precursors of modern psychopharmaceuticals, i.e. opium, hellebore and rauwolfia, cannot be considered in isolation but only by reference to their contemporary healing arts. Mental illnesses and their possible treatment have confronted people with the same questions at all times: where do the irrational ideas and impulses of the insane come from – their moods, notions, anxiety and illogical behavior? Have these people sinned so that God has now cast an evil spirit into them as a punishment? What is this evil spirit: a spirit of nature, the ghost of an ancestor, a devil? Or is it the patient's sick body that produces the delusions without an outside agent – an unknown disease, a poison from within?

In the history of psychiatry, sketched here in just a few paragraphs, the different views held of man at different times are reflected in the constant swings between naturalistic and spiritualistic concepts of disease and the corresponding therapeutic approaches (see Kirchhoff, 1912; Heiberg, 1927; Ackerknecht, 1967; Shorter, 1997).

In *Egypt* at the time of the Pharaohs, mental illnesses were a result of the wrath of gods, or even an expression of possession by demons. In agreement with this concept, the treatment given by the priest or doctor comprised: punishment or penance to appease the gods; exorcism and other means of driving out the demons; or the patient was isolated or banished to protect others from the frightening state. There is no record of the way in which opium, known in ancient Egypt, was part of the therapeutic procedures.

The *Old Testament* contains the impressive story about the first king of Israel, Saul, who was anointed by the prophet Samuel, whereupon "the spirit of God came over him", i.e. Saul had superhuman powers that even others could perceive. After the battle against the arch enemy, Amalek, in which Saul did not follow God's instructions, the spirit of God left him and "an evil spirit sent from God tormented him" (1 Samuel, 16: 14); Saul became depressed, suspicious and subject to outbursts of anger. David, the later son-in-law and eventual successor, could initially soothe the king with singing and harping, but Saul's state subsequently deteriorated and he broke down after a serious military reverse in Gilboa. His illness seemed to be a dark fate sent by God; Saul became increasingly entangled in guilt from which he found no way out, and even David's singing and all efforts to restore his mental balance remained ineffective.

The start of a scientific approach to mental health is generally attributed to the ancient Greeks. In the sixth century BC, Alkmaeon of Croton carried out systematic autopsies and discovered the pathways connecting the eye and ears with the brain. As a result, the brain was seen as the seat of reason and the soul. Around 400 BC, Hippocrates and his school placed natural, i.e. physical, causes in the foreground: mental illnesses are expressions or results of an imbalance between the body fluids (humors), which are normally present in harmonious proportions. The *humoral theory of Hippocrates*, certainly one of the most influential concepts in the history of psychology and psychiatry, counted on four basic fluids corresponding to four temperaments or character types and, in the case of pathological predominance of one component, to four mental illnesses (see Table 2.1).

Because mental illnesses are due to an imbalance between the body fluids, treatment must seek to restore the balance. Methods directed to the body were recommended, such as diet, bathing and showering, blood-letting and laxatives (hellebore).

The original writings of Hippocrates and his school have not been handed down to us. They reached Alexandria around 300 BC and were summarized by the Roman author Celsus in the first century AD. The need for individual adaptation of each therapy was stressed here: frightened patients are to be reassured in a friendly manner; manic patients should be chained and perhaps starved; music and poetry lift the melancholy; the mad should be shunned or brought to other thoughts by sudden noises; and adequate sleep should be ensured for all patients. Poppy (opium) and henbane were available for this, but rippling fountains could also have a calming and soporific action.

Table 2.1 Basis of the humoral theory of Hippocrates

Humor	Temperament: affectivity	Mental illness
Blood	Sanguine: lively and weak	Mania, insanity
Phlegm	Phlegmatic: slow and weak	Calm insanity
Black bile	Melancholic: slow and strong	Melancholy
Choler	Choleric: lively and strong	Hysteria, especially in women

The major authority for medicine in the Middle Ages was *Galen* of Pergamon, who worked in Rome in the second century AD. Galen adopted the humoral theory of Hippocrates, including the classification of mental illnesses, and his therapeutic recommendations were also based on the tradition of the Hippocratic school: diet, vomiting, blood-letting and the administration of soporifics.

The *Middle Ages* are not a high spot in the history of psychiatry. This was the time of possession by the devil and demons, of mass movements with a clearly pathological nature (flagellants, children's crusade), witch-burning and gruesome exorcism of spirits. Science and medicine did not develop further in Christian Europe because "the little that the Greeks knew was lost and an awful regression to earlier cultural stages occurred" (Ackerknecht, 1967, p. 18). However, this statement does not apply to the Islamic world: the Hippocratic–Galenic tradition was propagated further by Arabic doctors, and hospitals with separate departments for the mentally ill were available in Baghdad around AD 750 and in Cairo from AD 873. Treatment was based on the experience of the ancient world, so that measures directed to the body were predominantly used to overcome mental illnesses.

In the early Christian Middle Ages, however, a tradition arose that had a beneficial impact on the mentally ill, despite the fanaticism and incitement of later centuries: the tradition of *mercy*. Prayers were said for the possessed and the Church initially saw itself as a haven for the insane and epileptics also. Only in the eleventh century were some madmen considered to be envoys of the devil, to be combated by all available means; in the fourteenth century there was a change to isolating the insane from the healthy population in lunatic asylums and madhouses. Therapeutic measures for those isolated in this way were superfluous at that time, especially as those who knew about herbs and poisons were often themselves suspected of being witches (Duerr, 1979).

Between the Middle Ages and modern times stand physicians such as Paracelsus (1491–1541), Johann Weyer (1515–1588) and Felix Plater (1536–1614), who turned more or less clearly against the concepts of witches and spirits that prevailed at that time, and restored natural causes to the centre-stage of mental illnesses. They had no new treatments to offer and, true to the Galenic tradition, prescribed blood-letting and purging to clean the body fluids, baths and massages for relaxation and to strengthen the body, and soporifics and sedatives to stabilize excited minds.

2.3 THE MODERN AGE: PSYCHOPHARMACOLOGY BEFORE CHLORPROMAZINE

In the Age of Enlightenment and absolutism, psychiatry developed in different directions in the different European countries depending on local political and social circumstances (see Schrenk, 1973; Dörner, 1975; Foucault, 1978). The essential features of this development, which occurred in all countries sooner or later, are:

(1) The *spatial segregation of the insane* in houses that often lay outside the cities and towns, sometimes in one-time leper colonies.
(2) The gradual rediscovery of the *medical model* of mental illnesses, associated with research into pathological anatomical causes.
(3) Attempts to return the insane (the social outcasts) to a normal life by means of work, useful tasks and a regulated daily routine, and to support them as *members of society*.

It is clear that these trends are contradictory to some extent. A spatially segregated patient cannot lead a normal life in society. The medical model of mental illnesses, with its objective of detecting and, where applicable, correcting anatomical or functional disorders in the patient's body, contradicts a socially orientated concept of the illness underpinning treatment by educational methods. Modern psychiatry has grown up with these contradictions and still lives with them today (Rosen, 1969).

Psychopharmacology emerged very gradually in modern times. One of the earliest compendia of psychopharmacology to appear in German was written by P.J. Schneider (1824), and describes in some 600 pages the methods of psychiatric therapy used at the beginning of the nineteenth century. The description lacks discrimination in several respects and includes many measures that to us seem cruel or naive, insufficiently tested and often contradictory. Some 400 pages are devoted to 'Materia Medica' and it is here that the majority of medicinal recommendations are to be found. Many practices described in these Materia Medica are reminiscent of a torture chamber rather than of a hospital (Table 2.2) – and yet the author assures his readers that some of these measures were therapeutically effective in well-documented cases.

Psychotropic agents, in today's sense of the term, were classified by Schneider into the classes 'narcotic agents' and 'excitants, analeptics'. The list of allegedly useful substances, plants and extracts is extensive and colorful. Critical evaluation of the recommended active agents is hampered by the fact

Table 2.2 Materia Medica (after Schneider, 1824)

Antagonists (for use in cases of excessive nervous sensitivity and insufficient physical sensitivity)	Antiphlogistics (temperature-reducing measures)	Narcotic agents (calming agents)	Excitants, analeptics (nerve-invigorating agents)
A. Remedies promoting nausea and vomiting Internal: various emetics External: revolving machine, revolving chair, swing, red-hot iron, whips with nettles, cupping glasses; suppurating head wounds, gentle rubbing of the skin Enemas, mustard plasters, blistering plasters, ants, scabies Cold baths, snow baths, sudden immersion, ice bags, tepid baths B. Cathartics (laxatives) since psychic disturbances are often located in the abdomen Medicaments, some of which are still in use today	Medical Surgical (e.g. bleeding, cupping)	A. Narcotics: saffron, thorn apple, henbane, tobacco, alraun, prussic acid, opium B. Strong narcotics: belladonna, hemlock, foxglove, verbena C. External agents: sack, cupboard, hollow wheel, strait-jacket, strait-cradle	A. Internal remedies: camphor, sage, rosemary, lavender, balm mint, filix, valerian, green tea, arnica, cinnamon oil, nuniper oil, cumin, fennel, aniseed, peppermint and terpentine oil Musk, castoreum, Spanish fly Many spices Naphthalene, old wines B. External remedies: hot compresses on the head, sneezing powder, intake of irritants, electricity, galvanism, magnetism

that the author provides no proof of efficacy according to present-day standards and the reports of their effect are based on psychiatric terminology that nowadays is virtually incomprehensible. What does emerge clearly from this account is that Schneider numbered amongst the most effective medicaments the thorn apple (*Datura stramonium*), alraun, prussic acid, opium and belladonna. Alraun (*Mandragora*), henbane (*Hyoscyamus niger*) and belladonna (*Atropa belladonna*) are some of the traditional ingredients of witches' ointments and potions, to which was added the thorn apple at the beginning of the modern era (see Caldwell, 1978; Duerr, 1979).

Psychiatry as a discipline of medicine made considerable advances in England and France in the early nineteenth century. A classification of mental illnesses based on precise clinical observations and statistical comparison was developed by Philippe Pinel (1745–1826) and Jean Étienne Esquirol (1772–1840), and the cruellest of the treatment methods, including chaining the insane, had already been discontinued by the turn of the century in Paris. In 1818, Esquirol drew up an expert report on madhouses in France at the request of the French Home Office, and this shattering report led to a thorough reform of psychiatry. In his textbook of 1838, Esquirol spoke of "maladie mentale" ('mental illness') instead of the previously used term 'alienation', and thus announced the victory of the medical model over spiritualistic concepts of psychiatric diseases. With Wilhelm Griesinger (1817–1868), the German school of psychiatry underwent a similar transformation and, under Emil Kraepelin (1856–1926), a psychiatric classification was created, the essential features of which still remain valid today.

Griesinger's textbook of psychiatry (1861) gives extensive information on only a very few centrally acting medicaments; particularly recommended are opium, ether and chloroform narcoses, as well as prussic acid. Opium was observed in appropriate cases to "calm the sick, reduce hallucinations, dispel feelings of anxiety as well as delusions related thereto and occasionally to bring about their complete cure" (p. 488). Above all, younger patients whose ailment had not yet become chronic could, in Griesinger's experience, benefit from opium treatment – and interestingly enough no mention is made of the development of addiction.

Following narcoses, induced using either ether or chloroform, there was "often (but by no means consistently) a temporary remission of the melancholia and mania...now and then even a complete *lucidum inter-vallum*...but the earlier clinical picture soon reappeared" (p. 489). According to Griesinger's observations, repeated use of ether and chloroform leads to the remissions becoming briefer and soon disappearing completely. The hope that had been laid on the medical treatment of mental disorders with these new synthetic substances was thus not fulfilled. Prussic acid is a secondary remedy listed by Griesinger and was said to be capable of calming moderate exaltation, melancholic anxiety and similar states. The author made no further remarks concerning other remedies (datura, belladonna, quinine and hashish) listed in his book.

Griesinger devoted only little space to the use of medicaments in the treatment of mental illness, but Kraepelin's textbook of psychiatry (1899) made various references to the use of pharmaceuticals in the treatment of the mentally ill. Some of these are preparations having a certain tradition in psychiatry, whereas others were substances that had been discovered in the intervening period (Table 2.3). And yet, comparison of this list with Griesinger's recommendations shows how little progress had been made in the 40 or so years that had elapsed; although the number of hypnotics had grown somewhat, no fundamentally new types of activity had been found.

A similar stagnation is apparent when one compares the first eight editions of the *Lehrbuch der Psychiatrie* (*Textbook of Psychiatry*) by Eugen Bleuler, which appeared between 1916 and 1949. Although the heading 'Hypnotics' already appears in the index of the first edition, the concept 'Treatment with medicaments' only appears in 1949, in the eighth edition. All in all, Bleuler used pharmaceuticals much more restrictively than Griesinger and Kraepelin; he regarded opium as a risky remedy that should be avoided in view of the danger of habituation. He also rejects alcohol – which was still recommended by Kraepelin in 1899 – owing to the risk of alcoholism and in its place

Table 2.3 Psychopharmaceuticals listed by Kraepelin (1899)

1. *Narcotics: medicaments with calming action*

Opium: excitation, anxiety states and pain-induced unrest respond to it; also prolonged manic states
Morphine: similar to opium, but simpler to dose. Risk of toxic effects and/or morphinism. Codeine, another opiate, offers no advantages
Hyoscine (scopolamine): a useful medicament, induces deep sleep rapidly. Especially for manic patients
Hashish: hypnotic with unreliable action

2. *Hypnotics*

Chloral hydrate: induces longer sleep, sometimes with drowsiness in the morning. Mordant, unpleasant taste. Paraldehyde is similar but more of a soporific
Sulfonal, trional: Pleasant to take, but often give rise to tiredness and a feeling of weakness on the following day. Accumulation during prolonged use
Alcohol: mild hypnotic, recommended dose 40–60 g (corresponds to > 100 ml of cognac, whisky, etc.!); used in hysterical and neurasthenic, insomniac patients, and for insomnia in the elderly
Chloroform: for very severe states of excitation refractory to all other agents; the calming action does not last beyond the anesthesia

3. *Bromine salts*

Give valuable service in epilepsy and neurasthenia, eliminate inner tension and insomnia. Risks during prolonged use: motor dysfunction, apathy

Table 2.4 Psychopharmaceuticals recommended by Bleuler (1916). Reprinted with permission of Springer-Verlag GmbH & Co. KG

Hypnotics: sulfonal, trional, chloral hydrate, veronal, paraldehyde. Alcohol used as a hypnotic may be pleasant for the patient but the risk of habituation makes it dangerous and ineffective

Bromine: in nervous agitation and less severe depression

Opiates: can have a calming, sleep-inducing action. Less effective than expected in psychoses. To be avoided because of the risk of addiction

Hyoscine (scopolamine): useful in acute states of agitation and also in combination with morphine (Moscop)

recommends hyoscine (scopolamine) in states of pronounced agitation. As regards hypnotics proper, he advises against their prolonged use and suggests that the remedies be changed from time to time in order to prevent any habituation (Table 2.4). This reserved approach towards drug-based therapy remained unchanged throughout the following editions of his textbook and, as already stated, hardly any additions were made to Bleuler's list of recommended preparations between 1916 and 1949.

Apart from the slow progress in psychiatric pharmacotherapy it is striking that although Griesinger, Kraepelin and Bleuler cited a large number of sedatives and hypnotics their recommendation included no stimulating medicaments of any kind. Whereas several preparations were available that could be used to sedate raging, anxious, restless or sleep-disturbed patients, the psychiatrists of the time were virtually powerless in the face of depressive and stuporous states, if one discounts the not generally accepted use of opium. Here, a certain degree of progress was attained with the shock therapies: insulin-induced coma, cardiazole-induced shock and, in particular, electro-shock. Amphetamine was synthesized in 1927 and, owing to its stimulating properties, was used to a growing extent in the 1930s against narcolepsy and similar disorders. However, it never acquired any great importance in psychiatric pharmacotherapy because it only displayed a modest effect in states of exhaustion and slight depression, while remaining virtually ineffective in endogenous depression.

2.4 THE DISCOVERY OF MODERN PSYCHOPHARMACEUTICALS

2.4.1 CHLORPROMAZINE

Detailed accounts of the discovery of chlorpromazine as an antipsychotic drug have been given by two authors (Caldwell, 1970; Swazey, 1974); an abridged version is to be found in Caldwell (1978) and some personal memories are reported by Deniker (1988) and the Comité Lyonnais de Recherches Thérapeutiques en Psychiatrie (2000). It emerges clearly from all these descriptions that the discovery of the first neuroleptic drug was not the work of a single physician, scientist or research group. Nor did it emerge as the result of a planned research project aimed at finding a pharmacological therapy for schizophrenia. What in fact happened was that several initially unrelated developmental trends converged at the end of the 1940s in the most fortuitous fashion and, owing to precise clinical observations on the part of several doctors, led to the most significant advance in psychiatric therapy for many years. Swazey (1974) regards the following factors as critical:

- The efforts made by the French surgeon Laborit to find a safer anesthetic technique and to prevent surgical shock.
- A pharmacological development program embarked on by the drug company Rhône–Poulenc in Paris to screen for medicaments having an antihistamine action.
- The readiness to experiment displayed by several biologically interested psychiatrists trying out pharmacological remedies to more effective psychiatric therapy.

Of special interest is the contribution made by Henri Laborit, who had worked as an army surgeon during the Second World War and who, under the influence of his war experiences, devoted himself in subsequent years primarily to the problem of shock.

The term 'shock' when used in medicine relates to an acute state of general weakness and the restriction of many vital functions. Patients in shock are generally apathetic, their face is sunken and their expression is full of anxiety; skin is moist, cold and gray, pulse is rapid and faint, blood pressure is normally low, musculature is lax and superficial blood vessels are empty; respiration is superficial, basal metabolism is reduced and urine formation is considerably slower. Shock may be triggered by a variety of causes: severe physical injury with excessive loss of blood, surgery or severe psychic trauma; in predisposed persons it may also arise as a reaction to exogenous substances such as antibiotics or bee poison.

In the 1940s there were various current hypotheses as to the question of the biological or biochemical mechanisms underlying shock. In his own research Laborit arrived at the view that endogenous substances having a transmitter function (adrenaline, acetylcholine and histamine, see Chapter 4) are involved in the triggering and full-scale development of shock. In his view, shock is a consequence of excessively strong biological emergency reactions no longer adapted to the situation, and can be combated by blocking the effects of the transmitters using appropriate pharmacological agents, if possible at several points simultaneously. In light of this hypothesis, Laborit experimented with various substances known to have an inhibitory effect on adrenaline, acetylcholine and histamine. These included agents such as procaine, curare, atropine and – the class that was to decide future events – synthetic antihistamines.

This is where Laborit's interests coincided with those of the drug company Rhône–Poulenc, which had already embarked on a chemical and pharmacological program to develop antihistamine compounds several years before. An important point was reached when promethazine, an antihistamine with pronounced sedative and analgesic properties, was examined clinically by Laborit and other doctors. Not only was this medicament suitable, in combination with other substances, in preventing surgical shock, but Laborit observed that patients treated with promethazine were quieter and more relaxed and – even after major surgery – in relatively good spirits.

Impressed by this success, Rhône–Poulenc decided in 1950 to look for more antihistamines in the same chemical class as promethazine having an even more pronounced 'central' effect. This decision was by no means an obvious one, because the sedative effect of promethazine could barely be characterized using the contemporary methods of animal experiments. Furthermore, the sedating and sleep-inducing effect of promethazine was a distinct disadvantage in some therapeutic applications (hay fever, other allergies). In October 1950, disregarding these difficulties, P. Koetschet, one of the Rhône–Poulenc heads of research, suggested embarking on a goal-directed search for promethazine analogs with a greater effect on the central nervous system. Although it was not possible to foresee what therapeutic applications these substances would have, Koetschet envisaged their exploratory use in anesthesiology, in Parkinsonism, in psychiatry and possibly also in epileptic patients. As early as March 1951 a substance, given the number 4560 RP, was available that was chemically related to promethazine while revealing a considerably more pronounced central effect in pharmacological tests in animals. In April 1951 human trials of 4560 RP commenced and the first applications confirmed that the compound augmented the sleep-inducing action of barbiturates and also acted as a sedative when used on its own.

Laborit obtained 4560 RP in June 1951 and soon recognized the advantages of the new substance: it lessened the anxiety felt by patients prior to surgery, diminished surgical stress and made it possible to simplify the mixture of medicaments used by Laborit – the so-called lytic cocktails. Furthermore, the compound had a low toxicity and consequently could be used in a broader dosage rather than, for example, curare.

Under the effect of chlorpromazine, as 4560 RP was later to be named, patients did not lose consciousness but merely became sleepy and uninterested in everything going on around them and being done to them (Laborit *et al.*, 1952). Laborit and co-workers postulated that this strange central action suggested the use of chlorpromazine in psychiatry, e.g. in sleep therapy, where it was hoped to attain an improved effect and greater safety in comparison to hitherto known agents.

Laborit was not the only doctor conducting early clinical trials on chlorpromazine at the instigation of Rhône–Poulenc; it emerged from reports given by other clinicians that the substance produced a form of sedation in patients that previously had been unknown. Based on these observations, Rhône–Poulenc decided, at the end of 1951, to extend the research program to include the mentally ill and to use chlorpromazine, in combination with barbiturates, experimentally in sleep therapy and in the treatment of manic episodes. Independently of this, Laborit tried to encourage a few psychiatrists personally known to him to embark on clinical trials using chlorpromazine in restless patients. Eventually a group of doctors in a psychiatric military hospital decided to conduct an initial trial on a manic patient. After some three weeks of treatment with chlorpromazine in combination with other sedatives, the patient's condition improved to such an extent that he could be discharged and sent home. In a paper presented before the Société Médico-Psychologique, Hamon *et al.* reported on 25 February 1952 on their initial experiences with chlorpromazine, which they held to be interesting. However, because they did not consider the sedative effect of the new substance to be strong enough, they preferred the then customary electroshock therapy.

At about this time one of the best-known French psychiatrists of the day, Jean Delay, commenced his own studies with chlorpromazine in conjunction with a colleague, Pierre Deniker. Deniker had learnt, by private communications, of Laborit's experiments with chlorpromazine in anesthesiology, which were referred to as *hibernation artificielle*. He asked Rhône–Poulenc for drug samples and received them in February 1952. Unlike Laborit, who always used chlorpromazine in combination with other medicaments, Delay and Deniker decided to administer chlorpromazine without concomitant drugs to manically agitated patients. Their first findings were so beneficial that they presented an initial report to the Société Médico-Psychologique after 3 months, a report that appeared soon after in written form (Delay *et al.*, 1952). During the following months the same authors published a number of reports in rapid succession on the effect of chlorpromazine in various psychiatric conditions and thus helped to make the new medicament known in France and, in part, also abroad.

One of the first clinics outside France to show an interest in chlorpromazine was the Basel University Psychiatric Hospital. A young member of the clinic's staff (Felix Labhardt) had been in Paris for postgraduate training from summer 1951 to spring 1952 and had heard there of the application of the new substance 4560 RP in anesthesiology and psychiatry. An initial therapeutic trial commenced in Basel in January 1953 and was so successful that a rapid succession of patients with quite varied diagnoses underwent chlorpromazine cures. The first publication from the Basel clinic appeared in June 1953 (Staehelin and Kielholz, 1953): Largactil®, as the medicament was now named, was recommended in "all severe mental disturbances in which pronounced vegetative syndromes could be demonstrated", particularly in:

- emotional psychoses and other psychotic reactions
- detoxification cures for addicts
- severe neuroses, especially those with symptoms of anxiety and compulsion
- symptomatic psychoses tinged with anxiety
- certain forms of schizophrenia and manic–depressive psychosis

This list shows clearly the extent to which the fields of indication of chlorpromazine had broadened in barely one and a half years. Of special importance was its use in schizophrenia, which Labhardt presented shortly afterwards in a comprehensive lecture given at the First Largactil Symposium, held in Basel on 28 November 1953. According to the results presented by Staehelin (the then head of the Basel clinic) of the approximately 500 patients in the clinic, some 200 were on Largactil® and over 130 discharged patients were continuing to take the medicament. Figures cited by Staehelin's colleagues in their lectures were equally impressive: Kielholz reported on the results of treatment in 52 depressive patients, 16 drug addicts in withdrawal and more than 20 senile patients with nocturnal unrest. Labhardt presented data on the treatment of over 200 schizophrenic patients with chlorpromazine. To all this were added reports on therapeutic studies undertaken in other psychiatric hospitals in Switzerland and covering over 850 patients.

Particularly important consequences arose out of the findings presented by Labhardt (1954) on the treatment of schizophrenics: excellent results were obtained, not only in recently afflicted patients but also in those who had been hospitalized for several years. In the case of chronic patients in whom the illness went back over 5 years or more, significant improvements were observed in almost 60% of the cases, and some of the patients who had previously had an almost hopeless prognosis according to prevailing opinions could be discharged from hospital.

Spectacular findings were not just being recorded with chlorpromazine in Paris and Basel; other centres also achieved favourable results. Thanks to chlorpromazine, the character of psychiatric hospitals and of psychiatric care in general underwent a radical change. Lunatic asylums became peaceful hospitals and many patients who previously had to be institutionalized on account of the danger they presented to others and to themselves could be discharged and partially rehabilitated. There was a marked reduction in the average stay in psychiatric hospitals. Thanks to chlorpromazine it was recognized that not only is schizophrenia an illness that can be treated at least symptomatically by chemical means, but that it is in many cases an illness that can be cured – and the following years were to see a marked upswing in biologically orientated psychiatry.

2.4.2 ANTIDEPRESSANTS

The history of the first antidepressant, the monoamine oxidase (MAO) inhibitor iproniazid, is a complicated one for a number of reasons (Kline, 1970). Iproniazid was originally developed by the drug company Hoffmann-La Roche as a medicament for the treatment of tuberculosis, and attracted attention in 1951/52 during clinical trials on account of its stimulating and euphoriant effects; nervousness and sleep disorders occurred frequently and yet tubercular patients on iproniazid became cheerful and exuberant – moods strangely out of keeping with their condition. Initial applications in psychiatry, some in agitated and some in chronically apathetic schizophrenics, failed to lead to interpretable results, and the use of iproniazid against tuberculosis was increasingly being regarded as risky, mainly as a consequence of the stimulating effect of the preparation.

A more systematic clinical investigation of the antidepressant effect of iproniazid was only commenced in 1956 after animal experiments had suggested that the compound possessed an activity in this area. Pretreatment of animals with iproniazid prevented the so-called reserpine syndrome in mice and rats; instead of being calm and tame, as is normally the case after reserpine, animals pretreated with iproniazid became hyperactive and, in some cases, aggressive when given reserpine. Initial clinical trials revealed that iproniazid had a stimulating and mood-elevating effect in at least some of the patients with depression. On the other hand, reports kept coming in of side effects caused by the preparation and these impeded its broader use. The manufacturers ultimately withdrew the preparation in the USA and in some other countries but it remained on sale in further markets – a confusing situation that went on for years (Kline, 1970). Some subsequently introduced MAO inhibitors, such as isocarboxacid and tranylcypromine, were also withdrawn after a short time due to various types of side effects.

Another, and by no means always straightforward, path was followed by the discovery of the so-called *thymoleptics*, which eventually became more important as antidepressants than the MAO inhibitors. As in the case of Rhône–Poulenc, the firm Geigy in Basel had worked during the 1940s on antihistaminic substances that were chemically similar to promethazine and chlorpromazine. In animal experiments one of these compounds, number G 22150, had an antihistaminic as well as sedative action and was tested in 1950 by the Swiss psychiatrist Roland Kuhn in restless patients as a potential sedative and hypnotic. As Kuhn wrote in 1957: the "expected action was in most cases not found to be present . . . in the doses of 0.02–0.06 g used at that time. However, the preparation seemed to us to exert a pronounced calming effect in schizophrenics suffering from agitation, delusions and hallucinations". However, "this effect was assessed too much merely from the one-sided point of view of tranquillizing activity and hence the special interest of such substances was overlooked" (Kuhn, 1957, p. 1135).

In 1952 the first favorable results were obtained in psychiatry with chlorpromazine and Kuhn was among those psychiatrists to have access to the newly discovered neuroleptic. And yet, as Kuhn wrote in 1970, once chlorpromazine was on the market it was too expensive to be used in his hospital in large quantities. He therefore approached Geigy Pharmaceuticals in February 1954, pointing out the similarity between the effect observed with G 22150 and that of chlorpromazine. Further trial samples of G 22150 were supplied, but it became obvious that the Geigy preparation was inferior to chlorpromazine as an antipsychotic and, in addition, produced disturbing side effects. As a result, a further Geigy compound was selected for clinical trials – G 22355, which was chemically even closer to chlorpromazine than was G 22150. This substance was tested for about a year on some 300 patients with various mental illnesses and in spring 1956 Kuhn, to conclude his test series, also treated a few patients suffering from endogenous depression. It was discovered with surprise that the substance, later to be called *imipramine*, had a marked antidepressant effect that Kuhn (1957) described as follows:

- The patients' facial expression relaxes and regains expressivity. The patients become livelier, friendlier and more sociable. They talk more and louder.
- The moaning, crying and complaining stops; remarks relating to physical complaints decrease.
- The patients get up in the morning of their own accord and undertake activities under their own initiative; their lethargic pace of living returns to normal.
- The patients realize their improvement; feelings of heaviness, weakness and oppression decrease; feelings of guilt and depressive delusions disappear.
- Suicidal ideas and tendencies recede.
- Sleep disturbances and oppressive dreams become rarer. Daily mood swings with morning lows, lack of appetite and constipation cease.

According to Kuhn's observations, the effect of imipramine became apparent in some cases after a few days; in other cases several weeks passed before any therapeutic effect could be seen. He estimated his failure rate at 20–25%, but regarded his sample as too small for any reliable estimate to be made. If the medicament was discontinued too soon, there was said to be a danger of relapse. It was also not possible to ascertain from his observations whether imipramine shortened the natural duration of the depressive phase. The best therapeutic successes were recorded in "endogenous depression and in cases of depression which first appeared at the menopause, in cases where vital symptoms were clearly in the foreground". Kuhn also provided a comprehensive list of side effects of imipramine, which nevertheless in his view did not appreciably restrict use of the medicament. (None of the claims regarding the clinical pattern of action of imipramine made by Kuhn on the basis of open studies on 300 patients, 40 of whom suffered from endogenous depression, had to be withdrawn or significantly modified later.)

In contrast to iproniazid and imipramine, which were synthesized in the early 1950s and then tested in man, *lithium* had been known to medicine for almost 100 years before John Cade became aware of its specific antimanic action (see Cade, 1970). The starting point of this Australian psychiatrist's investigations was a hypothesis regarding the etiology of manic–depressive illness, according to which manic phases were triggered by poisoning due to a surplus of an endogenous substance, whereas the depressive phase was due to a deficiency of the same substance. In order to test this hypothesis, Cade injected the urine from manic patients into guinea pigs and found this urine to display greater toxicity than that of healthy subjects. He then began a search for substances that would protect the guinea pigs from the effects of the manic patients' urine. Via a few intermediate steps he came across lithium salts, which had the desired effect. In addition he noticed that, with the administration of lithium, the animals became lethargic and showed virtually no reaction to stimuli, although they did not lapse into a state of sleep. As Cade wrote later: "It may seem a long way from lethargy in guinea pigs to the control of manic excitement, but as these investigations had commenced in an attempt to demonstrate some possibly excreted toxin in the urine of manic patients, the association of ideas is explicable" (1970, p. 223). In any event, Cade conducted his first trials with lithium in manic patients in 1948 and reported very good therapeutic findings in 10 out of 10 patients.

Despite this favorable result, lithium was hardly considered as a psychopharmaceutical for many years. There were a variety of reasons for this. Firstly, mania is not a very common psychosis and there is spontaneous remission in many cases. There were thus not so many occasions where lithium treatment was indicated. Secondly, lithium salts were considered to be toxic because for some time they had been given in excessive doses to patients with heart failure and in this way, had led to a number of fatalities (Cade, 1970). Thirdly, a few years after Cade's first publication psychiatrists' attention had been claimed by chlorpromazine and the subsequent neuroleptics and antidepressants, thus explaining why lithium almost fell into oblivion. It was only in the 1960s that it once more attracted some interest, after the Danish psychiatrist Mogens Schou had shown that lithium salts were not only useful in the manic phase of manic–depressive illness but also could prevent depressive episodes in patients suffering from bipolar psychoses.

2.4.3 TRANQUILLIZERS

The discoveries of chlorpromazine and imipramine are generally regarded as greater scientific advances than that of the tranquillizers. However, in making the public aware of the fact that mental disturbances can be treated with chemical agents, tranquillizers – owing to their widespread use – played as important a role as neuroleptics and antidepressants.

Sedatives – above all, low dosages of sleep-inducing agents – were the historic precursors of tranquillizers but their use was severely restricted by serious disadvantages: a narrow therapeutic dose range and the risk of habituation and addiction. A first link in the chain leading to modern tranquillizers was forged by the compound *mephenesine*, which produced muscle relaxation, calm and a sleep-like state in animal experiments. Mephenesine was part of a chemical development program that had been started shortly after the Second World War in an English pharmaceutical company (British Drug Houses), aimed at finding compounds active against penicillin-resistant bacteria. The pronounced muscle-relaxing action of mephenesine became apparent during toxicological testing (Berger, 1970), as a result of which clinical trials commenced to examine the muscle-relaxant properties of this substance. It soon became evident that mephenesine was not only muscle-relaxing but also anxiety-relieving and psychically relaxing, leaving the patient's mind clear and free of any mental impairment.

Mephenesine is rapidly broken down in the organism and therefore its effect is only of short duration. At an early stage, therefore, chemists directed their efforts at finding longer-acting, i.e., more slowly metabolized, analogs of mephenesine. Many preparations were synthesized and some were even marketed (see Ban, 1969, p. 313) but *meprobamate* was the first to display the desired profile of action because it had pronounced muscle-relaxing and anxiolytic effects, adequate therapeutic safety margin and a long duration of action. Although the pharmacological profile of meprobamate was known as early as 1954, the substance was only accepted clinically as a tranquillizer in 1957. In the ensuing years, the practical application of meprobamate expanded to cover what was called neurotic tension and complaints of all kinds, and the compound enjoyed great commercial success only to be halted with the advent of the benzodiazepines.

The history of the *benzodiazepines* has been set down by their inventor, the Polish–American chemist L. Sternbach (1978). He tells how in the mid-1950s Hoffman-La Roche, in light of the success of the first psychopharmaceuticals, decided to investigate this field also. Of the possible approaches to chemical research and development – modification of already known and active molecules, synthetic work based on a specific biochemical hypothesis, synthesis of substances belonging to new chemical classes and their pharmacological screening in known experimental models – the firm chose the latter. Sternbach based his synthetic chemical work on a class of substances that he had examined earlier when working at the University of Cracow. Decisive in this choice was the fact that few scientists had concentrated on this class of chemicals and Hoffmann-La Roche consequently could expect to achieve a large number of patentable compounds. Furthermore, this class of substances was, as Sternbach emphasized, interesting for the chemist for scientific and technical reasons.

Regardless of these advantages, the newly synthesized compounds proved to be pharmacologically uninteresting and the program was consequently halted in 1957. Sternbach himself assumed new duties and was in the process of clearing the laboratory for new work when he came across two substances that had been synthesized earlier but had not yet been subjected to pharmacological tests. Without any great hopes, one of these substances was sent for pharmacological screening. Contrary to expectation, it proved to be effective in the series of tests designed to indicate a tranquillizing effect. In mice the compound was muscle-relaxing, sedating, anticonvulsant and antiaggressive, and these effects were confirmed in other species of animals. The molecule, later to be called chlordiazepoxide (Librium®), was more effective in all the pharmacological tests than the reference substance meprobamate. It was not hypnotic even at high doses, had no vegetative effects and its toxicity was very low. A taming effect was observed in rhesus monkeys, which can be very vicious in captivity.

Initial clinical trials were conducted in geriatric patients in spring 1958; although the substance clearly displayed the expected sedative properties, it led to severe ataxia and speech disturbances (Cohen, 1970), for which reason the clinical trials were interrupted for some months. A member of the Hoffmann-La Roche clinical research department then had the idea of having lower doses of the preparation tested by practising psychiatrists in outpatients suffering from neurotic disorders. The results of these additional studies were encouraging: chlordiazepoxide led to a reduction in tension and states of anxiety, without causing any significant side effects such as disturbed wakefulness and impaired mental functioning. The preparation had a broad therapeutic range and no toxic effects were observed in man. "This added up to an easily manipulated drug having a wide range of clinical application and minimal toxicity" (Cohen, 1970, p. 134). In view of these positive results, clinical trials were stepped up and as early as autumn 1959 a symposium was held in which reports were presented on experiences with chlordiazepoxide in several thousand patients. The US health authorities – the Food and Drug Administration (FDA) – approved the medicament Librium® in February 1960, 2 years after commencement of clinical trials.

2.5 DISCUSSION: HOW WERE MODERN PSYCHOPHARMACEUTICALS DISCOVERED?

All prototypes of modern psychopharmaceuticals (lithium, chlorpromazine, meprobamate, imipramine and chlordiazepoxide) were discovered in a period of about 10 years (Fig. 2.1). Neither before nor since has such a series of

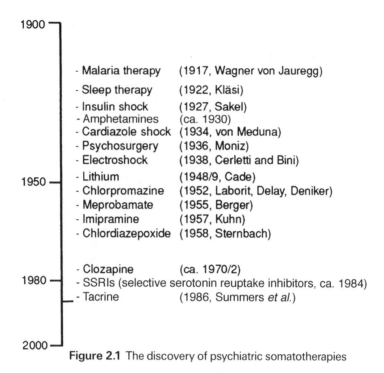

1900	
	- Malaria therapy (1917, Wagner von Jauregg)
	- Sleep therapy (1922, Kläsi)
	- Insulin shock (1927, Sakel)
	- Amphetamines (ca. 1930)
	- Cardiazole shock (1934, von Meduna)
	- Psychosurgery (1936, Moniz)
	- Electroshock (1938, Cerletti and Bini)
1950	- Lithium (1948/9, Cade)
	- Chlorpromazine (1952, Laborit, Delay, Deniker)
	- Meprobamate (1955, Berger)
	- Imipramine (1957, Kuhn)
	- Chlordiazepoxide (1958, Sternbach)
	- Clozapine (ca. 1970/2)
1980	- SSRIs (selective serotonin reuptake inhibitors, ca. 1984)
	- Tacrine (1986, Summers *et al.*)
2000	

Figure 2.1 The discovery of psychiatric somatotherapies

therapeutic advances been made in psychiatry. Several authors dealing with the history of modern psychopharmacology have thus raised the question of which factors made a decisive contribution to the discovery of modern psychopharmaceuticals within such a short time. Two partially negative answers can certainly be given: the discoveries followed no common pattern; and neither in the case of lithium nor in the case of chlorpromazine or imipramine can one speak of goal-directed developments whereby a substance was developed, on the basis of pathophysiological knowledge and a given pharmacological hypothesis, with a specific therapeutic indication in view. To recapitulate the sequence of events once more:

- Chlorpromazine emerged from a series of compounds that aroused interest mainly on account of their antihistaminic effects, and partly their anticholinergic effects.
- Imipramine also came from a class of substances having antihistaminic properties, and was earmarked and tested clinically as a possible competitor to chlorpromazine.
- Meprobamate was a further development based on another medicament (mephenesine), the muscle-relaxant effects of which had attracted attention as a side effect during toxicological trials.

- In the case of MAO inhibitors also, a side effect that had been observed in conjunction with their use for another indication (tuberculosis) was converted into a therapeutic effect for a different group of patients.

Only in the case of chlordiazepoxide can one speak in terms of goal-directed development; here the intention was to find tranquillizing compounds in a new and patentable class of substances. In no case, however, was there a biochemical hypothesis concerning the illness or symptoms to be treated that would have led to the rational synthesis and development of appropriate pharmaceuticals.

2.5.1 CHANCE DISCOVERY

Are the major discoveries in psychopharmacology based on *coincidence* and, if so, what is meant by coincidence? A stroke of luck, whereby some psychiatrist, somewhere, experimenting with some kind of substance unexpectedly hits on a major discovery, can certainly be ruled out in the case of chlorpromazine. For years Laborit had considered pharmacological ways of preventing shock, during which time he had systematically looked for suitable compounds and combinations of substances. Delay's and Deniker's efforts to alleviate psychoses by pharmacological means had had a long tradition; their experiments with chlorpromazine followed many trials using other sympathicolytic and anticholinergic substances. The same holds true for the Basel clinic, where the therapeutic indications of chlorpromazine were expanded systematically. An example to the contrary is given by Laborit's colleagues Hamon and co-workers, who were the first to test chlorpromazine in psychiatry (before Delay and Deniker) but did not recognize its potential.

How are the discoveries of imipramine, meprobamate, chlordiazepoxide and lithium to be judged in this context? According to their inventors, luck was always involved, albeit in quite different ways. In Cade's own version of the story the choice of lithium as a medicament against mania was made on the basis of unrelated factors; in his experiments on the toxic effect of the urine of manic patients he was looking for a water-soluble form of uric acid and, in so doing, came across lithium urate. This molecule quite unexpectedly reduced the toxicity of the uric acid. Instead of lithium urate, Cade subsequently used lithium carbonate, which also protected his guinea pigs from the toxic effects of uric acid, and this was the background against which the history of lithium as a psychopharmaceutical started. Had it not been for Cade's systematic method of working, the chance discovery of lithium might never have been made.

Looking back on it today, it would seem that chance played a smaller role in the discovery of the antidepressant effect of imipramine. The antimanic effect of lithium had already been recognized – although lithium was only being used in a few clinics – and the recently discovered antipsychotic effect of chlorpromazine suggested that major psychiatric disorders could be treated with pharmacological agents. Clinical trials in psychiatry with the chlorpromazine-like substances synthesized at Geigy Pharmaceuticals were therefore a logical step. The critical contribution here was the persistent way in which Kuhn, in close cooperation with scientific staff at Geigy (Broadhurst, 1998), conducted his clinical studies. Kuhn's personal conviction – a sort of magical belief that depression could be cured with pharmacological means – also played its part (Kuhn, 1970) and, taken together with the high price of chlorpromazine and the tight budget of a (non-university) psychiatric hospital in the mid-1950s, was probably decisive.

According to Sternbach's account of the discovery of chlordiazepoxide, chance was also at work in the laboratories of Hoffmann-La Roche, although in a different way; of the series of substances that Sternbach had synthesized, why should it have been chlordiazepoxide, of all others, that had been left behind untested in the chemist's laboratory? Rather than stressing this chance occurrence, the well-conducted clinical trial of the experimental preparation should be emphasized instead. This study was not restricted to a single indication or dosage range, but was extended – in the face of initial unfavorable results – into those indications within which the then standard preparation meprobamate achieved its best results (Cohen, 1970).

2.5.2 SERENDIPITY AND SPIRIT OF THE AGE (ZEITGEIST)

English-language authors, when referring to the discovery of the first psychopharmaceuticals, often state that '*serendipity*' was involved. This word, which comes from a Persian fairy tale, refers to the ability of a research worker to make a fortuitous and unexpected discovery while leaving open upon what this ability is based. Jeste *et al.* (1979) have set out the etymology of the word and at the same time spoke against overemphasis of the element of chance in the history of psychopharmacology. In their view, several impulses were needed to allow the development of the most important biological (pharmacological and other) methods of modern therapy in psychiatry:

- A strong individual motivation on the part of the research workers involved and the conviction that mental illnesses could be treated by physical methods.
- The ability to make precise observations and the persistence to follow up even unexpected results, and at the same time also the courage to extend laboratory observations to experiments in man.
- The *Zeitgeist* – the spirit of the times in which they worked, i.e. the cultural and, in the present case, the scientific views prevailing at a specific time and in a specific society.
- The availability of basic knowledge from several related disciplines.

At first sight we are quite willing to accept the importance of all four factors stated by Jeste *et al.*, but closer consideration raises several questions. There is no doubt that the discoverers of lithium, chlorpromazine, imipramine, etc. (Cade, Deniker, Kuhn) were highly motivated investigators and doctors, but there were also many highly motivated investigators at other times in psychiatry who were ready and able to check laboratory observations in clinical trials. The first two points put forward by Jeste *et al.* (1979) are thus quite non-specific. What characterized the scientific *Zeitgeist* of the late 1940s and how did this differ from that of the 1920s and 1930s? The question cannot be answered in this general form, but in the case of psychiatry it should be remembered that many physical and pharmacological methods of therapy had been introduced in earlier times without leading to the discovery of chlorpromazine, and the idea that mental illnesses could be caused or promoted by physical factors is a very old concept. What was decisive here was rather the circumstance that several pharmaceutical companies had started research and development programs after the Second World War, which, although aimed in different directions, resulted in pharmacologically active and relatively well-tolerated compounds that could be clinically tested for various, sometimes even speculative, indications.

The fourth point in the analysis by Jeste *et al.* (basic knowledge from allied disciplines) is also unconvincing. Did the improvement in basic knowledge really make a decisive contribution? Lithium was already known and in medical use in the nineteenth century, without its antimanic properties and prophylactic effect in depression being discovered. The synthesis of the chemical structures of phenothiazine and iminodibenzyl, from which chlor-promazine and imipramine, respectively, were developed, had also been known since the nineteenth century (Caldwell, 1978; Broadhurst, 1998) and although the benzodiazepine structure was new it was by no means so complicated that it could not have been synthesized far earlier. Finally, the pharmacological methods used to characterize the compounds in the laboratory were not based on newly acquired basic knowledge, despite the fact that the scientists at Rhône–Poulenc had to develop several new tests.

It follows that newly acquired basic knowledge in psychiatry, e.g. about the biochemistry of psychoses (which was essentially unknown around 1950), cannot have had a direct impact on the discovery of modern psychopharma-ceuticals. The neurophysiological, neurosurgical and neurochemical methods developed in the twentieth century played no part, either in the pharmacolo-gical or in the clinical characterization of lithium, chlorpromazine, imipramine, etc., and the minds of the then leading psychiatrists were directed primarily to psychoanalysis and not to the biological basis of psychiatry. On the contrary, major fresh impetus was given to neurophysiology, neuropharmacology, neurochemistry and to clinical research methodology *in the wake* of the discovery of these psychopharmaceuticals in the 1950s and 1960s.

2.5.3 QUANTITATIVE ASPECTS

Possibly too little attention is paid in the historical accounts of psychophar-macology to one quantitative factor: the number of research workers in the field of natural science who have at various times grappled with problems in psychiatry, and the numbers of substances used on the mentally ill at various periods in time. Both of these figures have grown very appreciably over the last 100 years, especially after the First and Second World Wars. It is probably no coincidence that the major discoveries – the shock therapies on the one hand and the psychopharmaceuticals on the other – fall within these periods. It is evident that the prospects of finding a suitable medication for an illness of unknown pathogenic mechanism increase with the number of novel substances tested – always assuming that the pharmacological and clinical-pharmacological work is properly conducted.

On the other hand, quantitative viewpoints alone are not sufficient to explain the sudden advance in the 1950s and the subsequent stagnation of psychopharmacology, with few new principles of action discovered in the following two or three decades (Fig. 2.1). In the 1960s and 1970s the number of researchers involved with psychopharmacology in hospitals, universities and industry increased considerably and an enormous number of substances were tested in the laboratory and on patients during that period, without awakening decisive advances in the pharmacotherapy of schizophrenia, depression and other mental disorders.

2.6. THE PAST 20 YEARS

More recent developments in psychopharmacology that are of interest include atypical antipsychotic drugs, new antidepressants, specifically selective serotonin reuptake inhibitors (SSRIs), and drugs for the treatment of Alzheimer's disease.

2.6.1 ATYPICAL ANTIPSYCHOTIC DRUGS

After the discovery of chlorpromazine as an antipsychotic drug many similarly acting compounds, later called typical neuroleptics (Chapter 1), were developed and marketed. Significant therapeutic progress was made when *clozapine*, the first atypical antipsychotic drug, was introduced in some European countries in the years 1971/1972. Clozapine had been synthesized as early as 1959 in the laboratories of a small Swiss drug company (Wander AG); its pharmacological profile was described for the first time in January 1961 (Schmutz and Eichenberger, 1983). A number of factors delayed the development of clozapine as an antipsychotic (Stille and Fischer-Cornelssen, 1988). Two open clinical studies in patients with schizophrenia were initiated in 1961/62 and produced contradictory findings. Subsequently, a multicenter study planned in Switzerland and Germany could not start because the amount of substance produced in a pilot plant was insufficient!

Clozapine was also tested as a potential analgesic, but had to be abandoned for this indication because patients were severely sedated even after small doses of the drug. Despite increasing scepticism about the future of the compound at Wander AG, clinical studies in schizophrenia were continued in 1965 on a small scale. A first publication highlighting clozapine's superior antipsychotic effects appeared in an Austrian medical journal (Gross and Langner, 1966) but had little impact. In the same year, a very positive account of the drug's clinical properties was given by a distinguished team of German psychiatrists at one of the first psychopharmacology congresses in Washington (Lehmann and Ban, 1997) – again with few immediate consequences.

It took almost 10 years to collect and consolidate clinical data sufficient for the registration of clozapine as an antipsychotic drug in Switzerland and elsewhere. Much of this delay was due to the fact that some leading psychiatrists of the time simply would not accept that a compound with marked peripheral side effects and strong sedative action, but not producing extrapyramidal motor symptoms, could be an effective or even superior antipsychotic drug. Based on clinical experience with the existing neuroleptics, there was a firm opinion that antipsychotic efficacy was tied to the propensity to cause extrapyramidal motor effects. The "strange story of clozapine" (McKenna and Bailey, 1993) is often quoted as an example to show how stereotyped scientific assumptions can hinder medical progress.

Once on the European market, clozapine rapidly gained a reputation of being clinically superior to other antipsychotic drugs; however its further expansion was stopped abruptly in 1974 when a rare but potentially fatal hematological side effect was detected in Finland. A number of patients developed granulocytopenia or agranulocytosis on clozapine; eight patients died from subsequent infections, causing an almost complete ban on the drug. Still, clozapine continued to be used in a few European countries as a last resort for severely ill patients not responding to any of the available neuroleptic drugs. The number of publications describing clozapine's clinical properties and discussing its mode of action increased steadily, causing the manufacturer of the drug to consider a re-launch of the product. In 1989, after a large controlled clinical study had confirmed the superiority of clozapine over conventional neuroleptics (Kane *et al.*, 1988), the drug was approved in the USA and other countries for use in treatment-resistant or neuroleptic-intolerant psychotic patients.

Compared with the history of clozapine, the development of the more recent atypical antipsychotics – risperidone and olanzapine – appears almost straightforward. *Risperidone* was introduced in the early 1990s as the second atypical antipsychotic drug after clozapine. Its pharmacological and clinical profile shows some overlap with properties of clozapine and those of typical neuroleptics like haloperidol (Owens and Risch, 1998). The compound was synthesized and developed by Janssen Pharmaceuticals in Belgium following an interesting clinical observation, i.e. that the serotonin 5-HT2 antagonist ritanserin, when added to typical neuroleptics like haloperidol, can lead to an improvement of negative symptoms, depression and anxiety in schizophrenic patients. The combination of haloperidol and ritanserin was also found to produce fewer extrapyramidal symptoms (EPS) than haloperidol alone. Risperidone, which is a potent blocker of central 5-HT2A receptors (like ritanserin) and dopamine D2 receptors (like haloperidol), was first tested in schizophrenic patients around 1986; as predicted from its pharmacological profile, the compound turned out to be equally effective as haloperidol with regard to positive symptoms, it showed some efficacy against negative symptoms and it caused fewer EPS than classical neuroleptics at clinically effective, low doses.

Olanzapine, a drug developed by Eli Lilly in England and the USA, is chemically and pharmacologically related to clozapine. It has high affinity to dopamine D1, D2 and D4, serotonin 5-HT2A and 5-HT3, histamine H1, α1-adrenergic and muscarinic M1 receptors. The compound was selected from a larger series of chemical analogs based on behavioral tests and not, as one would have expected at that time (in the late 1980s), on *in vitro* binding and other biochemical studies. Olanzapine blocked a conditioned avoidance response at lower doses than those needed to induce catalepsy in rats; this ratio was considered predictive for the relationship between antipsychotic and EPS-producing doses in patients. As stated by Tupper *et al.* (1999): "had binding studies been a primary method of selecting compounds, it is unlikely olanzapine would have been developed". According to information publicly available, the clinical development of olanzapine was uneventful. Registration documents were submitted simultaneously to health authorities in Europe and the USA in September 1995, with approval a year later. Together with risperidone, olanzapine is currently the most widely prescribed antipsychotic drug.

2.6.2 NEW ANTIDEPRESSANTS: SSRIs

Once the antidepressant effect of imipramine had been recognized, a large number of imipramine-like compounds with no really novel features were developed and marketed (Chapter 1). According to the Swedish pharmacologist Arvid Carlsson (1998), the next step occurred as follows: "During the 1960s the mechanism of action of imipramine was generally believed to be a blockade of norepinephrine reuptake. However, late in the same decade this picture started to change somewhat. In 1968, working with K. Fuxe and U. Ungerstedt,...I found that imipramine blocked not only the reuptake of norepinephrine but also that of serotonin. We then studied a large number of tricyclic antidepressants. Among them, clomipramine had the strongest action on serotonin uptake, more so than did imipramine... We then decided to try to develop a compound that was selective for serotonin reuptake... we synthetized and tested zimelidine and found it to be a selective serotonin uptake inhibitor... the first zimelidine patent was published in 1972. Later, zimelidine was tested clinically, and in several well-controlled clinical studies it was found to be a powerful antidepressant." Unexpectedly, zimelidine caused a severe, although rare, neurological side effect and the drug company involved (Astra AB in Sweden) decided to withdraw the product from the market.

At about the same time other drug companies, notably Ferrosan in Denmark, Beecham in England and Eli Lilly in the USA, had started their own programs to find and develop SSRIs for the treatment of depression. Drugs like fluvoxamine, paroxetine and fluoxetine reached the markets in relatively short sequence (in 1985) and were very successful, mainly due to their improved tolerability and safety but also to aggressive marketing. Important new clinical applications of SSRIs were anxiety disorders, once it had been recognized and widely publicized that benzodiazepines could cause tolerance and clinically significant withdrawal syndromes after prolonged use.

2.6.3 DRUGS TO TREAT ALZHEIMER'S DISEASE

The development of antidementia drugs such as donepezil (Aricept®), rivastigmine (Exelon®) and galantamine (Reminyl®) had its scientific origin in neurobiochemical discoveries made some 20 years earlier; Bowen *et al.* (1976) and Davies and Maloney (1976) reported on a marked decrease of cholinergic activity in the brains of patients who had died while suffering from Alzheimer's disease (AD). In the hippocampus – a brain structure critically involved in memory functions – and in some cerebral cortical areas of patients with AD they noted a significant reduction in enzymes required for the synthesis and breakdown of the neurotransmitter acetylcholine. As subsequently demonstrated by Perry *et al.* (1978), the cerebral cholinergic dysfunction in patients with AD was significantly correlated with the degree of cognitive decline.

The acetylcholine-deficiency hypothesis, also known as *cholinergic hypothesis of AD* (Bartus *et al.*, 1982), was supplemented by a host of pharmacological findings, all suggesting a close relationship between an intact cholinergic neurotransmission and cognitive functioning (for review, see Holttum and Gershon, 1992). Based on this body of knowledge, several possible approaches to treat AD could be envisaged (Spiegel 1996, p. 209):

- Enhancing cholinergic function in the brain by increased supply of the biological precursors of acetylcholine, lecithin or choline, similar to the treatment of Parkinson's disease with L-dopa, the precursor of dopamine. This approach, which was tried in dozens of short- and long-term studies, proved to be unsuccessful (Becker and Giacobini, 1988).
- Stimulation of postsynaptic cholinergic receptors with so-called cholino-mimetics, i.e. compounds that can mimic some functions of acetylcholine at cholinergic synapses. This approach, which included experimental compounds such as RS 86 (Wettstein and Spiegel, 1984), xanomeline (Sramek *et al.*, 1995) and AF 102B (Fischer *et al.*, 1996), failed, possibly due to a lack of specificity of the molecules tested (Marin and Davis, 1998).
- Administration of presynaptically active antagonists, i.e., substances that may trigger the synthesis and increased release of acetylcholine by presynaptic cholinergic neurons. It appears that this approach has not been tested systematically yet.
- Inhibiting the enzymes that break down the neurotransmitter acetylcholine (so-called cholinesterases) by the use of cholinesterase inhibitors. This approach, which bears some resemblance to the use of MAO inhibitors in depression (Chapter 4), turned out to be the only successful one still used today.

After a long series of clinical trials with inconclusive or negative results (Becker and Giacobini, 1988), the cholinesterase inhibitor approach attracted new interest following the publication of a clinical study in one of the most prestigeous medical journals (Summers *et al,* 1986). This paper described very positive therapeutic findings with the cholinesterase inhibitor tacrine in a group of 17 patients, some of whom were suffering from quite advanced AD. The response to tacrine was reported to last for many months in some cases and allowed the patients to continue a socially integrated and satisfactory life. Although the study was subsequently criticized for methodological short-comings and the positive findings could be confirmed only partially in better controlled trials (Davis *et al.*, 1992; Farlow *et al.*, 1992), its impact was great. Firstly, a pharmaceutical company took over the further development and clinical testing of tacrine and obtained a product licence (brand name Cognex®) in the USA and elsewhere. Secondly, several pharmaceutical companies started searching for more effective and better tolerated cholines-terase inhibitors than tacrine, resulting in the approval and marketing of donepezil (1997), rivastigmine (1998) and galantamine (2000). These drugs, whose full therapeutic potential is still being explored, produce some improvement in patients with AD having behavioral and psychiatric symptoms: they stabilize patients at their level of cognitive and daily life functioning and they may even delay progression of the disorder for one year or more (see Chapter 7).

2.7 CONCLUDING REMARKS

Following an extended period of stagnation, the last 20 years have witnessed the addition of several novel psychopharmaceuticals to the therapeutic armamentarium. Examples are the new antipsychotic drugs endowed with higher efficacy and/or partly better tolerability than conventional neuroleptics. Although these drugs do represent therapeutic progress, they are not usually perceived as a breakthrough in the treatment of schizophrenia comparable to the first neuroleptic agent, chlorpromazine. Development of risperidone, olanzapine and some more recent compounds was encouraged by the almost accidental discovery of clozapine's superior antipsychotic effect. The drug companies involved also profited from advances in medicinal chemistry, pharmacology and toxicology, which facilitated preclinical drug discovery and development. It is worth mentioning, however, that neither clozapine nor risperidone or olanzapine were found and developed based on significant new insights into the pathophysiological mechanisms underlying schizophrenia.

Similar observations can be made with regard to the antidepressants introduced in the last 15 years or so. Both SSRIs and serotonin norepinephrine reuptake inhibitors (SNRIs) represent some quantitative progress from the earlier antidepressants in that they are less toxic, cause fewer medically significant adverse events and support treatment compliance. As is the case for antipsychotics and schizophrenia, the development of these newer antidepressants was not based on fundamentally new insights into the pathophysiology of affective disorders.

The development and introduction of the more recent antidementia drugs occurred in a different context because effective drug treatment of dementia was not available when the first cholinergic agents were tried in patients with AD. On the other hand, a large body of scientific findings regarding cholinergic drugs and their impact on cognitive processes had been collected, and a coherent scientific hypothesis supported the experimental use of cholinergic compounds in AD. Given these factors, it is perhaps surprising that almost 20 years had to pass between the original descriptions of a cholinergic defect in brains of patients with AD and the approval of the first cholinesterase inhibitor for this indication. Having personally participated in some of these developments, I would suggest that at least three factors prevented fast progress:

(1) The typically advanced age of patients with AD and their often frail health state, setting strict limits to clinical experimentation.
(2) The small therapeutic margin of cholinergic drugs, i.e. their propensity to cause nausea, vomiting and other side effects early in treatment, necessitating slow and individualized dose escalation.
(3) Our initial ignorance regarding the beneficial effects one could realistically expect from cholinergic drugs in patients with AD.

Most of the early trials with cholinergic drugs in AD were limited to a few days or weeks, producing predominantly negative results. It took many failed studies to realize that the test paradigm familiar in clinical psychopharmacology, i.e. placebo-controlled trials of a few weeks' duration (Chapter 5), was not appropriate in a degenerative, progressive disorder such as AD. Researchers and clinicians will now agree that the therapeutic benefit of cholinesterase inhibitors consists of cognitive and functional stabilization, and that controlled trials of several months' duration are necessary to demonstrate reliable and clinically significant effects of these drugs. Once again, it was necessary to overcome some preconceived ideas in order to reach progress in a sub-area of psychopharmacology.

3

Effects of Psychotropic Medication on Healthy Subjects

3.1 INTRODUCTION

Psychotropic medication is meant to be used therapeutically in patients with serious emotional problems, mental disorders or with deficits in neurological or cognitive functioning. What kind of useful information can one possibly expect from experiments on subjects who do not suffer from similar symptoms or disorders? As will be seen in this chapter there is indeed useful information originating from such studies, whose scientific objectives can be one or more of the following:

(1) *Drug-orientated.* Here the interest lies primarily in the compounds being studied and their specific profiles of activities with regard to a variety of psychological and physiological parameters. It is assumed that information coming from studies in healthy volunteers is relevant because it allows a 'clean' assessment of drug effects without the confounding effects of an underlying illness. Typical questions addressed are: What profile of activities does a new, clinically unknown compound display in healthy persons? Does a given compound that improves learning and memory in animal experiments display similar effects in man? Do drugs used in different clinical indications also show characteristic differences with regard to their effects on healthy people? – This field of investigation is sometimes termed *human pharmacology*, i.e. pharmacological studies performed on human subjects, and investigations of this kind are often carried out in early phases of development of new drugs (Chapter 5).

Psychopharmacology, Fourth Edition. By R. Spiegel
© 2003 John Wiley & Sons, Ltd: ISBN 0 471 56039 1: 0 470 84691 7 (PB)

(2) *Methodology-orientated.* Interest is directed primarily to the assessment methods, particularly their sensitivity with regard to drug effects. The characteristic effects of the substances used in these experiments are presumed to be known, i.e. the drugs serve as readily usable and easily quantified tools for modifying the mental state of the subjects. Some authors use the term *pharmacopsychology* to designate this type of study.

(3) *Understanding clinical drug effects.* Here the goal is to understand the therapeutic efficacy of a drug based on some or all of its effects seen in healthy subjects. A typical question would be whether hypnotic drugs produce effects in healthy people, e.g. sleepiness during daytime or deeper sleep at night, which may be seen as homologous to the therapeutic action of these drugs in patients with insomnia.

(4) *Theory-orientated.* Some questions regarding brain–behavior relationships may be approached by the application of pharmacologically well-defined substances to healthy volunteers. For instance, if one is interested in the relationship between brain dopaminergic function (Chapter 4) and specific aspects of attention and motivation, it may be useful to use antipsychotic drugs or some of the psychostimulants with their known effects on dopaminergic function to affect brain dopaminergic activity and to study the impact of these interventions on selected psychological parameters. Of course, this type of study can only be performed if it is safe and ethically justifiable to do so and if methods are available to assess specifically the physiological or mental functions of interest.

(5) *Practice-orientated.* Some drug experiments in healthy volunteers also serve a very practical purpose, namely to assess the effects of specific drugs on everyday activities, e.g. driving a car or operating complicated machinery. Such studies, which are easier to perform in a controlled fashion on healthy volunteers than on psychiatric patients, are based on the assumption that results from healthy subjects can be extrapolated to the conditions prevailing in patients, or at least to those who have recovered from their most severe symptoms and are still kept on medication.

A brief comment is in order regarding the 'healthy subjects' volunteering for drug studies. It is usually understood that they are persons who are medically and mentally healthy and do not take any medicines at the time of the experiment. Health therefore means 'absence of a detectable illness' and generally implies that the subjects have also not suffered previously from severe mental disturbances. Many of the older drug experiments reported in this chapter were conducted in university laboratories and the healthy subjects were typically students, i.e. a group that is in several ways not representative of the general population. More recently drug experiments have often been performed at commercially directed private institutes, so-called contract research organizations (CROs), especially in the testing of new substances. The healthy subjects in these cases are often unemployed people, sometimes even destitute tourists passing through the country, or pensioners, all of whom wish to improve their financial situation by participating in drug trials. The term 'healthy subjects' can thus mean a number of different things, and attention needs to be paid to the subject selection criteria used in a study when interpreting its findings.

3.2 STUDIES CONDUCTED BY EMIL KRAEPELIN

Early pharmacopsychological experiments were conducted by the renowned German psychiatrist Emil Kraepelin (1892), although this area of research only really began to acquire quantitative importance in the years following the discovery of chlorpromazine (e.g. Uhr and Miller, 1964). Kraepelin's studies 'Ueber die Beeinflussung einfacher psychischer Vorgänge durch einige Arzneimittel' (On the influence of some medical drugs on simple mental processes) related in particular to the psychotropic effects of alcohol. In addition, Kraepelin studied the then available hypnotics paraldehyde and chloral hydrate, as well as the 'inhalation poisons' ether and chloroform. The stimulants tested were caffeine and tea and some of his experiments related to morphine. Kraepelin's expectations were twofold. On the one hand, he regarded it as a forward step "to be able to set out, in numerical terms, those changes in our mental life which we could otherwise only describe in quite general terms using the deceptive method of self-observation and to attribute these to certain very simple, elementary disturbances through the use of experimental methods" (1892, p. 227). On the other hand, he hoped to acquire new knowledge for psychology, because drugs can be used to act repeatedly on normal mental processes and thus enable one to better study their 'true nature'.

Kraepelin performed his studies under Wilhelm Wundt at the University of Leipzig, using the objective methods newly developed in this first laboratory of experimental psychology. Reaction time was measured as an indicator of 'mental performance in general'; reading speed was assessed with the aid of standardized printed texts, and calculation performance by means of the addition of single-digit numbers over 5-min periods. Sequences of 12-digit numbers had to be learnt off by heart, the number of repetitions until a sequence could be recited without error being used as a measure of memory performance. Time-estimation trials were intended to indicate inner mental speed, and association experiments were used to record the speed and wealth of verbal association processes.

Apart from some technical refinements, many of the methods described by Kraepelin in his 1892 monograph are still used today in psychological experiments dealing with various aspects of mental performance. What has evolved substantially in the intervening period is the experimental design and set-up of such studies. Kraepelin's trials were mostly conducted in the evenings because he himself and some of his colleagues served as test persons at the end of their normal working day. Kraepelin was often his own experimenter and in all cases the subjects knew what dosage of which substance they were taking. Repeated blank trials (without medication) were run in order to obtain reference values, yet no-substance and active-ingredient days were not balanced, and the use of a placebo for experimental purposes was unknown. Kraepelin ensured that no subject consumed tea, coffee or alcohol for 5–6 h preceding a trial and saw that the last meal was taken 2–3 h before an experiment commenced. What he could not prevent, however, was that many of the trials took place under unfavorable circumstances; his subjects and he himself were occasionally overtired or indisposed for other reasons, which may explain why one repeatedly reads references to the difficulty of establishing the drug effects over and above spontaneous fluctuations. A further obvious difference in comparison to present-day experiments is the absence of formal statistical comparisons; Kraepelin confined himself to the presentation of mean or median values and to descriptive comparisons between treatment conditions. Tests of significance and statistical test procedures in the present-day sense were unknown at the end of the nineteenth century.

Despite many shortcomings in trial design and execution, the results reported by Kraepelin are interesting:

- After 30–50 g of *alcohol* (consumed as 70–110 ml of cognac or whisky or 250–400 ml of wine) a biphasic action was observed. Some 30–45 min after the alcohol had been ingested, simpler mental activities such as reading and speed of simple reactions were often improved but there was no change in the more difficult tasks. Later on, i.e. more than 45 min after intake, performance was in general reduced, particularly for higher doses of alcohol and more complex activities (choice reaction times, wealth of word associations).
- After 3–5 g of the hypnotic *paraldehyde* a qualitatively similar pattern of action was observed as with alcohol, although the stimulation phase was briefer and less pronounced and the 'paralysing' action of the preparation was stronger. Following the intake of *chloral hydrate* and with the inhalation poisons the paralysing effect was still more pronounced.
- Only very few experiments were conducted using *morphine* (10 mg subcutaneously) owing to poor tolerability, and no conclusions could be drawn.
- Following 500 mg of *caffeine* and after tea (10 g of yellow China and black East Indian tea, allowed to infuse for 5 min), improved performance was observed in a number of areas: an increase in the number of additions in the

arithmetic test and in the number of word associations but not in the inventiveness of the words produced.

In the 'Summary of the results', which he formulated with great caution, Kraepelin made the following comments:

(1) He was "very gratified" to note that "the results of our studies show that each of the substances discussed herein exert an entirely characteristic effect on our spiritual life" (p. 228).
(2) His "aim was exclusively to develop methods for a precise determination of the actions of drugs on the mind, and to demonstrate the possibility of their practical application and the utility of their results in selected examples" (pp. 229–230). This aim was achieved, even though some questions could not be answered definitively, such as that concerning 'individual differences' in response to drugs.
(3) It was possible to link the results achieved experimentally with everyday experience, e.g. in the use of alcohol, and to gain a better understanding of the mode of action of the substances used.

Whereas the care devoted by Kraepelin to the individual assessment methods was in some contrast to the more loosely handled experimental design and conditions, great importance nowadays is laid on details of design and statistical analysis of human pharmacological studies. The most important elements in the organization of such trials are:

- Selection of subjects commensurate with the purpose of the study.
- Consideration of the constitution and disposition of the subjects: age, gender, body weight; health condition during preceding days; medication taken in the last 2 weeks; sleep during the preceding night.
- Standardization of experimental conditions: time of day; personnel in charge.
- Balanced administration of test substances and placebo.
- Blinding of the subjects and experimenters with regard to treatment given on a particular day.
- Use of statistical methods appropriate to the data level.

The studies reported and discussed in the following sections of Chapter 3 considered most or all of these methodological issues.

3.3 ASSESSMENT METHODS USED IN DRUG EXPERIMENTS ON HEALTHY VOLUNTEERS

Psychotropic drugs exert effects that are usually noticed by the subject and in principle can be described in words – these are termed *subjective effects*. In addition, effects are produced that may be noted by an observer – a subject appears to slow down, his performance deteriorates, his thoughts seem to wander; such changes – termed *behavioral effects* – can be assessed using methods known in neuropsychology. Psychotropic drugs may also produce changes in brain electrical and chemical activity, which can be recorded by means of appropriate technology; these will be summarized under the heading of *neurophysiological effects*.

3.3.1 METHODS FOR RECORDING SUBJECTIVE DRUG EFFECTS

The method that appears to be the simplest for recording subjective drug effects is to ask a subject how he feels before a substance is given and then to repeat the question at suitable times after the drug has been ingested. This approach allows the subject to describe his current condition in his own words. The experimenter then can ask some specific questions designed to help a subject to compare his current state with his state before ingestion of the drug. Based on these *free descriptions*, one can record individually perceived, and qualitatively possibly very differentiated, subjective drug effects. The problems posed by this approach lie in the semantic and metric areas: what is the meaning of such remarks as "I feel all closed up" or "It is like being behind a smoke-screen" to the individual subject? What do they mean to the investigator and how can one collate and quantify such individual declarations into standardized terms and dimensions?

A more standardized method for determining subjective drug effects is that of *structured questioning*: here, the subject is asked specific questions as to his mood, state of wakefulness and physical freshness or any other aspects of his condition of interest in the context of a study, and should then quantify his answers wherever possible into 'somewhat', 'slight', 'of medium intensity', etc. An advantage of this procedure is that ambiguous answers can be clarified immediately by further questioning; a disadvantage is that the experimenter loses much time (and may get bored) in trials with larger groups of subjects and several repetitions on the same test day. Moreover, the experimenter's questions may be unduly influenced by his personal impressions of the real or presumed state of the subject.

For reasons of expediency and objectivity, and particularly in the case of more extensive studies, questions are preferably submitted in writing, i.e. in some form of *self-rating scale*. Here one can distinguish between symptom checklists, adjective checklists, semantic differentials and visual analog scales.

Symptom checklists are often formulated as alternatives, i.e. the subject is asked whether or not he is experiencing a symptom, e.g. headache, at a given point in time. The list of symptoms presented to subjects can either be compiled on the basis of previous knowledge of the substances being tested, or a standardized list can be used. Symptom checklists may also be formulated in

The words below can be used to describe an individual's mood. Please rate yourself according to what you are feeling *at this moment*, using the extreme terms given and placing a cross in the appropriate box: ☒

At this moment I feel . . .

	very					very	
concentrated	☐	☐	☐	☐	☐	☐	absent-minded
sleepy	☐	☐	☐	☐	☐	☐	wide-awake
talkative	☐	☐	☐	☐	☐	☐	silent
sad	☐	☐	☐	☐	☐	☐	cheerful
attentive	☐	☐	☐	☐	☐	☐	inattentive
anxious	☐	☐	☐	☐	☐	☐	confident
interested	☐	☐	☐	☐	☐	☐	uninterested
confused	☐	☐	☐	☐	☐	☐	lucid
irritable	☐	☐	☐	☐	☐	☐	well-balanced
sociable	☐	☐	☐	☐	☐	☐	withdrawn
over-worked	☐	☐	☐	☐	☐	☐	refreshed
serious	☐	☐	☐	☐	☐	☐	frivolous
active	☐	☐	☐	☐	☐	☐	passive
tired	☐	☐	☐	☐	☐	☐	fresh
self-controlled	☐	☐	☐	☐	☐	☐	boisterous
bad-tempered	☐	☐	☐	☐	☐	☐	good-tempered

Should you wish to provide additional information on your condition, please do so here:

Figure 3.1 Example of a semantic differential

grades, i.e. the subject is asked if a given symptom is absent, mild, moderate, severe or intolerable. An example of this format is the Revised 90-Item Symptom Check List (SCL-90-R; *ECDEU Assessment Manual*, 1976). There is no general rule as to which procedure is preferable, but short lists are best if several evaluations are to be made on the same test day.

Adjective checklists can be formulated as alternatives or in grades. In both cases the subjects seek to describe their current subjective state by means of

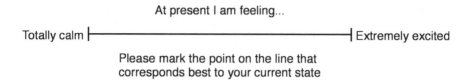

Figure 3.2 Example of a visual analog scale

predetermined adjectives. Well-known instruments for use in English-speaking countries are the Clyde Mood Scale (Clyde, 1963) and the POMS (Profile of Mood States; see *ECDEU Assessment Manual*, 1976). Adjective checklists can be arranged in the format of *semantic differentials* (Fig. 3.1) and subjects are required to check one of the boxes placed between two extreme terms and corresponding best to their current state. V*isual analog scales* (VAS; Fig. 3.2) have become very popular and can be adapted individually to suit specific questions. These enable a subject to pinpoint his current condition somewhere along a 10 cm line, the ends of which usually denote extreme states (Bond and Lader, 1974; Maxwell, 1978).

In general, standardization of questionnaires and their items helps to simplify quantitative comparisons between individuals and conditions but simultaneously curtails each individual statement and may force it into inappropriate categories. Moreover, allocating the same weight to all the items in a questionnaire, such as all pairs of opposite terms in a semantic differential, may iron out the effects of substances and obscure interesting individual effects. A freely formulated description of drug action, be it in oral or written form, should therefore be included in studies of this kind.

3.3.2 METHODS FOR RECORDING BEHAVIORAL DRUG EFFECTS

In principle any form of human activity capable of being observed and recorded objectively and reliably can serve as a basis for assessing the effect of psychotropic drugs. Behavior in social situations (e.g. in small groups), behavior in situations where a specific performance is required and behavior at times of relaxation or pleasure all vary according to the degree of wakefulness and state of motivation of an individual and could provide valuable opportunities for observations of drug effects. Review of the literature shows, however, that almost all studies published in the last 20 years focus on performance-related behavior and that there have been very few studies of drug effects on social behavior and virtually none of drug effects on behavior during relaxation and pleasure. This one-sidedness may be a result of the difficulty in creating standardized, relevant and ethically acceptable situations in which specific forms of social behavior can be studied. It should be noted, however, that older 'sociopharmacological' studies summarized by McGuire *et al.* (1982) provided only minimal insights into relevant drug effects.

In the following paragraphs the emphasis has consequently been laid on studies using a variety of *performance tests*. There are many ways to classify such methods, e.g. by the specific mental function a task is thought to tap or simply by test duration. Similar to a classification used by Deutsch Lezak (1995) for neuropsychological tests, we will distinguish the following areas of mental performance:

- attention and concentration
- perception
- learning and memory
- verbal functions and language skills
- concept formation and reasoning
- motor performance and executive functions

There are no sharp borderlines between some of these areas of mental performance (elements of attention, perception and some motor function are involved in all forms of performance), and allocation to a specific area is debatable for many tests. When studies are planned in practice this will be considered by compiling a battery of tests containing some redundancy while still retaining parameters from various areas of performance.

Attention and Concentration

No special abilities such as verbal intelligence or motor dexterity are usually needed to perform tests of attention and concentration. Popular methods include cancellation and coding tests, simple arithmetical tasks and tasks designed to assess vigilance (Table 3.1). Tests of attention and concentration not only differ with regard to the nature and difficulty of the tasks to be performed, but also in respect of their duration. Thus, most cancellation tasks last only a few minutes but vigilance tests usually take longer, in extreme cases such as the Mackworth Clock (Mackworth, 1965) up to 1 h. By using longer lasting tests it is possible to measure fluctuations of performance in time, although long-lasting tests cannot be repeated more than two or three times on the same experimental day.

Perception

The term perception designates physiological and mental processes that serve to absorb and classify information from our internal and external environments. Speed, extent and quality of perception not only depend on the condition of the sensory organs but they are also a function of such factors as wakefulness, attentiveness or concentration, emotional and motivational state

Table 3.1 Typical tests of attention and concentration (for details see Deutsch Lezak, 1995, p. 352)

Assessment	Test procedures	Duration
Short-term attention, concentration	• Cancellation tests: picking out and marking numbers, letters and geometric shapes according to a given criterion	A few minutes
	• Digit symbol substitution tests (DSST): allocation of given symbols to numbers. Contains short-term memory component	A few minutes
	• Calculation tests of different complexity and duration. More complex tests (with calculation of intermediate results) also assess short-term memory	Variable
	• Reaction time tasks (see Table 3.3)	
Sustained attention	• Continuous performance test (CPT): usually discrimination tasks of long duration	20–60 min
	• Vigilance tests: long series of identical sounds with rare sounds of slightly longer duration interspersed – these have to be reported	Up to 60 min
Divided attention	• Keeping track of more than one task at the same time, e.g. dichotic listening	Variable
	• Trail Making B	A few minutes

and short-term memory. A distinction may be made between procedures for the determination of:

- thresholds of perception
- speed of perception
- extent of perception
- qualitative characteristics of perception

Only a small proportion of the methods available, mainly for diagnostic purposes (Lezak, 1995, p. 385), have been used in drug experiments. Special mention should be made of the determination of *critical flicker fusion frequency* (CFF) and of tachistoscopic trials, i.e. of methods directed at the characteristics of visual perception. In contrast, drug effects on hearing have rarely, and those influencing senses of touch, smell and taste have hardly ever, been investigated (Turner, 1971).

In studies of CFF the frequency of a discontinuous (flickering) light source is increased until the subject reports seeing a continuous light. The corresponding frequency is termed the CFF, measured in cycles per second (cps) or hertz (Hz). Another procedure, which is usually combined with the first, consists of gradually reducing the frequency of a light source until that threshold is attained at which the previously continuous light begins to flicker. The CFF is thought to reflect "cortical function and more specifically may reflect occipital/parietal lobe activity" (Curran and Wattis, 1998), although the underlying neuronal mechanisms are poorly understood. Interpretation of CFF findings may be complicated if drugs affect pupil diameter, as is the case for many psychotropic compounds (Schmitt et al., 2002).

Tachistoscopic trials serve to record speed and extent of perception. In the course of such experiments visual stimuli are shown for a very short time and the subject has to name the items presented as far as he has recognized them. Tests with simple configurations of stimuli (colors, single letters or objects) primarily record speed of perception, whereas experiments with more varied content also investigate elements of short-term memory. Tachistoscopic experiments are nowadays hardly used in pharmacopsychology, presumably because of their low sensitivity to the effects of substances.

Learning and Memory

The processes of learning and remembering can be broken down into stages that follow each other in time: information intake (registration), processing (encoding), storage and retention and retrieval (reproduction). In addition, a division into memory files or 'stores' has been proposed, involving, depending on the author, two or more components: ultrashort-term, short-term and long-term stores are constructs that can be operationalized and quantified experimentally. The concept of a 'working memory' (Baddeley, 1986) also comprises a short-term storage and a number of executive processes that operate on the transiently stored material.

Regardless of the specific model of memory used, the time at which a pharmacological agent is administered and develops its action is crucial (Fig. 3.3):

(1) If a drug is administered before the material to be learned is presented, i.e. *before the registration phase*, its effects on wakefulness, alertness and motivation of the subject are obviously confounded with a possible specific action on learning, i.e. on the processes linked with registration and encoding. It is therefore to be expected that stimulant substances administered at low doses before the registration phase will show a 'memory-promoting' effect as a result of their action on attentiveness, whereas sedative compounds will have the opposite effect.

(2) Drugs can be administered *after the registration phase* with the purpose of studying their action on encoding processes. Trials of this type in humans are difficult to interpret, mainly because encoding processes of various types and levels may last for seconds, minutes or hours, whereas the time at

Registration	Encoding	Storage	Reproduction
(Ultra) Short-term storage	Long-term storage		(retrieval)

↑   ↑   ↑ ↑ ↑   ↑
(1)   (2)   (3) (3) (3)   (4)

(1) Administration of a drug before the registration phase.
(2) Administration after the registration phase, at the time of encoding.
(3) Chronic administration during long-term storage.
(4) Administration before the retrieval phase.
(1) and (4): Experiments on state-dependent learning and memory.

Figure 3.3 Possible timing of drug administration during the learning and memory process

which a drug reaches and affects the relevant brain structures cannot be controlled precisely.

(3) Drugs can be administered *after the completion of the encoding processes*, i.e. at a time when the acquired information is thought to be stored in long-term memory. A drug may then counteract or promote the spontaneous decay of previously learned information. This is a particularly interesting question in cases of long-term drug administration, which is typical for the therapeutic use of most medications.

(4) A drug may be administered when a subject tries to remember previously learned material, i.e. *before the reproduction phase*, in order to study its action on the retrieval of stored information. Also in this case, the effect of a substance on wakefulness, motivation, etc. may be confounded with a possible specific drug effect on retrieval.

Another area of interest are studies on so-called *state-dependent learning and memory*, i.e. the registration and retrieval of information occurring under the same or different drug treatment conditions. This constitutes a special case of context-dependent learning and memory because it concerns the question of whether information acquired under the influence of a drug (case (1) above) can be retrieved better or worse when this same substance or placebo is administered before the retrieval phase (case (4)).

Studies of drug action on learning and memory are attractive in several respects, yet they make particularly great demands on the planning and interpretation of a trial. This is the case particularly for cases (2) and (3), whereas case (1) is relatively straightforward. Some well-known test methods for learning and memory are summarized in Table 3.2, only a few of which are regularly used in pharmacopsychology (e.g. digit span, word list learning and paired associate learning tests).

Table 3.2 Typical tests of learning and memory (for details see Deutsch Lezak, 1995, p. 429)

Procedure	Activity required	Usual duration
Digit span	Repetition forwards or backwards of a series of single-digit numbers of increasing length	3–5 min
Word list learning, e.g. Rey's 15 words	Repetition of a series of 15 words, five repetitions until criterion	~5 min
Selective reminding	Repetition of a series of 10–12 words, only missed words are repeated by the tester	~10 min
Benton visual retention test	Geometric shapes drawn from memory (drawing version) or picked out from several similar shapes (multiple-choice version)	5 min
Paired associate learning	Learning of words, numbers, etc. paired to a stimulus word or number, shape, etc. (recall of the associated items may be tested after minutes, hours or days)	5–10 min
Logical memory	Recall of stories with specific numbers of elements (recall may be tested after minutes, hours or days)	5 min

Verbal Functions and Language Skills

Vocabulary and word fluency tests provide subjects with an initial letter for which they should name as many nouns as possible, or they are asked to name as many four-legged animals as possible within a given time limit. Other tasks tend rather to call for logical thinking, such as finding communalities, similarities and exceptions within a series of words. Several equivalent parallel forms of these tasks must be available if the same subject needs to be tested more than once or a few times on the same day.

Concept Formation and Reasoning

Although of great value in functional psychodiagnostics, tests of concept formation and reasoning, such as the Wisconsin Card Sorting Test (WCST), are only little used in drug experiments with healthy volunteers. This is probably due to their complex administration and interpretation. In contrast, the Digit Symbol Substitution Test (DSST) from the Wechsler Adult Intelligence Scale (WAIS), which some include in the category of concept formation tasks, has been used in many studies; this is mainly due to its brevity and to the fact that one can easily devise parallel forms. If used several times on the same subject, coding tasks assess attention and concentration (Table 3.1) rather than concept formation or reasoning.

Motor Performance and Executive Functions

There are numerous methods for recording motor performance (Table 3.3), drawn mainly from occupational and traffic psychology. A comprehensive account of the methods available is given in Kunsman *et al.* (1992) and Deutsch Lezak (1995, chapter 16). Some of these tasks are subject to a pronounced practice effect and, if repeated several times by the same subject, turn into tests of attention and concentration rather than of motor performance.

Executive functions can be sub-classified into volition, planning, purposive action and effective performance. Volition, "this most subtle and central realm of human activity" (Deutsch Lezak, 1995, p. 651), is not usually assessed in drug experiments. Typical tests to assess planning are mazes of different complexity and brain teasers such as the Tower of London or Hanoi. In drug experiments with healthy volunteers, purposive action and effective performance are usually measured by means of the methods listed in Tables 3.1 and 3.3.

3.3.3 NEUROPHYSIOLOGICAL PARAMETERS

Psychotropic drugs exert their intended actions on the brain, and it is therefore logical to study brain functions as directly as possible in order to understand the actions of these substances. The possibilities for studying drug effects *in situ* in the human brain are limited because: so-called invasive techniques used in animal studies (removal of tissues, insertion of electrodes or cannulas into the brain) cannot be considered for research purposes in humans, and the newer non-invasive procedures such as positron emission tomography (PET) and functional magnetic resonance imaging (fMRI) have their own limitations (see Chapter 6). For these reasons some of the neurophysiological techniques developed several decades ago are still in use today.

The *electroencephalogram* (EEG), first described by H. Berger in the late 1920s, makes it possible to record electrical correlates of brain activity in human subjects in a non-invasive manner. The EEG patterns alter in relation to the degree of wakefulness, and drugs such as cocaine, scopolamine and chloroform were already used by Berger (1931) in order to manipulate the "degree of consciousness" of his subjects and to investigate the electrical correlates of the conditions brought about. Computerized procedures to evaluate EEGs quantitatively arose in the 1960s, allowing longer EEG traces to be analyzed more easily and objectively and thus permitting more extensive

Table 3.3 Methods for testing motor performance and executive function

Procedure	Activity required	Usual duration
Dynamometer	Pressing a handle, etc. repeatedly against resistance	15–60 s
Tapping	Tapping on a pad as quickly as possible	30–60 s
Aiming	Placing a dot, the beam of a light pen, etc. into circles or squares arranged in various patterns	A few minutes
Peg board	Inserting pegs into rows of holes in a board	
Saccadic eye movements	Fast conjugate eye movements, e.g. when reading or following moving objects	A few minutes
Visual pursuit, tracking	Tracking a regularly or irregularly moving light spot with the eyes; or, using a light-pen, following a point describing simple or complex trajectories on a screen	Up to 5 min
Reaction time	Motor reaction to simple or complex acoustic or optical stimuli (complex reaction time tasks are also subsumed under tests of attention and concentration)	2–10 min
Car driving, flight simulator	Appropriate reaction to and behavior in simulated road or air traffic situations	10–30 min

pharmacological investigations. Experiments of this type, involving waking subjects and the administration of drugs, are termed *pharmaco-EEG* studies.

The 1960s also saw the rapid growth of psychophysiological sleep research. It was noticed that psychotropic drugs not only affect the pattern of wake EEGs but also alter the electrophysiological correlates of the sleep state, as recorded in *sleep polygrams* or *hypnograms*. Thus it became possible to study the actions of drugs on the brain over a broad range of vigilance states from deep sleep to the active waking state. At about the same time investigators started to examine the effects of drugs on *evoked potentials* (EPs), i.e. the electrical correlates of brain responses to sensory stimuli. As is the case for the EEG in wake and sleep states, EPs can be recorded from the surface of the skull and provide information on the functional state of the brain in response to standardized tactile, visual or auditory stimulation.

Recordings of the wake EEG, sleep polygram and EPs are all based on the principle of sampling, amplifying and filtering the changes in electrical potential arising on the cranial surface as indicators of brain activity. In spite of some technical similarities, the three approaches differ very much with regard to time-related and other characteristics, thus allowing the study of different aspects of a drug's effect in the brain. All three approaches offer several advantages that still support their use in human psychopharmacology:

(1) The recordings are non-invasive and inconvenience the subject only slightly, mostly in the beginning or not at all.
(2) Once the subjects have become adapted to 'being wired', the recordings are usually very stable.
(3) Recordings require no special attention or effort on the part of a subject and consequently do not alter the processes they are designed to study (some EP paradigms are an exception in this respect; see below).
(4) Recordings can be made while subjects are engaged in other activities, and it is then possible to relate aspects of the ongoing performance and the subjective state to neurophysiological parameters.
(5) The EEG recordings can in principle be continued over hours, days and even weeks, particularly when telemetric instrumentation is available.

Pharmaco-EEG

Most techniques used to analyze pharmaco-EEGs are based on the averaging of a number of artefact-free recordings, assuming that a subject's state of vigilance does not change significantly during the time interval studied, which is usually a few minutes. The EEG signals recorded are characterized by their frequency (measured in cps or Hz) and amplitude (in microvolts, μV). Pharmaco-EEG studies make use of the classification and interpretation of EEG waves by their frequency that was introduced by Berger and his successors (Table 3.4). So-called topographic EEGs, also termed EEG- or brain-mapping procedures, are concerned with the distribution of EEG frequency components over the entire cranial surface and not just at individual lead points. Such EEG mapping is used in some centers for diagnostic purposes (Szelies, 1992; John et al., 1994) but applications in pharmacopsychology have not become widespread.

Historically, and in the context of psychopharmacology, Bente (1961) assumed that there are 'regular correlations' between the changes occurring in the EEG of healthy subjects after a single dose of psychotropic drugs and those occurring in patients under therapeutic conditions. Fink (1981), Itil (1981) and other authors subsequently published a number of studies concerning the classification of psychotropic drugs on the basis of quantitative EEG criteria. Much of this work was based on two hypotheses: (1) the differential therapeutic effects of antipsychotics, antidepressants, anxiolytics, etc. are also expressed in the form of differential EEG effects in patients as well as in healthy persons; (2) it must therefore be possible to allocate new and clinically as yet unknown substances tentatively to a therapeutic class on the basis of their EEG effect in healthy subjects, and then to confirm this allocation in clinical trials.

Table **3.4** EEG rhythms in man

Name, frequency and amplitude	Localization	Appears under the following conditions
Alpha activity 8–13 Hz 20–60 µV	Occipital, parietal (posterior area on the skull)	Eyes closed, relaxed wake state. Disappears when eyes are opened, when concentrating on a task
Beta activity 14–30 Hz > 20 µV	Central, frontal (upper, anterior area on the skull)	Eyes open, alertness, concentration on a task; often in combination with low-amplitude theta waves
Delta activity 0.5–3.5 Hz Up to 300 µV	All regions on the skull	During wake: rare and of low amplitude. During sleep: with higher amplitude and synchronized. Indicates very low level of activation
Theta activity 4–7.5 Hz Up to 150 µV	Central, temporal (upper and lateral areas on the skull)	Sleepiness, light sleep; in young children also during wakefulness. Mostly in combinations with superimposed beta waves

Polygraphic Sleep Studies

Sleep polygrams, i.e. simultaneous recordings of the EEG, eye movements (electro-oculogram, EOG) and the activity of representative muscles (electromyogram, EMG), are performed through entire nights and are classified, via visual inspection or computerized analysis, into so-called sleep stages. The sleep of man and of many species of animal is a cyclical process, the individual segments (sleep stages) of which follow a regular sequence in time (Fig. 3.4).

The relationships between the stages of sleep and its subjective aspects, such as the feeling of depth of sleep, the state of recovery and mood in the following morning, have been investigated in hundreds of studies without fully clarifying the biological and psychological relevance of sleep and its stages. It is generally agreed that the duration of slow-wave sleep in a given person is mainly a function of the prior time spent awake: the longer a person has been awake, the greater is the slow-wave sleep fraction of total sleep time in a subsequent night of undisturbed sleep. Rapid eye movement (REM) sleep designates periodically appearing phases of 10–40 min duration, characterized by fast and large eye movement recorded in the EOG and generally accompanied by dreams (although dreams also occur in other sleep segments, primarily in stages 1 and 2).

Ian Oswald is to be considered a pioneer in this field of research, having taken up sleep polygraphic investigations of the action of barbiturates, amphetamines, antidepressants, benzodiazepines and other substances in the early 1960s (Oswald, 1968). He and others found that almost all psychotropic

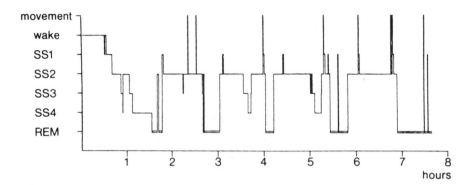

Figure 3.4 Schematic representation (hypnogram) of the course of sleep. The hypnogram of a 25-year-old healthy subject illustrates the temporal sequence of polygraphic sleep stages (SS) in a single night. Each non-REM–REM cycle begins with non-REM sleep (stages 2, 3 and 4) and ends with a REM period that lasts from a few up to 40 or more minutes. Slow-wave sleep stages 3 and 4 mainly occur during the first two to three non-REM–REM cycles; as the night wears on, sleep becomes more superficial (from Spiegel, 1981, p. 41)

substances have effects on the sleep pattern of healthy subjects and mentally ill patients after single and repeated administrations, and that there are systematic relationships between the assumed mechanism of action of a substance and its effects on the sleep polygram.

Evoked Potentials (EPs) and Event-related Potentials (ERPs)

When a subject is exposed to sensory stimuli it is possible to record evoked potentials, i.e. changes in electric potential that arise as a function of the nature and intensity of the stimuli and other conditions of the experiment. The naked eye is hardly able to detect EPs individually in the wake EEG because they are concealed by spontaneous EEG waves with higher amplitudes. Evoked potentials are made visible by repeatedly presenting the same standardized stimuli and then mathematically averaging the respective EEG segments. In this manner it is possible to 'average out' spontaneous EEG activity, and the EP, the amplitude of which lies between 5 and 30 µV, emerges. Evoked potentials consist of several components: in the case of visual EPs (Fig. 3.5) and similarly for EPs of other sensory modalities, a distinction is made between a primary response, i.e. changes in potential that appear with particular clarity above those parts of the cortex onto which the stimulus in question is projected, and secondary responses, which may be observed somewhat later and are presumably phenomena linked to the associative or cognitive processing of the stimulus in the brain (Hillyard and Kutas, 1983). Primary responses (also termed stimulus-correlated potentials) with a latency of up to about 100 ms depend largely on the objective, physical features of the stimuli used. Secondary responses (also called event-related potentials, ERPs) depend primarily on the mental disposition of the subjects, i.e. their expectations and alertness at the time of the experiment.

Evoked potentials with latencies below 100 ms are used clinically for functional testing of the optic, auditory and various somatosensory nerve pathways; they are not influenced by factors such as motivation and tiredness, including drug-induced changes of alertness, and are considered to be uninteresting for psychological questions.

The situation is different with EPs having longer latencies, especially waves N200 and P300. The (negative) N200 wave (also called N2) appears about 200 ms after a suitable stimulus, and the (positive) P300 wave (also called P3) appears after about 300 ms on average. Both N2 and P3 can be elicited in so-called odd-ball (two-stimuli differentiation) paradigms: the subject is presented with a sequence of frequent and rare stimuli, e.g. frequent high tones and rare low tones, and is given the task of observing and counting only the rare stimuli. Both N2 and P3 arise after the noted rare stimuli; their amplitude depends on the stimulus probability and the relevance of the stimulus in the experiment. Wave P3 can also be induced by creating an expectancy in the subjects that is

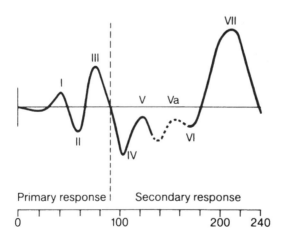

Figure 3.5 Classification of the components of visually evoked potentials (VEPs). The two negative peaks I and III and the positive peak II were termed the primary response by Cigánek (1961), peaks IV–VII (negative peaks = 'upwards' pointing peaks) being termed the secondary response. The amplitude of these peaks lies in the region of 10–30 μV. In addition to amplitudes (e.g. between peaks I and II), latencies are determined, i.e. the time in milliseconds between the stimulus and the appearance of a peak, e.g. peak IV

then not fulfilled, e.g. by omitting a stimulus in an otherwise unchanged stimulus sequence.

Another electric signal recorded from the surface of the skull is termed *contingent negative variation* (CNV). This is a very late potential fluctuation in the parietal region that arises when a subject participating in a reaction time experiment is advised, through a warning stimulus, of the imminence of another stimulus to which he or she has to respond.

Historically, Saletu (1976) performed a series of EP experiments in healthy subjects to study the action of several antipsychotics, antidepressants, anxiolytics and psychostimulants. Similar to Fink and Itil for the pharmaco-EEG, he reported on systematic, drug-type-related changes in EP latencies after somatosensory stimulation of his subjects.

3.4 FINDINGS IN DRUG EXPERIMENTS ON HEALTHY VOLUNTEERS

The following paragraphs, which are organized by drug classes, provide summaries of numerous, with few exceptions placebo-controlled, double-blind experiments with psychotropic drugs in healthy subjects. The number of published studies in this area is huge and only a small selection of references, some of them in German or French, plus a number of 'classical' studies and review articles dealing with early work will be given. References to studies before 1995 will be found in Chapters 3 and 4 of previous editions of the current book (Spiegel and Aebi, 1983; Spiegel, 1989, 1996).

3.4.1 ANTIPSYCHOTIC DRUGS (Table 3.5)

Subjective Effects

Two early publications (Delay *et al.*, 1959; Di Mascio *et al.*, 1963) deal with the *subjective effects* of the first antipsychotics in relatively high doses. Chlorpromazine at single doses of 100–200 mg gave rise to the following effects in healthy volunteers:

- pronounced tiredness, wish to sleep, but no pleasant relaxed feeling
- slower and confused thinking, difficulties in concentrating, feelings of clumsiness
- dejection, anxiety, irritability

Dryness of the mouth, visual disturbances, sweating and similar peripheral effects were also experienced by the subjects after single doses of 50 mg or more of chlorpromazine and contributed to a subjectively quite disagreeable state. Lower doses (12.5 and 25 mg) lead to milder sedation and fewer peripheral

Table 3.5 Effects of antipsychotic drugs in healthy subjects

Area of assessment	Clinically sedative antipsychotics, e.g. chlorpromazine, clozapine, olanzapine		Less sedative antipsychotics, e.g. haloperidol, perphenazine, pimozide, sulpiride	
	Low dose[a]	High dose[b]	Low dose[a]	High dose[b]
Subjective effects	Tiredness, sleepiness	Urgent need to sleep, unpleasant state	Little if any effect	Unpleasant state, inner unrest, sedation
Attention, concentration	Performance impaired	Performance strongly impaired	No effect	Some impairment
Perception	CFF: decrease	CFF: decrease	No effect	CFF: decrease
Learning, memory	No effect	Impairment (very few data)	No effect	No effect (very few data)
Verbal, logical functions	Some decline	Decline	No effect	No data
Motor, executive functions	Some slowing	Slowing	No effect	Slowing
Wake EEG	Delta, theta ↑ Alpha ↓	Delta, theta ↑ Alpha ↓	Enhanced alertness (?)	Delta, theta ↑ Alpha, beta ↓
Sleep polygram	WASO, unrest ↓	Sleep duration ↑	No effect	No effect
Early EPs	No data	No data	No data	No data
Late ERPs	No data	No data	No data	No data

[a] Up to about 20% of average daily clinical dose.
[b] More than 20% (up to 100%) of average daily clinical dose.
For detailed results with individual drugs, see text and earlier editions of this volume (Spiegel, 1996, Chapters 3 and 4).

effects. Perphenazine and trifluoperazine, which were administered in rather high doses in the study conducted by Di Mascio *et al.* (1963), and haloperidol, which has been tested in single doses up to 6 mg (King *et al.*, 1995; Lynch *et al.*, 1997), do not induce sleep in healthy subjects but produce a subjectively unpleasant state. After each of these drugs, some of the subjects felt dysphoric; in the case of haloperidol, a state is described that is characterized simultaneously by inner restlessness and external sedation. No significant subjective effects were reported after 1.0 or 2.0 mg of flupenthixol, 1.0 and 2.0 mg of pimozide (Brauer and de Wit, 1996) or after 400 mg of sulpiride, compounds with only weak sedative or sleep-inducing action in patients. A single dose of 300 mg of sulpiride could not be distinguished from placebo in a study reported by Meyer-Lindenberg *et al.* (1997).

Of the atypical antipsychotics, clozapine produced tiredness and a desire to sleep in healthy volunteers at very low single doses of 5 and 10 mg; a dose of

50 mg of clozapine induced significant reductions in self-rated 'alertness' and 'contentedness' (Pretorius *et al.*, 2001). Single and repeated doses of 3 mg of olanzapine given to healthy elderly volunteers resulted in reduced self-rated alertness on day 1, with some attenuation of the effect on day 4 (Beuzen *et al.*, 1999). Amisulpride was found to be free of subjective effects in healthy young volunteers at single and repeated doses of 50 and 400 mg (Ramaekers *et al.*, 1999), and 50 as well as 200 mg of this compound did not produce any measurable subjective changes in a group of elderly healthy volunteers (Legangneux *et al.*, 2000).

Behavioral Effects

Whereas the effects of chlorpromazine on various areas of performance have been studied thoroughly and over a wide dosage range, only fragmentary results are available for other antipsychotics. At single doses of 50 mg or more, chlorpromazine may cause a drop in performance in several areas (attention/ concentration, perception, motor performance), whereas learning and memory functions were not significantly affected up to 50 mg. Less sedative antipsychotics such as flupenthixol, haloperidol, perphenazine or trifluoperazine reduced performance in individual tests but did not display a uniform pattern of activity at relatively low single doses. In one study in elderly subjects 3 mg of haloperidol produced a late-appearing cognitive impairment (Beuzen *et al.*, 1999). Rather high doses of haloperidol (up to 6 mg) impair performance on the DSST and reduce peak saccadic velocity; in contrast, performance on the CPT was not significantly affected (Lynch *et al.*, 1997). Sulpiride at single doses of 300 mg was found to decrease CFF and to prolong choice reaction decision times, although time estimations and choice reaction movement times were unaffected (Meyer-Lindenberg *et al.*, 1997).

A significant decrease of CFF was noted after 50 mg of clozapine; sedation after this dose was so strong that some subjects fell asleep during the study (Pretorius *et al.*, 2001). Single and repeated doses of 3 mg of olanzapine produced detectable impairment in all areas of cognitive and psychomotor performance assessed in a group of healthy elderly volunteers (Beuzen *et al.*, 1999); the impairment was very much attenuated but still noticeable on day 4 of drug administration. Amisulpride at a dose of 50 mg had no significant impact on any performance parameter assessed in a study by Ramaekers *et al.* (1999); however, 400 mg of the compound was found to have negative effects on some psychomotor and cognitive measures of performance on day 5 but not on day 1 of drug administration. In the healthy elderly volunteers studied by Legangneux *et al.* (2000) neither 50 nor 200 mg of amisulpride was associated with any signs of cognitive impairment.

Neurophysiology

Chlorpromazine and clozapine at low doses lead to an increase in slow (delta, theta) waves and a decrease in alpha activity in the *pharmaco-EEG* of healthy subjects. Findings regarding beta activity are less uniform. Rohloff *et al.* (1992) reported on an increase in slow frequency components and a decrease of alpha and beta activity after 4.0 mg of haloperidol. Low doses of amisulpride (up to 50 mg) were reported to display an 'alertness-enhancing' effect (Rosenzweig *et al.*, 2002).

There are no striking effects on *sleep polygrams* of healthy subjects after the intake of low doses of antipsychotic drugs shortly before sleep onset: sedative drugs such as chlorpromazine and clozapine stabilize sleep, i.e. there is less wake time after sleep onset (WASO in Table 3.5) and there are fewer brief interruptions in the course of sleep (unrest in Table 3.5); in larger doses these drugs may prolong the duration of sleep. Haloperidol and pimozide are unremarkable with regard to their effects on sleep. The effects of antipsychotics on REM sleep are not uniform, and the impact upon other sleep stages is slight.

Only isolated reports on the effects of antipsychotic drugs on EPs have appeared in the literature: an early study by Saletu (1976) describing prolonged latencies to primary and secondary responses after several neuroleptics was not reproduced by other authors. Sulpiride at doses of 150 and 300 mg induced increases of P200 and P300 latencies (de Visser *et al.*, 2001). Contingent negative variation amplitudes were found to be attenuated after 50 mg of chlorpromazine (Tecce *et al.*, 1978). It appears that there are no studies with neurophysiological techniques dealing with the newer atypical antipsychotics.

3.4.2 ANTIDEPRESSANT DRUGS (Table 3.6)

Subjective Effects

Amitriptyline was reported to have a calming action at doses of 6.25 and 12.5 mg, whereas drowsiness is usually experienced by healthy volunteers at somewhat higher doses (25 mg and above). Various authors have described a sleep-inducing effect with single doses of over 25 mg of imipramine; at yet higher doses a subjectively unpleasant state of sedation and lethargy, sometimes accompanied by dullness and confusion and associated with pronounced vegetative symptoms, occurs. Some of the older antidepressants, which are more markedly sedating in clinical use (dothiepin, maprotiline, mianserin, trimipramine), were found to induce tiredness or drowsiness in healthy subjects at doses considerably below those used in depressed patients.

Reports are on hand relating to more recent antidepressants such as bupropion, citalopram (Fairweather *et al.*, 1997), fluoxetine (Gelfin *et al.*, 1998), moclobemide (Dingemanse *et al.*, 1998) and paroxetine (Brauer *et al.*, 1995). These products, in agreement with their clinical profiles, produce fewer subjective effects and generally less sedation in healthy subjects than the older

Table 3.6 Effects of antidepressant drugs in healthy subjects

Area of assessment	Clinically sedative antidepressants, e.g. amitriptyline, mianserin, trimipramine		Less sedative antidepressants, e.g. bupropion, fluoxetin, moclobemide, nefazodone	
	Low dose[a]	High dose[b]	Low dose[a]	High dose[b]
Subjective effects	Relaxation, drowsiness	Drowsiness, unpleasant state	No effect	Weak effects if any
Attention, concentration	Performance impaired	Performance strongly impaired	No effect	Weak effects if any
Perception	CFF: decrease	CFF: decrease	No effect	CFF: increase (?)
Learning, memory	Weak effects if any	Some impairment	Enhanced long-term memory	No effect
Verbal, logical functions	No data	Decline	No effect	No data
Motor, executive functions	Slowing	Slowing	No effect	No effect
Wake EEG	Delta, theta ↑ Alpha ↓	Delta, theta ↑ Alpha ↓, beta ↑	No effect	No or little effect
Sleep polygram	WASO, unrest ↓ REM sleep ↓	Sleep duration ↑ REM sleep ↓↓	REM sleep ↓	Sleep unrest ↑ REM sleep ↓↓
Early EPs	No effect (few data available)	No data	No data	No data
Late ERPs	No data	Latencies increased	No effect	No effect

[a] Up to about 20% of average daily clinical dose.
[b] More than 20% (up to 100%) of average daily clinical dose.
For detailed results with individual drugs see text and earlier editions of this volume (Spiegel, 1996, Chapters 3 and 4).

tricyclic compounds. In some instances, the doses tested in volunteers approached clinical dose levels, thus supporting the absence of pronounced subjective effects of these compounds. Nefazodone at doses of 100 and 200 mg showed opposite effects in two experimental models of anxiety: it attenuated subjectively rated anxiety in a conditioning paradigm but enhanced unconditioned fear in a simulated public speaking situation (Silva *et al.*, 2001).

Behavioral Effects

Clinically sedative compounds such as amitriptyline, dothiepin, mianserin and trimipramine produce a decline in almost all areas of performance at relatively low single doses; less sedating antidepressants such as bupropion, citalopram, fluoxetine, fluvoxamine (Fairweather *et al.*, 1996), moclobemide, nefazodone (van Laar *et al.*, 2002), paroxetine (Robbe and O'Hanlon, 1995) and trazodone (Rush *et al.*, 1997) did not significantly impair performance in healthy subjects. Some studies reported slight improvements of performance after SSRIs (e.g. citalopram: Harmer *et al.*, 2002; paroxetine: van Laar *et al.*, 2002). Curran and Wattis (1998) reviewed CFF findings for 20 different antidepressants: eight were reported to decrease, five to increase and seven to have no effect on CFF. Some caution is required in the interpretation of these findings because many antidepressants, e.g. the SSRIs citalopram and sertraline, induce an increase in pupil size and may then mask actual decreases of CFF (Schmitt *et al.*, 2002).

The 'natural antidepressant' hypericum perforatum is reported to have only few effects on cognitive and psychomotor performance in healthy volunteers: after single doses of 900 and 1800 mg only one test (DSST) within a large battery was significantly affected (Timoshanko *et al.*, 2001). The effects of single doses of lithium on healthy volunteers are small. This also holds true when the substance is given over a period of several weeks.

Neurophysiology

Amitriptyline, imipramine and mianserin were found to cause an increase in delta and theta and a decrease in the alpha bands, indicative of their sedative properties, in *pharmaco-EEG* studies. An increase in beta power around 20 Hz also seems to be typical for these older antidepressants. Variable effects of different antidepressants have been reported for yet faster EEG frequencies; these may be due to methodological differences between studies. Little or no effect on EEG frequencies was seen after bupropion and viloxazine, and findings reported for fluvoxamine are controversial: Curran and Lader (1986) noted no changes in quantified EEG parameters after 50 mg; Nishimura *et al.* (1996) observed an increase of slow and fast as well as a reduction of alpha waves after the same dose of fluvoxamine. Taking all reported data together, a common pharmaco-EEG pattern does not seem to exist for antidepressant drugs from different pharmacological classes. Lithium at single doses had no significant effects on quantified EEG parameters; after repeated administration for 2 weeks some increase in slow waves at the expense of alpha waves was detected.

Polygraphic sleep studies with antidepressants have traditionally been of great interest since certain forms of depression are characterized by common features in the sleep polygram (very short REM sleep latency, i.e. time until appearance of first REM phase; frequent sleep interruptions) and it was found that many antidepressants affect the sleep pattern of healthy subjects in the opposite way to that observed in endogenous depression (Vogel *et al.*, 1990). Typically, many antidepressants lead to a dose-dependent prolongation of REM latency and an overall reduction in the duration of REM sleep. However, this effect is not seen after trazodone and nefazodone (Sharpley *et al.*, 1996), and REM sleep findings reported for hypericum perforatum are controversial (Schulz and Jobert, 1994; Sharpley *et al.*, 1998). Sedative antidepressants such as amitriptyline, dothiepin (Wilson *et al.*, 2000), doxepine and trimipramine stabilize sleep (less wake time after sleep onset, fewer brief interruptions of the course of sleep) and, in larger doses, prolong its duration; antidepressants with little or no sedative properties, such as fluvoxamine (Wilson *et al.*, 2000), moclobemide and paroxetine (Sharpley *et al.*, 1996), intensify sleep unrest in normal subjects and can lead to a decrease in the duration of sleep when given in larger doses (Fig. 3.6).

An early report by Saletu (1976) suggested that latencies of primary EP responses are shortened and those of secondary responses are prolonged after antidepressant drugs. In studies by Tomotake *et al.* (1997), Hanano *et al.* (1997) and Matsuoka *et al.* (1997), clomipramine at a dose of 0.5 mg/kg was reported to have no effect on early and middle AEP and VEP latencies, but to shorten P2 and N2 SEP latencies. Mianserin at a dose of 0.3 mg/kg was found to prolong P3 latencies of the auditory, sensory and visually evoked potentials (AEP, SEP and VEP); late AEP and SEP latencies were also increased. The authors interpret their findings as being indicative of the stronger sedative effect of mianserin. Van Laar *et al.* (2002) performed an extensive study with amitriptyline (25 plus 50 mg/day), nefazodone (200 mg twice a day) and paroxetine (30 mg/day): amitriptyline had thorough effects on a number of ERP components, notably the P3 latency on day 1, but nefazodone and paroxetine did not significantly affect these parameters. Hegerl *et al.* (1990) found increases in amplitudes and latencies of early AEP components (P1, N1) after 10 days of lithium administration to healthy volunteers. They did not interpret the finding but stated that similar effects are observed in bipolar patients treated with lithium.

3.4.3 ANXIOLYTIC AND HYPNOTIC DRUGS (Table 3.7)

Subjective Effects

In some experimental paradigms of situational anxiety, benzodiazepines were shown to have relaxing or even anxiolytic effects in healthy subjects. However, this observation has not been confirmed in all studies and seems to be restricted to a narrow dose range: just a slight increase in dose leads to feelings of tiredness, drowsiness and languor in healthy subjects. Similar effects are experienced by healthy subjects after taking usual doses of sleep-inducing agents of the benzodiazepine group. Instead of relaxation, either no effect or general sedation is experienced after administration of the non-benzodiazepine anxiolytic buspirone and the hypnotic drugs zolpidem (Rush *et al.*, 1996) and zopiclone.

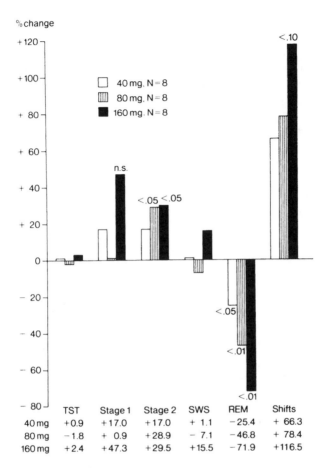

	TST	Stage 1	Stage 2	SWS	REM	Shifts
40 mg	+0.9	+17.0	+17.0	+ 1.1	−25.4	+ 66.3
80 mg	−1.8	+ 0.9	+28.9	− 7.1	−46.8	+ 78.4
160 mg	+2.4	+47.3	+29.5	+15.5	−71.9	+116.5

Figure 3.6 Effect of a tricyclic antidepressant on polygraphic sleep stages. The characteristic effect of many antidepressants is a dose-dependent reduction in REM sleep. The present trial included eight healthy male volunteers who slept in the laboratory on five successive nights. After allowing one night for adaptation, they received placebo, 40, 80 and 160 mg of the antidepressant dibenzepine (Noveril®) in a balanced sequence. Sleep was recorded polygraphically for 7.5 hours. The figure shows the mean percentage changes after dibenzepine from the individual placebo values; statistical comparisons were performed by means of three-way analyses of variance and subsequent pair comparisons (from Spiegel, 1981, p. 50 reproduced with kind permission of Kluwer Academic Publishers)

Behavioral Effects

There are hundreds of published studies on the effects of benzodiazepine anxiolytics and hypnotics on *performance parameters* in healthy subjects, and it is generally recognized that these drugs cause a dose-related reduction in most areas of performance. Tasks that appear to be particularly sensitive to the effects of benzodiazepines are those calling for complex motor or psychomotor coordination, such as simulated traffic situations. Vigilance tests of longer duration are also considered to be very sensitive. In the hands of many investigators, reaction times to different configurations of stimuli were not very sensitive; in contrast, Wesnes and collaborators have performed a number of studies with simple and more complex reaction time paradigms (e.g. Thompson *et al.*, 1999) and found them very sensitive to the effects of benzodiazepines. In the case of the anxiolytic buspirone, no adverse effects on performance are usually detected after single doses corresponding to the therapeutically used ones, whereas the sedating action of the non-benzodiazepine hypnotics zolpidem (Rush *et al.*, 1996) and zopiclone manifests itself in various areas of performance. Benzodiazepines (with the exception of clobazam) and the non-benzodiazepine hypnotic zolpidem decrease the CFF but buspirone does not affect it (Curran and Wattis, 1998).

Great interest has traditionally been shown in the amnestic effects of the benzodiazepines, which are also utilized in anesthesiology. When given prior to surgery, higher doses of these compounds lead to amnesia covering the period immediately preceding, during and – depending on the dose and the duration of action of the preparation used – after an operation. This led to the question as to whether amnestic effects of benzodiazepines also occur in their use as

Table 3.7 Effects of anxiolytic drugs in healthy subjects

Area of assessment	Benzodiazepines and related drugs	Non-benzodiazepines (buspirone)
Subjective effects	Relaxation; tiredness with higher (therapeutic) doses	No effect at lower, possibly sedation at higher doses
Attention, concentration	Impairment at higher (therapeutic) doses	No effect
Perception	CFF reduced	No effect
Learning, memory	Impairment	No effect
Verbal, logical functions	No clear effects	No data
Motor, executive functions	Slower saccades. Some impairment, especially in complex tasks	No effect
Wake EEG	Alpha ↓, beta ↑	No effect
Sleep polygram	WASO and unrest ↓, stage 2 and sleep duration ↑, REM sleep ↓	No data
Early EPs	No effect	No data
Late ERPs	Latencies increased	No data

For detailed results with individual drugs see text and earlier editions of this volume (Spiegel, 1996, Chapters 3 and 4).

anxiolytics, i.e. at non-anesthetic doses. Curran *et al.* (1998) reported findings from a study with lorazepam, which, in their interpretation, "provide strong evidence for a dissociation between the effects on episodic memory and on arousal" of the benzodiazepine anxiolytic. Given its clinical importance, this controversial issue is treated more extensively in Chapter 7 (Section 7.4.2).

Neurophysiology

Benzodiazepine anxiolytics and hypnotics lead to a decrease in alpha and an increase in beta activity in pharmaco-EEG trials. With regard to theta and delta activities, the results of different studies vary. Buspirone at the usual therapeutic doses induces no or only a very weak EEG effect (Greenblatt *et al.*, 1994) and is thus differentiated from the benzodiazepine anxiolytics.

In polygraphic sleep studies benzodiazepines stabilize and, at higher doses, increase the duration of sleep. Also at higher doses benzodiazepines are reported to reduce the proportion of REM sleep and the number of eye movements during REM sleep (REM density). A striking feature emerging in polygraphic sleep studies is the increase in spindle activity, i.e. groups of waves arising phasically in the 12–14 Hz band, after benzodiazepines at higher doses or after repeated administration. Another feature of the benzodiazepines, not shared by zolpidem and zopiclone, is a reduction of slow-wave sleep after single doses, and even more pronounced after repeated administration (Parrino and Terzano, 1996).

Early work by Saletu (1976), which suggested that latencies of primary EP responses are prolonged and those of secondary responses are shortened after benzodiazepines, has not been replicated by other authors. Urata *et al.* (1996) observed prolonged P300 latencies and reduced P300 amplitudes after small doses of triazolam. This was similar to a report by Pooviboonsuk *et al.* (1996) about prolonged P300 latencies and reduced P300 amplitudes after two doses of lorazepam. In contrast, van Leeuwen *et al.* (1995) observed reduced amplitudes of the P1, N1, P2N2 and P3 waves but no changes of latencies to these potentials after two doses of oxazepam given to healthy volunteers.

3.4.4 PSYCHOSTIMULANT DRUGS (Table 3.8)

Subjective Effects

Amphetamines and related psychostimulants, modafinil and caffeine (ingested as capsules or as caffeinated drinks), produce feelings of increased energy and activity. These effects are particularly pronounced if subjects are engaged in strenuous or monotonous activities of longer duration. According to some reports, there seems to be a minority of subjects who show negative responses to stimulants and may feel tired, listless and occasionally even depressed (Corr and Kumari, 2000).

Table 3.8 Effects of psychostimulant drugs in healthy subjects

Area of assessment	Amphetamine and related drugs	Non-amphetamines (caffeine)
Subjective effects	Increased energy, activity, interest, well-being	Increased energy, activity; at higher doses, nervousness
Attention, concentration	Improved performance	Improved performance
Perception	CFF: no consistent results	No data
Learning, memory	Evidence of improved performance, mainly acquisition	Some evidence of improvement
Verbal, logical functions	Improved performance	Some evidence of improvement
Motor, executive functions	Improved performance	Improved performance
Wake EEG	Inconsistent findings	Inconsistent findings
Sleep polygram	Sleep unrest ↑, sleep duration ↓, REM latency ↑, REM sleep ↓	Sleep unrest ↑, sleep duration ↓
Early EPs	No data	No data
Late ERPs	No data	No data

For detailed results with individual drugs see text and earlier editions of this volume (Spiegel, 1996, Chapters 3 and 4).

Behavioral Effects

The effects of stimulants on *performance criteria* have been studied extensively and may be summarized as follows:

(1) Improvements in performance after amphetamine in dosages of 2.5–20 mg are particularly marked in tasks where prolonged attentiveness and concentration are called for. With increasing test duration the positive effect of amphetamine on performance in tests of cancellation, arithmetics and vigilance becomes more pronounced.

(2) A few studies involving amphetamine suggested improved learning and memory performance. These effects presumably may be attributed to improved alertness during the acquisition phase (Chapter 7).

(3) Performance involving a motor component is improved only slightly in rested subjects, but improvements are more pronounced when the test persons are exhausted, e.g. after sleep deprivation.

A frequently used test to assess the effect of psychostimulants is the CPT. Methylphenidate at doses of around 0.3 mg/kg usually improves performance, i.e. reduces the number of errors, on the CPT whereas the effects of *d*-amphetamine (at doses between 5 and 20 mg) and pemoline (10–60 mg) appear to be less reliable (Riccio *et al.*, 2001). The stimulating effect of caffeine in various areas of performance is of shorter duration than that of amphetamine and methylphenidate. Doses tested and found to be effective usually lay between 75 mg (corresponding to two cups of coffee) and 750 mg. Significant improvement in the Wilkinson vigilance test and in a complex reaction test was seen after just 32 mg of caffeine, i.e. after an amount corresponding to a cola drink or a cup of coffee. Single doses of 250 and 500 mg/70 kg caffeine attenuated the negative effects of the benzodiazepine lorazepam on a number of performance tasks (Rush *et al.*, 1994). Improvement in psychomotor performance and vigilance results from the administration of modafinil (another catecholaminergic stimulant) in subjects previously fatigued by sleep deprivation. Thus, after 40-h periods of continuous wakefulness, pilots in a helicopter simulator performed significantly better when given 600 mg of modafinil than on placebo, with the greatest effect seen between 0330 and 1130 hours when the combined impact of sleep loss and the circadian trough was most severe (Caldwell *et al.*, 2000).

Neurophysiology

Published pharmaco-EEG trials provide a heterogeneous picture: some studies with *d*-amphetamine and methylphenidate reported a reduction in delta and theta waves; other authors found either an increase in delta and theta activity or no effect at all on the quantified EEG. There is also no agreement in the case of changes in the alpha and beta bands after several stimulants. Some of the contradictory findings are most likely to be due to different experimental conditions, particularly the duration of EEG recordings (for details see Spiegel, 1996, p. 90).

Stimulants, if taken in the evening, delay sleep onset, impair the continuity of sleep at low doses and curtail its duration at higher doses (Fig. 3.7). Amphetamine-like stimulants and caffeine have different effects on REM sleep, which is unchanged after caffeine but dose-dependently reduced after amphetamine. Modafinil at single doses of 100 and 200 mg has only weak effects on the sleep polygram, with a pattern similar to that of amphetamine.

According to Saletu (1976), latencies of primary and secondary responses are shortened after stimulants. Methylphenidate was reported to enhance P300 amplitudes in children with attention deficit hyperactivity disorder (Jonkman *et al.*, 2000), and whether the compound has similar effects in healthy volunteers is not known. The amplitude of the CNV was reported to be increased after stimulants, although the opposite effect has also been observed in some studies.

3.4.5 NOOTROPICS AND ANTIDEMENTIA DRUGS

Subjective Effects

Few results are available from experiments in healthy volunteers involving the use of the older nootropic drugs, such as co-dergocrine mesylate, piracetam or

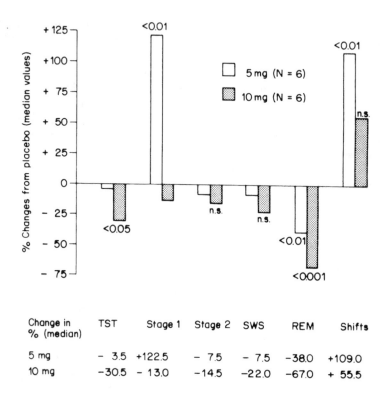

Change in % (median)	TST	Stage 1	Stage 2	SWS	REM	Shifts
5 mg	− 3.5	+122.5	− 7.5	− 7.5	−38.0	+109.0
10 mg	−30.5	− 13.0	−14.5	−22.0	−67.0	+ 55.5

Figure 3.7 Effects of *d*-amphetamine on polygraphic sleep stages. A decrease in REM sleep, an increase in sleep unrest (shifts from sleep stages 2, 3 and 4 into the waking state and into stage 1) and an increase in stage 1 are typical effects seen after amphetamine-like stimulants used at small doses. After larger doses REM sleep is even more markedly reduced and total sleep time (TST) is shortened (reproduced from Spiegel, 1982, with permission from S. Karger AG, Basel)

vincamine; findings reviewed some years ago suggested that single doses of these substances in the therapeutic dose range have no subjective stimulant or other effect in healthy young volunteers (Spiegel, 1992). Cholinergic drugs, such as the muscarinic agonist RS 86 (Azcona *et al.*, 1986) and the cholinesterase inhibitor rivastigmine (Enz *et al.*, 1991), were found to have unspecific effects in healthy volunteers: they produce some drowsiness at lower doses and dizziness and nausea at higher doses.

Behavioral Effects

There are only isolated reports on studies in healthy volunteers with the old nootropics. On the basis of a report by Hindmarch *et al.* (1990) on pyritinol and our own results with co-dergocrine mesylate, piracetam and vincamine (Spiegel, 1992), it is safe to assume that a single administration of these products at usual therapeutic doses has no effect on the performance of healthy subjects. Cholinergic agents such as the muscarinic agonist RS 86 and the cholinesterase inhibitors donepezil and rivastigmine did not have an impact on cognitive or behavioral parameters at well-tolerated single doses (Azcona et al., 1986; Enz et al., 1991; Nathan et al., 2001). Another cholinesterase inhibitor, pyridostigmine, given three times a day for five consecutive days, was associated with an improvement in reaction time on tests of memory and attention and fewer errors on a tracking task (Cook et al., 2002).

Neurophysiology

Nootropics induce very weak or no EEG effects at all in single-dose experiments in healthy subjects. A lack of significant effects was also found in sleep polygraphic studies with several nootropic drugs (Maggini et al., 1988; Spiegel, 1992).

Compounds with direct or indirect agonistic effects on cholinergic receptors facilitate the appearance of REM sleep early in the night: shorter REM sleep latencies were noted after the cholinesterase inhibitors physostigmine (Gillin and Sitaram, 1984) and tacrine (Riemann et al., 1996). The muscarinic agonists RS 86 (Spiegel, 1984) and pilocarpine (Berkowitz et al., 1990; Seifritz et al., 1998) also shortened the REM latency of healthy subjects. The cholinesterase inhibitor rivastigmine was found to increase REM density early in the night but had no significant effect on REM latency (Holsboer-Trachsler et al., 1993).

3.5 DISCUSSION

3.5.1 DIFFERENTIAL DRUG EFFECTS

Psychotropic drugs induce a variety of subjective and objective effects that can be detected and quantified using psychometric and neurophysiological methods. With regard to the first question posed in Section 3.1 – i.e. whether psychotropic drugs used in different clinical indications produce differential and perhaps specific patterns of activity when given to healthy subjects – the findings summarized in the foregoing paragraphs suggest the following:

(1) *Antipsychotic drugs* with strong sedative clinical effects (e.g. chlorpromazine, clozapine, olanzapine) produce subjective and objective sedation and impair most areas of performance in healthy volunteers, usually at doses far below those typically used in patients. Antipsychotic drugs with little sedative clinical action (e.g. pimozide, sulpiride, amisulpride) produce few subjective and objective effects in healthy

subjects, even if given at doses that are close to those used clinically. Thus, as in therapeutic use, antipsychotic drugs do not show a uniform pattern of activity in healthy subjects, but the clinically more and the less sedative representatives of the class also differ with regard to their effects on healthy volunteers. It should be noted that the less sedative antipsychotics are relatively pure D2 dopaminergic antagonists (Chapter 4), whereas the sedative, sleep-promoting compounds also have effects on muscarinic, noradrenergic and histaminic receptors. Neurophysiological techniques, notably pharmaco-EEG studies, generally confirm the distinction between more and less sedative compounds, although there does not seem to be a specific neurophysiological pattern of activity of antipsychotic drugs.

(2) *Antidepressant drugs* with more and with less sedative clinical action show similarly different effects in healthy volunteers to those seen with more and less sedative antipsychotics. Studies in healthy volunteers do not reveal a specific subjective or behavioral profile of antidepressants and, based on their effects in such experiments, it would not be possible to distinguish reliably between sedative antipsychotics and antidepressants or between non-sedative antipsychotics and antidepressants. As is the case with antipsychotics, antidepressants with strong sedative action in patients and healthy subjects affect muscarinic, noradrenergic and histaminic receptors (Chapter 4). Pharmaco-EEG studies also help to differentiate between sedative and non-sedative antidepressants but, in contrast to some claims by earlier authors, there does not appear to be a specific 'antidepressant EEG profile'. Furthermore, although many antidepressants do suppress REM sleep in polygraphic sleep studies in healthy volunteers, this effect is not shared by all clinically effective antidepressants, and there are many other drugs, with no recognized antidepressant activity, that also delay the onset of REM sleep and reduce its duration.

(3) *Anxiolytics* of the benzodiazepine type produce dose-dependent subjective sedation; they also impair a wide range of performance parameters in healthy volunteers, usually at doses identical or close to those used in patients with anxiety syndromes. Some anxiolytics may be qualitatively different from sedative antipsychotics and antidepressants with regard to their subjective effects noted by healthy volunteers (benzodiazepines are perceived by many subjects as being pleasantly relaxing), but nuances of this kind have not been studied in direct comparative trials. With regard to its subjective and behavioral effects the non-benzodiazepine anxiolytic buspirone and its derivatives may be more similar to the non-sedative antipsychotics and antidepressants than to benzodiazepines, but here again there are no direct comparative trials. A striking feature of the benzodiazepines is their effect on some neurophysiological characteristics, in particular the marked increase of slow beta waves (12–14 Hz) seen in wake EEGs and in the EEG recorded during sleep. This effect is not shared

by the non-benzodiazepine anxiolytics, indicating that it is not related to the anxiolytic effect but rather to some specific pharmacological action of the benzodiazepines.

(4) *Psychostimulants* of the amphetamine type (which have been little studied in the last 10 years) as well as caffeine can be clearly distinguished from the other classes of psychotropic drugs on the basis of their subjective and objective effects: in no other drug class is there a consistent pattern of subjective and objective improvements in drive, mood and performance as in the case of stimulants. Sustained wakefulness (or vigilance) after amphetamine, caffeine, etc. can also be demonstrated in EEG trials: although none of these compounds displays a specific pattern of EEG effects, they keep subjects awake in longer recordings and can thus be distinguished from placebo and other drugs (Fig. 3.8). In polygraphic all-night recordings, stimulant drugs interfere with the onset and duration of sleep; furthermore, amphetamine-like drugs suppress REM sleep in a dose-dependent fashion.

(5) The so-called *nootropics* have no actions in healthy volunteers that characterize them as clearly active in the brain or as an independent class of psychotropic substances.

(6) Although there are only few published data with *antidementia drugs*, the effects of cholinesterase inhibitors in healthy awake volunteers appear to be unspecific. In contrast, the REM-sleep facilitating effect of these compounds appears to be a property not shared by other psychotropic drugs.

3.5.2 SENSITIVITY OF THE ASSESSMENT METHODS USED IN PHARMACOPSYCHOLOGY

Dose–effect studies with well-known drugs can be used to determine the sensitivity of different assessment methods: in experiments of this kind the lowest dose of a given drug that leads to reliable changes from baseline on a particular parameter can be considered a marker of its sensitivity. An assessment method is recognized as being particularly sensitive when it indicates a drug effect at doses that do not yet induce effects on other parameters measured at the same time.

Kraepelin (1892, p. 88) assumed "that the course of very simple mental processes which have furthermore become almost automatic through long practice is less changed by the influence of medicaments than are those more complex processes which always represent a special mental performance". Accordingly, a complex task such as driving a car should be a more sensitive indicator of drug effects than the simple tapping task. However, inspection of Tables 3.5–3.8 shows that Kraepelin's assumption is not so generally applicable: for example, in some of the older experiments with antipsychotic

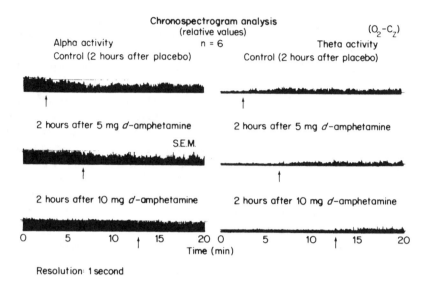

Resolution: 1 second

Figure 3.8 Effects of d-amphetamine on the wake EEG. Mean EEG spectral values for six healthy male subjects who took placebo, 5 mg and 10 mg of d-amphetamine on separate occasions in a balanced crossover trial are shown. Whereas the EEG trace 2 h after placebo (upper third) shows a rapid decline in alpha waves and an increase in theta waves (see arrows pointing to the alpha decrease and the theta increase), the corresponding changes occurred later after 5 mg (middle third) and 10 mg (lower third) d-amphetamine. The decay of alpha and increase of theta activities occurred after 2 min on placebo, but only after 7 min on 5 mg d-amphetamine and after 12 min on 10 mg of d-amphetamine, thus reflecting a vigilance-stabilizing effect of d-amphetamine (Matejcek, 1979, with permission)

drugs, doses that induced reliable changes on several other parameters of performance had little effect on more complex verbal and logical tasks, and the relative insensitivity of intelligence tests to sedative drug effects was also found in studies with anxiolytics. With regard to psychostimulants, Weiss and Laties (1962) stressed that the performance-improving effect of these drugs is clearer in the simple and repetitive than in the more intellectually demanding tasks. Latz (1968), in another thorough review of early studies with psychostimulants, reached a similar conclusion.

The issue of sensitivity of different objective assessment methods has been discussed extensively in earlier editions of this volume (Spiegel and Aebi, 1983, p. 75; Spiegel, 1989, p. 72). The – somewhat updated – conclusions were as follows:

(1) Methods that focus on attention and concentration are particularly sensitive to the actions of drugs, even though impairments caused by sedative substances are not always detected in tests of short duration.

Vigilance tests and continuous performance tests (Table 3.1), which usually last for more than 15 min, take first place with regard to sensitivity (see also Koelega, 1989, 1993). More recent work (e.g. Thompson *et al.*, 1999) suggests that computerized reaction time tasks of short duration may be equally as sensitive as some of the older, longer tests.

(2) Except for the CFF technique, methods that assess perception have found little use in recent studies. The CFF seems to respond very sensitively to sedative substances, especially benzodiazepines (see also Curran and Wattis, 1998).

(3) Motor and so-called psychomotor tasks, e.g. reaction-time tests of varying complexity, also respond reliably to sedative and stimulant drug effects (Kunsman *et al.*, 1992); however none of the procedures shows particularly great sensitivity.

(4) Methods that assess thought processes or aspects of intelligence have not been used in more recent studies; their sensitivity to the effects of psychotropic drugs seems to be low.

(5) Learning and memory processes may be impaired by sedative substances, especially benzodiazepines and related drugs; this topic will be discussed further in Chapter 7.

An important and also practical question concerns the relative sensitivity of subjective and objective assessment instruments used in pharmacopsychology and elsewhere: If subjects are negatively affected by drugs with regard to their cognitive or motor performance, will this always be reflected in their self-assessment? This issue was studied in a systematic way some time ago by Bye *et al.* (1973, 1978), Clubley *et al.* (1979) and Peck *et al.* (1979). Among the subjective methods, the VAS stood out as being particularly sensitive; among the objective procedures the Wilkinson vigilance test was the most sensitive. At very low doses of sedative or stimulating substances, both of these methods were about equal in terms of their sensitivity, suggesting that objective impairment (or improvement) of performance is generally perceived by test subjects in an experimental situation. Whether this conclusion can be extrapolated to everyday life, e.g. to traffic or complex professional situations, is a different question. Thus, Wesnes (personal communication) quotes the example of a study by Beuzen *et al.* (1999), which showed that self-rated alertness by healthy subjects clearly underestimated the extent of impairment recorded in tests of vigilance and attention. Still, subjective methods such as the VAS are time-economical and they also make it possible to determine substance effects outside the stimulation–sedation continuum.

Whether any of the neurophysiological approaches is more or less sensitive than psychological instruments to delineate drug effects in healthy volunteers is difficult to judge because only a few studies used both types of methodology in parallel. Nevertheless, in order to provide a rough overview, Table 3.9 sets out those doses of some older psychotropic drugs that were found to produce statistically significant effects in a diversity of separate studies using psychological and electrophysiological measurement methods. The picture that arises is incomplete (particularly in the absence of usable information concerning EPs and ERPs) but does reveal that electrophysiological and psychological parameters generally respond to drug doses of the same order of magnitude. In the case of sedative substances, i.e. some antipsychotics, antidepressants and anxiolytics, the minimum effective doses at the various levels of measurement are similar, and the same applies to psychostimulants. Sleep polygraphic studies appear to be particularly sensitive to the actions of many antidepressants, mainly those that suppress REM sleep. Sleep polygraphic studies also indicate a facilitatory effect of some antidementia drugs (cholinesterase inhibitors) upon REM sleep, although this class of compounds will not produce significant effects in other areas of assessment.

In a review article published in 1986, Münte et al. expressed their surprise at the fact that the effects of psychotropic drugs on ERPs had not received great attention. The few studies of P300 cited by Münte et al. suggested that compounds such as methylphenidate and scopolamine could influence certain components of the P300 complex. However, because the corresponding experiments were mostly performed with specific experimental–psychological rather than pharmacological orientation, it is not possible to assess the sensitivities of the various P300 paradigms for pharmacological questions. Because only isolated EP and ERP drug studies have been published in the meantime, it is still not possible to judge the sensitivity of these neurophysiological approaches for psychopharmacology.

3.5.3 UNDERSTANDING AND PREDICTING CLINICAL DRUG EFFECTS

As shown in the foregoing paragraphs, it is possible to delineate sedative and stimulant drug effects in healthy subjects and to relate them to the effects and side effects seen with the same drugs in a clinical situation. A variety of partly complementary methods is available for this purpose. On the other hand, there do not seem to be reliable experimental equivalents ('surrogate markers') of antipsychotic or antidepressant drug effects in healthy subjects that could be used to distinguish between representatives of these two classes of drugs or to predict the clinical indication of novel compounds. In other words, it is not possible to understand or predict the specific therapeutic effects of antipsychotic and antidepressant drugs from their effects occurring in healthy subjects.

Beyond the possibility of characterizing stimulant and sedative drug effects in a controlled setting, what is the relevance of performing studies with psychotropic drugs in healthy volunteers? From a pragmatic standpoint one could argue as follows: drug experiments in healthy subjects make it possible to detect subjective, behavioral and neurophysiological drug effects after small,

Table 3.9 Sensitivity of psychological and electrophysiological parameters to psychotropic drug effects

Substance class	Compound	Subjective criteria	Performance parameters	effect	Wake EEG	Sleep polygram
Antipsychotics	Chlorpromazine	25–50 mg	25–50 mg	↓	50 mg	12.5 mg
	Clozapine	5 mg	No data	0	5, 10 mg	5, 10 mg
	Haloperidol	2 mg	Up to 4 mg		Up to 4 mg	1 mg
Antidepressants	Amitriptyline	6.25–12.5 mg	6.25–12.5 mg	↓	25 mg	12.5 mg
	Imipramine	50 mg	75 mg	↓	35 mg	25 mg
	Mianserin	No data	15 mg	↓	15 mg	5, 10 mg
Anxiolytics	Chlordiazepoxide	10–30 mg	20 mg	↓	No data	35 mg
	Diazepam	5–10 mg	5 mg	0	5 mg	5 mg
	Meprobamate	Up to 800 mg	Up to 800 mg		600 mg	400 mg
Psychostimulants	d-Amphetamine	5 mg	2.5 mg	↑	5 mg	2.5–5 mg
	Caffeine	75 mg	75 mg	↑	100 mg (?)	200 mg
	Methylphenidate	No data	10–20 mg	↑	30 mg	5 mg

The table shows the smallest single dose producing significant changes in the respective area of measurement. Doses given are from tables 3.4–3.8 and 4.2–4.4 in Spiegel (1996): ↑ and ↓ stand for significant improvement or deterioration in performance assessments.

i.e. safe doses; the exact timing of the onset, peak and duration of a drug action on the brain can be determined under laboratory conditions; in addition, correlations between the blood concentration of a substance and its effects, as well as pharmacological interactions between several concomitantly or successively administered compounds, can be studied. Thus, drug studies in healthy subjects can be useful at several stages of drug development (see Chapter 5): in early stages, as so-called screening trials, i.e. to roughly characterize novel, clinically yet unknown substances with regard to their effects on the human brain; in later stages, for studying aspects of drug safety and for the investigation of other major practical questions.

In our own work with potential antidementia drugs we have made use of psychological as well as neurophysiological techniques to study the effects of cholinergic agents in healthy volunteers. Once the REM-sleep enhancing properties of muscarinic agonists and cholinesterase inhibitors had been demonstrated (see Section 3.4.5), we used polygraphic sleep recordings to test a number of such drugs (e.g. Hohagen et al., 1993) in healthy volunteers. Rivastigmine (ENA 713), a dual cholinesterase inhibitor, was found to increase the density of rapid eye movements during REM sleep (Holsboer-Trachsler et al., 1993) at doses that were well tolerated by healthy subjects in preceding trials (Enz et al., 1991). The REM-enhancing doses (1–2 mg) were considered the minimum CNS-active ones and were included as single starting doses in the first clinical trials in patients with Alzheimer's disease. Clinically effective doses of Exelon® (rivastigmine) in Alzheimer patients were determined at 3–6 mg given twice a day, with some individuals also responding to 2 mg twice a day – thus providing a positive example for the practical relevance of drug experiments in healthy subjects.

3.5.4 THEORY-ORIENTATED ISSUES

A number of authors, notably Wilhelm Janke, have referred to the possibility of using psychotropic drugs experimentally for theory-orientated objectives: "The administration of drugs represents a central research strategy for physiological psychology. It is distinguished from other classical methods, such as lesions, by the reversibility and quantifiability (by using different doses) of the effects achieved. In humans, the administration of drugs is often the only feasible method for modifying somatic processes directly and thus to study them as independent variables" (Janke and Erdmann, 1992, p. 121). An example of the use of psychotropic drugs in physiological psychology would be the administration of a neuroleptic of the haloperidol type (as a dopamine D2 antagonist) and of d-amphetamine (as an indirect dopamine agonist) to study relationships between the dopaminergic activity in the brain and psychological constructs such as attentiveness, mood, etc. Prerequisites for experiments of this type are: the availability of pharmacologically well-characterized, safe and well-tolerated drugs with specific actions; and the confidence that suitable instruments are available to determine complex mental functions such as attentiveness or mood (e.g. King and Henry, 1992).

Theory-orientated objectives in the context of differential psychology focussed on the relationships between so-called personality features (e.g. neuroticism or extraversion according to Eysenck, 1962) and drug actions, a topic of great interest in the 1960s. It was repeatedly shown that subjects with higher levels of 'anxiety' could respond to sedative substances in a different way from less anxious test subjects. This differential response was explained on the basis of a theory of activation (Claridge, 1967), i.e. as the consequence of different baseline 'levels of arousal' of anxious and less anxious subjects. Janke, Debus, Kohnen and other German authors also examined the question of how far the test situation in pharmacopsychological experiments could be modified in the directions of 'stress accentuation' or 'relaxation', and how manipulations of this type would influence the responses of healthy subjects to drugs. Studies of this kind, which do not seem to be fashionable at the present time, are discussed extensively and with the appropriate literature references by Debus and Janke (1986), Janke and Erdmann (1992) and Kohnen (1992).

3.6 CONCLUSIONS

Many, and quite differentiated, drug effects can be shown and quantified in healthy volunteers under standardized and thus reproducible conditions. The information gathered in these experiments can be usefully applied in a number of theoretical and practical contexts. This chapter has not dealt with some of the herbal medicines, and we also omitted discussion of older studies with simultaneous or consecutive administration of more than one drug, e.g. the so-called scopolamine model to study cognition enhancers (see Spiegel, 1989, p. 180). As will be noted in Chapter 5, experiments in healthy volunteers still play their role in the development of new drugs, some of them under the new name of 'proof of concept' (PoC) or 'proof of effect' (PoE) studies.

4

Preclinical Research in Psychopharmacology

By
CONRAD GENTSCH

4.1 INTRODUCTION

This chapter deals with a fact that may be hard to understand at first sight, namely that psychopharmaceuticals – chemical compounds administered in the form of tablets, capsules or injections – can act on mental phenomena such as feelings, mood, behavior and positive and negative symptoms. The term *mechanism of action* expresses the fact that the effects of drugs on mental processes do not occur directly but via a chain of intermediate links. Some of these links, i.e. biochemical, neurobiological and electrophysiological processes, are discussed in the first four sections of this chapter.

Psychopharmaceuticals are most frequently taken in the form of tablets, capsules or coated tablets, i.e. orally. Parenteral presentations are also available for some psychopharmaceuticals, i.e. injection or infusion solutions that can be administered directly into the bloodstream and thus circumvent the gastrointestinal tract. Questions of absorption, metabolism and absorption of these drugs will be discussed in Chapter 5, which deals with clinical trials in psychopharmacology.

Psychopharmaceuticals exert their intended effects in the central nervous system (CNS), where they primarily affect those processes that are involved in the transmission of information between nerve cells. All these drugs act via one or several mechanisms that are thought to be impaired or functioning suboptimally in patients with mental disturbances. Such malfunctioning may

Psychopharmacology, Fourth Edition. By R. Spiegel
© 2003 John Wiley & Sons, Ltd: ISBN 0 471 56039 1: 0 470 84691 7 (PB)

be transient and caused by specific circumstances and/or genetically determined. By specifically interfering with these mechanisms, readjustment of the processes underlying mental functioning is achieved and this represents the drug's therapeutic benefit. We will describe the most important hypotheses, some historical, that were formulated to explain the effects of antipsychotic, antidepressant and anxiolytic drugs.

Psychopharmaceuticals may be of natural origin (e.g. phytotherapeutics extracted from plants), chemically modified natural products or they may have an entirely new, purely synthetic chemical structure. Identification and preclinical development of new psychotropic drugs involve several major steps: once a compound has been synthesized in medicinal chemistry, it is submitted to extensive *in vitro* characterization prior to its initial testing in living animals. If rated as being of potential interest based on *in vitro* findings, the compound will be evaluated in initial *in vivo* studies for brain penetration and brain and plasma pharmacokinetics and, if applicable, *in vivo* tests of functional agonism or antagonism are performed. Indication-finding studies follow, in which the candidate compound is compared with clinically known, effective compounds for potential anxiolytic, antidepressant, antipsychotic or other psychotropic properties. Once a dose–response relationship and, ideally, also a minimal effective dose have been established, additional *in vivo* studies mainly deal with the likely side-effect profile of the drug candidate. These latter studies aim at demonstrating superiority of the novel compound over the best available drugs with regard to tolerability because even a drug with similar efficacy to existing medication may be a successful therapeutic agent if it has a superior side-effect profile. Assuming that the extensive toxicological tests that terminate the preclinical evaluation of the compound do not point to any prohibitive findings, the compound's clinical development (Chapter 5) can be initiated.

Much of the preclinical work with a new compound deals with so-called animal models, i.e. experimental set-ups thought to provide relevant information on the mechanism of action of a drug and to allow predictions about its potential clinical use. Sections 4. 5 and 4. 6 of this chapter provide descriptions of typical models used in many of these studies. Although some of these models are based upon hypotheses concerning the mechanisms of action of existing psychopharmaceuticals, the emphasis of these sections is on behavioral models that appear to be of greatest interest in the current context.

4.2 THE TARGET

4.2.1 THE NERVOUS SYSTEM

The nervous system is probably the most important organ system of higher organisms. Anatomically, a distinction is made between the CNS and the peripheral nervous system: the CNS consists of the brain and the spinal cord, the peripheral nervous system comprises all nerves outside these two structures. Within the peripheral nervous system additional distinctions are made either between the efferent part (the part involved in transmitting information from the CNS to the periphery of the body) and the afferent part (the part involved in transmitting information from the periphery to the CNS) or between the sensory–somatic and the autonomous system.

For efferents linking the CNS with skeletal muscles the term 'motor efferents' is used, whereas those efferents linking the CNS with glands and smooth- and cardiac muscle are named 'vegetative efferents'. Afferents are distinguished into 'somatic afferents' and 'visceral afferents', depending on whether the information flow towards the CNS stems from joints, muscle or skin or the viscera, respectively. The term 'viscera' designates organs of the digestive, respiratory, urogenital and endocrine systems as well as the spleen, heart and great vessels.

4.2.2 NEURONS

Like all the other organs the nervous system is built up of individual cells. In the brain mainly two types of cells are found: neurons, which conduct action potentials, and *glia cells*. The neurons are still the main focus of neurobiological research and much less attention has been paid to the glia cells, because they are considered to be the brain's packing material (glia in Greek originates from the word for glue) with the primary function of delivering nutrition for the neurons. Today, astrocytes, one dominant type of glia cells, are considered to be much more important, having control over neurogenesis, the generation of new neuronal cells (Song *et al.*, 2002).

As depicted in Fig. 4.1, neurons, despite a high region-dependent variability in shape, have a common basic structure. Each neuron consists of the cell body (soma, which contains the cell nucleus), several dendrites and an axon that spreads out distally into axon branches.

Neurons are the material units of information processing in the nervous system. Each individual neuron is connected to dozens up to several thousands

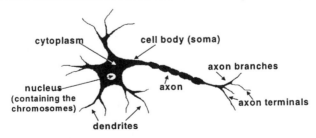

Figure 4.1 Diagram showing the structure of a neuron

of other neurons. It is the sum of all the impulses (stimulatory or inhibitory) arriving at a given moment from all connected neurons that ultimately determines the current activity of a neuron. This activity level then determines which information is propagated to a large number of other connected neurons. Given this high interconnectivity it is evident how complex the flow of information, in the form of electrical impulses (see below) within groups and between groups of neurons, can be. Keeping in mind that the number of neurons in a human brain is 10^{10}–10^{13}, this certainly adds ample evidence for the impressive dimension of neuronal complexity and the capacity of our brain (see Box 4.1). It is thus becoming clear that suboptimal connectivity as well as any changed sensitivity of neurons may be detrimental and lead to altered functionality, reflected in less efficient mental processing and ultimately mental deficiency and/or illnesses.

Box 4.1 A Metaphor for the Brain's Complexity
Within our brains there are some hundred billion neurons

To get an idea of just how big a hundred billion is, the Amazon rain forest offers an appropriate analogy. The Amazon rain forest stretches for 2 700 000 square miles and contains a hundred billion trees. There are about as many trees as neurons in the brain. Considering the huge number of connections between neurons, there are about as many as the leaves on the trees in the Amazon jungle.

4.2.3 SYNAPSES

Synapses are the contact points of two nerve cells or of a nerve cell with an effector cell (such as a muscle, glandular or sensory cell). It is at the synapse, exactly at the synaptic cleft, where the transfer of information from one cell to the next takes place. It is estimated that the diameter of a synaptic cleft, i.e. the distance between the presynaptic membrane (part of the first cell) and the postsynaptic membrane (part of the second cell), is about 100–300 µm. Depending on the carrier of information, electrical and chemical synapses can be distinguished:

• In an *electrical synapse* the electrical signal is transferred directly because the membranes of the two cells are in close vicinity. This is the fastest possible intercellular propagation system of information. Electrical synapses are present and have been studied mainly in lower animals.

- In a *chemical synapse* the two adjacent membranes are not sufficiently close to each other and, in order to pass the information from one cell to the next, the electrical signal is converted transiently into a chemical signal. Most of the synapses in vertebrates are chemical synapses.

The Electrical Part of the Cross-talk between Neurons

In its resting state every neuron has a negative electrical membrane potential – a voltage difference of about $-70\,mV$ between the inside and the outside of the cell, i.e. the inside is electrically negative relative to the outside. The difference in electrical charge is generated as follows: inside the cell there is a lower concentration of positively charged sodium ions (Na^+) and negatively charged chloride ions (Cl^-) and a higher concentration of positively charged potassium ions (K^+) compared with the extracellular space. Depending on the efflux and influx of these ions (due to their size, only the positively charged ions can cross the cell membrane) the electrical net charge of a cell is changeable. Influenced by the input from other neurons, the membrane potential of a neuron is briefly shifted away from its resting state. In an *excitatory synapse* the membrane potential tends to shift to positive, whereas in an *inhibitory synapse* the membrane potential tends to shift to negative. Because any neuron receives synaptic input from many connected neurons, an integration of the excitatory and inhibitory inputs takes place, and if the resulting change in the membrane potential rises above the positive threshold then the neuron produces an impulse, the so-called *action potential*. The action potential travels down the axon of this neuron and either causes a synaptic input to another neuron (if the firing neuron is an interneuron) or a muscle contraction (if the neuron is a motoneuron).

The Chemical Part of the Cross-talk between Neurons

Once the electrical signal has arrived at a chemical synapse (see Fig. 4.2) a cascade of events is triggered: with the arrival of an electrical impulse (an action potential), a chemical compound known as a neurotransmitter is released from the presynaptic side into the synaptic cleft. The released neurotransmitter then reaches the membrane of the second cell (postsynaptic membrane) where it interacts with a macromolecule, a so-called receptor. It is this neurotransmitter–receptor interaction that triggers another cascade of (chemical) reactions within the second cell and this ultimately leads to the generation of an electrical signal within this cell. This signal then is transferred along this second cell's axon towards another synapse.

Once a neurotransmitter is bound to the postsynaptically located receptor a change in the electrical potential of the postsynaptic membrane occurs. Depending on both the type of transmitter and the properties of the postsynaptic receptor involved, the membrane potential of the second cell is

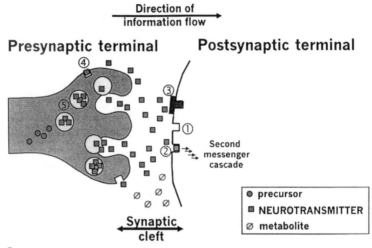

①   Receptor located on the postsynaptic membrane (postsynaptic receptor)
②   Agonist bound to the postsynaptic receptor, triggering second messengers
③   Antagonist bound to the the postsynaptic receptor, inhibiting an agonist from
         interacting at this receptor site
④   Receptor located on the presynaptic membrane (presynaptic receptor)
⑤   Vesicles, containing the neurotransmitters

Figure 4.2 Schematic representation of a chemical synapse, the location within a neuronal network where the transfer of information from one neuron to the next takes place by means of neurotransmitters

either *hyperpolarized*, i.e. its electrical charge is shifted to negative, or *depolarized*, i.e. its electrical charge is shifted to positive. When the membrane potential reaches a critical value (threshold), an action potential is generated and transported along the axon.

Activation of the postsynaptic receptor also leads to activation of the enzymes involved in the formation of so-called 'second messengers' (see Box 4.2 for explanation of this and other terms used in this section). Best-known 'second messengers' are cyclic adenosine monophosphate (cAMP), cyclic guanosine monophosphate (cGMP) and cleavage products of phosphatidylinositol. These molecules are formed at the cell membrane and migrate into the cell where they affect the activity of other enzymes.

Receptors are also located on the presynaptic membrane. These *autoreceptors* regulate the release and synthesis of the neurotransmitter and are part of a feedback mechanism that aims to keep the activation or inhibition within the synapse for a discrete time interval and to terminate the signal transfer once the information has reached the adjacent cell via removal (inactivation) of the neurotransmitter from the synaptic cleft.

Box 4.2 Definitions of Some of the Terms Used

Synapse: Location where two neurons are in closest contact and where the chemically mediated information propagation takes place

Synaptic cleft: Gap of about 100–300 μm in diameter between two neurons. A neurotransmitter is released from the first neuron into the synaptic cleft and may interact with a receptor located on the membrane of the second neuron to trigger reactions leading to the propagation of information

Presynaptic membrane: Part of the first neuron facing a synapse

Postsynaptic membrane: Part of the second neuron

Neurotransmitter: A chemical entity that transmits an electrical signal generated by one neuron to the next by being released and, following interaction with a receptor, generating an alteration in the electrical state (action potential) of the next neuron. The best known neurotransmitters are the monoamines (amine-containing chemical entities) and peptides (conjugates of several amino acids)

Vesicle: Small membrane-walled containers (50 nm diameter) present at the presynaptic terminal of the neuron in which neurotransmitters are stored and from which neurotransmitters are released into the synaptic cleft

Release: Liberation of the neurotransmitter from vesicle: electrical firing of a nerve leads to fusion of vesicles with the cell wall, allowing the neurotransmitter to be released into the synaptic junction

Metabolism: Building up (synthesis) and breaking down of a compound, also of neurotransmitters

Enzyme: A protein molecule that catalyzes specific metabolic reactions without being permanently altered or destroyed itself

Precursor: A chemical entity that is part of the reaction leading to the formation of another molecule (e.g. a neurotransmitter)

Metabolite: A chemical entity formed as a breakdown product of, for example, monoamines. In most cases metabolites are no longer active at the original compound's target

> **Degradation**: Breakdown into (in most cases) biologically inactive molecules (metabolites), aiming at stopping/inactivating information transfer via neurotransmitters
>
> **Receptor**: A macromolecule or a polymeric structure in or on a cell that specifically recognizes and binds a compound acting as a molecular messenger (e.g. neurotransmitters, hormones, drugs)
>
> **Second messenger**: An intracellularly present substance or ion that increases or decreases in response to the stimulation of a receptor by its agonist

4.2.4 RECEPTORS

Receptors are macromolecules of peptidic structure (a three-dimensionally arranged sequence of amino acids) that are predominantly located within cell membranes. One common structural form is the so-called seven-transmembrane receptor, which consists of seven domains located within the membrane plus an extracellular (top of Fig. 4.3) and an intracellular (bottom of Fig. 4.3) part. Within the receptor molecule there is also a specific binding pocket (not shown in the figure) for a message molecule (a neurotransmitter or any other ligand) and this part of the three-dimensionally arranged receptor molecule is named the binding site.

The interaction between a ligand and its receptor can be characterized by the metaphor of a key (the ligand) and a lock (the binding site of a receptor). Because one can lock and unlock a door only with a specifically tailored and thus closely fitting key, it is only when the ligand is tightly fitting into the binding site that the receptor will be activated. Subsequent to this event, an activation or an inhibition of a neuron will occur.

Receptors are generally named after their ligand, e.g. dopaminergic, serotonergic, noradrenergic and γ-aminobutyric acid (GABA)-ergic receptors. Another distinction of receptors concerns the impact of their activation: *ionotropic* receptors directly regulate ion channels; *metabotropic* receptors are linked to an intracellular enzyme via an intermediate G-protein.

The GABA-A receptor (Fig. 4.4) constitutes an example of an ionotropic receptor. It is composed of five different protein subunits – two alpha-1, two beta-2 and one gamma-2 – and is therefore called a pentamer. The benzodiazepine binding site is located at the $\alpha1/\gamma2$ interphase, whereas the activation sites for GABA are located at the $\alpha1/\beta2$ interphase. Once a benzodiazepine molecule has bound, the receptor will change its shape so that it responds more to GABA. Upon activation of the GABA-A receptor the ion channel opens and chloride ions can pass.

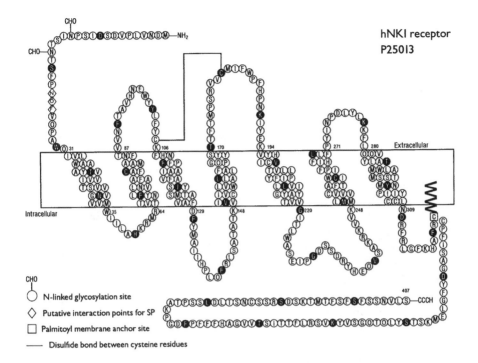

Figure 4.3 Schematic representation of a 7-transmembrane receptor, exemplified with the human neurokinin-1 receptor (hNK₁). The extracellular elements of the receptor are shown in the upper part: the amino-acid chain ends with a free amino-residue (NH2) and is called the amino-terminal of the receptor. The longer amino acid chain of the intracellular part (lower part) ends with a free acid-residue (COOH) and is called the carboxylic end. The seven transmembrane domains are 'lined up' within the box, which represents the membrane

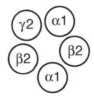

Figure 4.4 View from above onto a GABA-A receptor. The GABA-A receptor is composed of five subunits, i.e. two α1, two β2 and one γ2 subunits. Following activation of the receptor, the chloride ions will enter the cell through the channel formed by the pentamer

4.2.5 LIGANDS

Depending on their effects at receptors, ligands can be separated into two categories:

- Compounds that trigger an action specific for the receptor, e.g. a polarization or an opening of an ion channel, are named *agonists*. Agonists can be endogenous, i.e. naturally occurring in the respective organism, or exogenous, e.g. a synthetic substance having the same effect at the receptor as the endogenous agonist. Agonists also can be subdivided into full agonists and partial agonists. Whereas *full agonists* always induce maximal activation, *partial agonists* will cause a partial rather than a maximal activation, irrespective of the amount applied.
- Compounds that do not activate a receptor but oppose the effect normally induced by another bioactive agent, such as an agonist, are named *antagonists*. Binding of an antagonist to a receptor causes the cell to lower its function and this may cause an inhibition or activation (via inhibition of an inhibition) within a neuronal circuit. Antagonists can be subdivided into two types: *competitive antagonists* bind at the same site as do the agonists whereas *non-competitive antagonists* bind at a site on the receptor that differs from the agonist's binding site. Both interactions, however, prevent further binding of the agonist, be it by direct competition at the binding site (in the case of a competitive antagonist) or via a conformational change of the

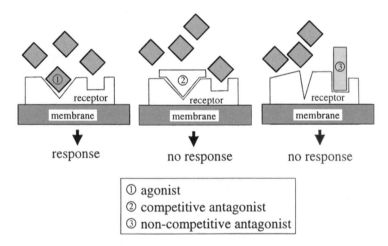

Figure 4.5 In competitive antagonism and non-competitive antagonism the agonist is no longer able to bind to the binding pocket, so the activity of the cell is attenuated (=no response). The agonist binding site is either occupied (by the competitive antagonist) or has undergone a conformational change (by the non-competitive antagonist).

agonist binding pocket (in the case of the non-competitive antagonist) (see Fig. 4.5).

4.2.6 INTERACTION BETWEEN THE LIGAND AND RECEPTOR

The strength ('*affinity*') with which a ligand, be it an agonist or antagonist, binds to a target varies and depends largely upon the chemical structure of the ligand. It is the shape and the physicochemical properties that determine how closely a molecule fits into the binding pocket. Like all chemical reactions, the ligand–receptor interaction is governed by the law of mass action: an equilibrium between the free concentrations of the ligand and receptor and the concentration of the receptor/ligand complex is established. At equilibrium, the amounts of ligand going onto (association) and going off (dissociation) the receptor site are identical (Fig. 4.6).

$$\text{Ligand} + \text{receptor} \underset{\text{dissociation}}{\overset{\text{association}}{\rightleftharpoons}} \text{Ligand / receptor complex}$$

Figure 4.6 The interaction between any ligand and a receptor is governed by the equilibrium according to the law of mass action

Studying ligand–receptor interactions is one of the most widely used approaches during the *in vitro* period of drug selection, because *in vitro binding studies* provide crucial information about a compound's affinity to receptors as well as about its selectivity among several binding sites. The following Internet links provide more details about such studies:

- http://www.biotrend.com/pdf/radiochemrev.pdf
- http://www.unmc.edu/pharmacology/receptortutorial

In addition to *in vitro* binding studies, another experimental approach to evaluate a compound's interaction with receptors is becoming more and more widely used. The technique is known as *positron emission tomography* (PET) and necessitates that the molecule of interest be labeled with a radioisotope of short half-life (ideally ^{18}F). Positron emission tomography is used in neuropsychiatry to determine the distribution of a radioactively-labeled compound ('*radiotracer*') within the brain following peripheral injection of the radiotracer into a vein. Studies with PET provide information as to where in the brain a compound is concentrating and possibly acting. By investigating how a novel compound displaces a radioactively labeled radiotracer with known mechanism of action (e.g. a dopamine antagonist), valuable information on the therapeutic potential, receptor occupancy and effective dosing of a drug candidate can be made available at an early stage of development (see Appendix to Chapter 5).

4.2.7 NEUROTRANSMITTERS

Neurotransmitters are defined as chemical substances that:

(1) Are present in presynaptic terminals.
(2) Are released from presynaptic terminals into the synaptic cleft (synapse) upon stimulation of the neuron.
(3) Cause an effect (activation or inhibition) at the postsynaptic site.
(4) Are inactivated either by a metabolic (enzymatic) mechanism or by removal from the synapse through a presynaptically located mechanism ('re-uptake').

Figure 4.7 gives some basic information on the best known neurotransmitters, their precursors, the enzymes involved in their synthesis, their principal receptors and their metabolites. Drugs that modulate any of the steps involved will affect the availability of the respective neurotransmitter and thus might be used as a potential therapeutic principle to affect the aberrant functioning of one or several neurotransmitter systems.

Serotonin, dopamine, noradrenaline, acetylcholine and GABA are the best characterized neurotransmitters but the list of known and putative neurotransmitters is much longer, including:

• Amino acids such as glutamate, aspartate, and glycine.
• Smaller and larger peptides ('*neuropeptides*') such as substance P, somatostatin, vasopressin, corticotropin-releasing factor (CRF), neuropeptide Y or cholecystokinin (CCK).

For many of the neuropeptides the receptors are known, and more recently non-peptidic, small-molecule antagonists have become available. Application of these antagonists will help to elucidate further the involvement of peptidic neurotransmitters within the nervous system, as well as their contribution to mental disturbances. It is also expected that some of the recently developed antagonists may become useful therapeutic agents.

For additional reading on neurotransmitters, the following Internet links provide useful information:

• Dopaminergic: http://www.biotrend.com/pdf/dopa.pdf
• Serotonergic: http://www.biotrend.com/pdf/serot.pdf
• Adrenergic: http://www.biotrend.com/pdf/adren.pdf
• GABA-ergic: http://www.biotrend.com/pdf/gabarev.pdf

4.3 HYPOTHESES RELATING TO THE MODE OF ACTION OF PSYCHOPHARMACEUTICALS

As described in Chapter 2, much serendipity was involved in the discovery of the first modern psychopharmaceuticals. When the antipsychotic action of

Serotonin (5-HT)

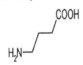

- Precursors: L-tryptophan, 5-hydroxytryptophan (5HTP)
- Enzymes involved in synthesis: tryptophan hydroxylase, aromatic amino acid decarboxylase
- Principal receptors: 5-HT1, 5-HT2, 5-HT3, 5-HT4, 5-HT6, 5-HT7, including subtypes
- Enzymes involved in degradation: monoamine oxidase (MAO), aldehyde dehydrogenase
- Metabolite: 5-hydroxyindolacetic acid (5-HIAA)

Dopamine (DA)

- Precursors: L-tyrosine, L-dihydroxyphenylalanine (L-dopa)
- Enzyme involved in synthesis: tyrosine hydroxylase
- Principal receptors: D1, D2, D3, D4, D5
- Enzymes involved in degradation: MAO, catechol-*O*-methyl-catechol-*O*-methyltransferase (COM⁻
- Metabolites: homovanillic acid (HVA), 3,4-dihydroxyphenylacetic acid (DOPAC), 3-methoxytyramine (3-MT)

Noradrenaline (NA)

- Precursors: L-tyrosine, L-dopa, dopamine
- Enzymes involved in synthesis: tyrosine hydroxylase, dopamine-beta-hydroxylase
- Principal receptors: alpha- and beta-adrenergic, including subtypes
- Enzymes involved in degradation: MAO, COMT
- Metabolites: 3-methoxy-4-hydroxyphenylglycol (MHPG), vanillylmandelic acid (VMA)

Gamma-amino-butyric acid (GABA)

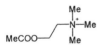

- Precursors: L-glutamate
- Enzyme involved in synthesis: glutamate decarboxylase (GAD)
- Principal receptors: GABA-A, GABA-B
- Enzyme involved in degradation: GABA transaminase
- Metabolites: succinic semialdehyde, succinate

Acetylcholine (ACh)

- Precursors: choline, acetyl coenzyme A
- Enzyme involved in synthesis: choline acetyltransferase (CAT)
- Principal receptors: muscarinergic and nicotinic
- receptors
- Enzyme involved in degradation: acetylcholinesterase, butyrylcholinesterase Metabolites: choline, acetate

Figure 4.7 Chemical structures of the principal neurotransmitters

chlorpromazine was noted in the years 1952/53, this effect could not be explained in terms of the pathophysiological concepts of schizophrenia prevailing at that time. Speculation certainly concerned possible biological or biochemical disturbance in the brain of schizophrenic patients but analytical methods necessary to confirm or refute these assumptions were not available. The same was true when, a few years later, the antidepressant efficacy of imipramine was discovered. All hypotheses regarding the mode of action of psychopharmaceuticals evolved slowly, and some of the most recent theories still contain elements from the very early times of modern psychopharmacology.

4.3.1 HYPOTHESES RELATING TO THE MODE OF ACTION OF ANTIPSYCHOTICS

The Serotonin Hypothesis of Schizophrenia

In 1954, i.e. about 2 years after the discovery of chlorpromazine in Europe, two American biochemists (Woolley and Shaw) published the hypothesis that schizophrenia and similar psychoses could be based on a disturbance of serotoninergic neurotransmission in the brain. This hypothesis was supported by some facts that had become known shortly beforehand: the spectacular psychotropic actions of LSD (lysergic acid diethylamide), which can trigger disturbances in perception, thought and feelings as well as hallucinations in healthy subjects (Stoll, 1947); and the serotonin-antagonistic effects of LSD, i.e. its ability to block the actions of serotonin in various pharmacological tests.

Although it was not known at this time that serotonin occurs in the brain and acts as a neurotransmitter, Woolley and Shaw speculated that the psychotropic effects of LSD were the result of its ability to block serotonin effects in the brain; they then suggested that a disturbance in serotoninergic neurotransmission underlies schizophrenic psychoses, which, among other things, are characterized by disorders in perception and thought processes.

It became known in the same year (1954) that the substance reserpine, derived from the Indian plant *Rauwolfia serpentina*, had antipsychotic effects similar to those of chlorpromazine. This finding was of interest for two reasons: the molecular structure of reserpine has some similarity to that of serotonin and LSD; and it was found that reserpine liberates serotonin from presynaptic stores in the CNS and thus produces a short-lived excess supply of functionally available serotonin at the synapse. In the context of a serotonin hypothesis of schizophrenia, it could be postulated that the antipsychotic effect of reserpine was due to its ability to liberate serotonin presynaptically and make it functionally available. However, despite its scientific appeal, the serotonin hypothesis of schizophrenia did not last long because it was in conflict with both psychopathological and pharmacological findings:

(1) The 'psychotic' symptoms produced by LSD in healthy persons differ qualitatively and quantitatively from the symptoms typical of schizophrenia (Bleuler, 1956). Thus, the hallucinations experienced by schizophrenic patients are predominantly acoustic in nature, whereas LSD mainly gives rise to visual phenomena.

(2) LSD is not a specific serotonin antagonist but also exerts agonistic effects at serotonin receptors. On the other hand, many serotonin antagonists, which are more effective than LSD, are not hallucinogenic.

(3) In addition to serotonin, reserpine also releases other neurotransmitters, especially dopamine and noradrenaline, from their stores in presynaptic nerve endings. Furthermore, the action on the synapse of the neurotransmitters released in this way is limited because they undergo intracellular enzymatic degradation.

(4) The administration of biological precursors of serotonin, which can be converted to serotonin in the CNS, was found to have no clear-cut antipsychotic effect in acute schizophrenic patients (in contrast to what had been predicted by Woolley and Shaw).

(5) Unlike reserpine, chlorpromazine has neither a serotonin-like chemical structure nor does it release serotonin from nerve endings.

Despite its relatively fast and thorough rebuttal, the serotonin hypothesis of schizophrenia was fruitful in two respects: it gave rise to the development of sensitive serotonin assay methods and proof that serotonin does occur in the brain (Carlsson, 1987); and it served as the prototype for other simple and thus readily testable biochemical hypotheses of mental illnesses. Interest in serotonin has been reawakened in recent years in relation to the mechanism of action of some antipsychotics (see below); however, this development had little to do with the serotonin hypothesis of schizophrenia in its original version.

The Dopamine Hypothesis of Schizophrenia

Although the serotonin hypothesis of schizophrenia was formulated at approximately the same time as the discovery of the first neuroleptics, it had no direct connection with the pharmacological properties of these drugs. The situation is different in the case of the dopamine hypothesis because all known neuroleptics have some inhibitory action on dopaminergic neurons, even though they vary considerably with regard to other pharmacological effects.

At the time of the discovery of chlorpromazine, dopamine could not be assayed directly and its role as a neurotransmitter was unknown (Carlsson, 1987). Chlorpromazine exerts a large number of pharmacological effects, all of which could, in principle, be considered responsible for its clinical action. Thus, it was first assumed that the antipsychotic action of chlorpromazine and similar neuroleptics depends directly on their cataleptic potency, i.e. their ability to induce catalepsy in animal experiments, as well as the extrapyramidal symptoms in clinical use. This assumption first lost credibility when thioridazine, a neuroleptic with weak extrapyramidal effects but good antipsychotic activity, became available; the assumed connection was definitively refuted with the introduction of clozapine.

In the late 1950s it was found that patients with Parkinson's disease have a dopamine deficiency in the basal ganglia that can be treated with L-dopa, a biological precursor of dopamine. This and the simultaneously observed similarity between some symptoms of Parkinson's disease and the dyskinesias noted during neuroleptic treatment led to the assumption that the 'neuroleptic parkinsonoid' of schizophrenic patients could be due to a disturbance of dopaminergic neurotransmission. The postulated mechanism of the disturbance and the significance of dopamine as a neurotransmitter were clarified further in animal experiments. Carlsson and Lindquist (1963) found that chlorpromazine increased the turnover of dopamine in mouse brain, whereas no such effect arose on promethazine, a compound chemically related to chlorpromazine but devoid of antipsychotic efficacy. Carlsson and Lindquist interpreted the effect of chlorpromazine on dopamine turnover as being the consequence of a hypothetical blockage of dopamine neurotransmission through the action of the neuroleptic. They assumed that presynaptic dopaminergic neurons tend to compensate for the blockade of postsynaptic receptors through increased dopamine synthesis and release in order to restore the functional balance that had been disturbed by the antagonist.

Chlorpromazine and other neuroleptic drugs were thus recognized as dopamine antagonists, and the next step was to clarify whether and to what extent the anti-dopaminergic action of various neuroleptics is related to their antipsychotic efficacy. *In vitro* receptor binding studies indicated that the affinities of various neuroleptics for dopamine receptors in the brain are highly correlated with their antipsychotic potencies (Creese *et al.*, 1976), which again supported the dopamine hypothesis of neuroleptic action. However, a close correlation existed only with affinity to the dopamine D2 receptor, whereas affinities for the D1 receptor showed hardly any correlation with the strength of antipsychotic action (Seeman, 1980).

Despite a number of necessary refinements in later years, the dopamine hypothesis in its simple original version ('neuroleptics act via blockade of postsynaptic dopamine receptors') is still consistent with many pharmacological and clinical observations, such as:

• Parkinson patients treated with L-dopa or dopamine agonists sometimes suffer from hallucinations and other psychosis-like states, and these abnormalities are most likely a consequence of dopaminergic overstimulation.

- Amphetamine used at high doses can provoke a toxic syndrome ('amphetamine psychosis') in healthy subjects that shows certain similarities to schizophrenic psychoses. Like cocaine, high-dose amphetamine is known to trigger a massive release of dopamine and noradrenaline from presynaptic sites and thus to produce a temporary excess supply of both neurotransmitters at the respective synapses.
- Even at smaller doses, amphetamine can exacerbate psychosis in schizophrenic patients, and similar symptom provocation may arise with other dopaminergic substances.

Some further observations also supported the dopaminergic mechanism of antipsychotic drugs. Alpha-methyl-*para*-tyrosine (AMPT), which interferes with the synthesis of dopamine and noradrenaline from their biological precursors (and thus also inhibits dopaminergic neurotransmission), augments the antipsychotic efficacy of neuroleptics. Furthermore, the toxic psychosis occurring in healthy subjects after large and repeated amphetamine doses can be antagonized by administration of (antidopaminergic) antipsychotics but not noradrenaline antagonists. Some other empirical findings could not, however, be incorporated unequivocally into the dopamine hypothesis:

(1) The blockade of dopamine receptors by antipsychotic drugs is an immediate effect that can be detected even after a single dose, whereas the therapeutic action of these drugs becomes apparent only after several days or weeks of treatment.
(2) Dopaminergic agonists such as bromocriptine and apomorphine, which act directly on postsynaptic receptors, do not provoke psychosis-like states in healthy subjects.
(3) Some schizophrenic patients respond to amphetamine administration not with a deterioration but with an improvement in their state (Angrist *et al.*, 1982).
(4) There is no evidence for an elevated dopamine content or hypersensitivity of dopamine receptors in the brain of schizophrenic patients. Breakdown products of dopamine and noradrenaline are elevated neither in the urine nor in the blood or cerebrospinal fluid of schizophrenic patients. In some patients with chronic schizophrenia there is even evidence of dopamine hypofunction (Karoum *et al.*, 1987).

Despite some unexplained or contradictory findings, the dopamine hypothesis still represents the best developed overall theoretical basis on which to explain many biochemical, animal experimental, human pharmacological and clinical findings (McKenna, 1987). Criticism is often directed at the overemphasis on one individual neurotransmitter, i.e. disregard for the fact that the transmitter systems in the CNS work in close mutual interdependence. From the viewpoint of drug research, one might criticize the fact that the dopamine hypothesis is a retrospective theory and has not facilitated the search for fundamentally novel antipsychotic drugs.

Further Development of the Dopamine Hypothesis

A *two-factor theory of schizophrenia* proposed by Davis in 1974 takes into account the fact that although neuroleptics exert a dopamine antagonistic effect from the very start, their antipsychotic action becomes evident with a delay of several weeks. According to the two-factor theory, schizophrenic disorders originate from a defect other than dopaminergic overactivity, although the latter is involved as a second factor and augments the intensity of the psychotic process. This dopaminergic factor responds to treatment with antipsychotics so that the disorder becomes attenuated and, ultimately, intrinsic repair processes may bring about complete remission. The two-factor theory does not clarify the nature of the structural, biochemical, psychological or other factor(s) that are thought to lie at the origin of the pathological process.

Another hypothesis (Crow, 1982) involves a division of schizophrenias into two types: "Type I corresponds to acute schizophrenia or schizophreniform disorder in which one observes more positive symptoms of hallucinations and delusions with a good prognosis and excellent response to neuroleptics... Type II represents chronic schizophrenia with affective flattening, poverty of speech and loss of drive, the so-called negative symptoms of schizophrenia. Type II patients respond less well to neuroleptics..." (Snyder, 1982). Type I patients would fit into the dopamine hypothesis whereas a pathophysiological basis other than dopaminergic hyperactivity must be assumed for type II patients. However, as pointed out by Snyder (1982), "one should be cautious about drawing such a distinction."

More recent variants of the dopamine hypothesis have been derived mostly from the profile of actions of the atypical antipsychotic clozapine and seek to relate pharmacological findings to the clinical actions of this product. At the same time the pharmacological profile of clozapine is being used as a starting point for obtaining safer and more effective antipsychotics. Comparison of the major clinical and pharmacological effects of clozapine provides the picture shown in Table 4.1.

Although it was (and still is) not known which pharmacological effects are responsible for the unique clinical action of clozapine, two new hypotheses were put forward: the so-called 5-HT2:D2 and the D1:D2 equilibrium hypotheses. According to the former, the beneficial actions of clozapine are the result of simultaneous blockade of (serotonin) 5-HT2 and (dopamine) D2 receptors (Meltzer, 1989). According to the latter hypothesis, the clinical effects of clozapine and particularly the absence of extrapyramidal side effects are due to the balanced action of clozapine on dopamine D1 and D2 receptors

Table 4.1 Clinical and pharmacological properties of clozapine

Clinical features	Effects observed in animals
Strong antipsychotic efficacy also in patients refractory to conventional neuroleptics	Inhibition of motor activity and conditioned avoidance
Action on negative symptoms	Relatively strong binding to (dopamine) D1 receptors
Beneficial effects on mood and well-being	Blockade of (serotonin) 5-HT2 receptors
No extrapyramidal side effects	No catalepsy, no marked antagonism of apomorphine
Anticholinergic side effects, marked sedation at start of therapy	Anticholinergic effects, sedation

(Markstein, 1994). Both hypotheses have given rise to dozens of preclinical and clinical studies but it is still open as to which of the two or any other hypotheses, such as that of frontal dopaminergic underactivity with compensatory mesolimbic hyperactivity (Davis *et al.*, 1991), is closer to the truth. Practical use was made of the 5-HT2:D2 hypothesis during the development and marketing of risperidone (p. 52), although the occurrence of extrapyramidal symptoms at higher doses of this drug would rather argue against this hypothesis. Olanzapine, on the other hand, has a complex pharmacological profile similar to that of clozapine and thus the question as to which pharmacological features are responsible for the atypicality of the more recent compounds, including their antipsychotic efficacy, is still open.

The Glutamatergic Hypothesis

At therapeutically effective doses all antipsychotic compounds, including the atypical ones, are antagonists of central D2 receptors. However, the late onset of the antipsychotic activity suggests that another still largely unknown mechanism must be involved. Thus, the observation that blockade of *N*-methyl-D-aspartate (NMDA) receptors, e.g. by means of *phencyclidine*, induces a psychosis-like state in healthy volunteers led to the NMDA hypofunction theory, which states that a hypoglutamatergic state at postsynaptic NMDA receptors is involved in schizophrenia. Unfortunately, testing of the hypothesis through the use of direct glutamatergic agonists is hampered by a concern that excessive activation of the NMDA receptors might cause excitotoxic damage to neurons (Olney, 1990). As an alternative, indirect modulation of NMDA receptors via, for example, the AMPA or glycine site, might become an important treatment strategy for schizophrenia. Preliminary clinical experience suggests that adding glycine, D-serine or cycloserine to ongoing antipsychotic medication may reduce negative and positive symptoms and improve cognitive functioning of schizophrenic patients (Heresco-Levy *et al.*, 1996; Tsai *et al.*, 1998). Furthermore, preclinical studies suggest that AMPA/kainate receptor antagonists and group II mGluR agonists such as LY-354740 might develop into novel therapeutic principles of schizophrenia (Moghaddam and Adams, 1998). It is currently considered that the glutamate hypothesis represents a wide new avenue to explore compounds that interact subtype-specifically with receptors involved in glutamatergic neurotransmission for their potential as antipsychotic treatments (for review see Sawa and Snyder 2002; Tsai and Coyle (2002).

For additional reading, see Internet link

- http//kore.psy.du.edu/manakata/csh/neuron_minirvw_lewis&leiberman.pdf

4.3.2 HYPOTHESES RELATING TO THE MODE OF ACTION OF ANTIDEPRESSANTS

After the discovery of drugs with antidepressant activity in the late 1950s, an intensive search was undertaken for pharmacological models that would provide an understanding of the therapeutic effects observed and at the same time assist in the development of other, still more effective and specific antidepressants. In pharmacological tests then available, the prototype imipramine showed sedative, antihistaminic and anticholinergic effects and thus did not differ fundamentally from other medicaments with no antidepressant activity, e.g. antihistamines. The following observations then led to a further step forward in the development of hypotheses:

- The behavioral syndrome induced in mice and rats by reserpine – sedation, catalepsy and ptosis – can be reversed by imipramine.
- The effect of noradrenaline at various organs is potentiated by imipramine.
- Imipramine inhibits the reuptake of previously released noradrenaline in isolated tissues.

Taken together, these findings suggested that imipramine augments the action of noradrenaline ('*amine potentiation*') or is able to correct a state brought about through noradrenaline deficiency. It was also known that reserpine (which was mainly used as an antihypertensive at that time) could trigger clinically relevant depressions in some patients. A subsequent observation – that reserpine released neuronal noradrenaline, dopamine and serotonin from their protecting presynaptic stores and thus exposed them to inactivation by intracellular enzymes – led to the first hypotheses concerning the relationship between depressive syndromes and disturbances in the metabolism of these neurotransmitters: the catecholamine and serotonin hypotheses of depression.

The Catecholamine Hypothesis of Depression

This was put forward in 1965 by J. Schildkraut and states that "some, if not all, depressions are the consequence of an absolute or relative deficiency of catecholamines, particularly norepinephrine, at functionally important adrenergic receptor sites in the brain" (Schildkraut, 1965, p. 509). The evidence brought forward in support of this hypothesis was impressive (Table 4.2) because it covered both clinical and multifarious pharmacological findings. The antidepressant effect of imipramine and of the monoamine oxidase (MAO) inhibitors was attributed to the fact that these medicaments bring about an increased supply of functionally available catecholamines at the synapse:

- Imipramine prevents the reuptake (and hence the inactivation) of previously released noradrenaline from the synaptic cleft into the presynaptic nerve ending.
- The MAO inhibitors prevent the breakdown of the released and functionally available catecholamines by the MAO present in the extracellular space (within the cells, monoamines are protected by the vesicles).

The catecholamine hypothesis brought several pharmacological findings together in an illuminating relationship but contradicted a number of clinical observations, in particular the delayed onset of action of antidepressant drugs. This also applies to the serotonin hypothesis, which was formulated at about the same time.

The Serotonin Hypothesis of Depression

This hypothesis states that some or all depressions are due to a lack of serotonin in certain parts of the brain stem (Coppen, 1967). Older and newer arguments to support the serotonin hypothesis are:

- Imipramine and other tricyclic antidepressants inhibit not only the reuptake of catecholamines into presynaptic nerve endings but have the same effect on serotonin.
- Monoamine oxidase inhibitors inhibit serotonin inactivation in the extracellular compartment, just as they inhibit catecholamine inactivation.
- Reserpine, which can trigger depressions, releases not only catecholamines but also serotonin from the presynaptic stores.
- Serotonin and its metabolites are reduced in the cerebrospinal fluid of some depressive patients, which suggests reduced serotoninergic activity in the brain of these individuals.
- Serotonin precursors (L-tryptophan, 5-hydroxytryptophan) have some antidepressant action, whereas a reduction in the blood levels of tryptophan in remitted depressed patients can provoke clinical relapse.

Table 4.2 Elements of the catecholamine hypothesis of depression

Substance	Psychological effects in man	Effects on behavior in animals	Effects on catecholamines at brain synapses
Reserpine	Sedation; in some cases depression	Sedation, catalepsy, hypothermia	Intracellular release, hence rapid degradation and less availability
Amphetamine	Stimulation, mood improvement	Stimulation; at higher doses stereotypy	Release and inhibition of re-uptake
MAO inhibitors	Antidepressant effect	Stimulation; prevent sedation after reserpine	Prevent degradation after release into synaptic cleft
Imipramine	Antidepressant effect	Prevents sedation after reserpine; potentiates effect of amphetamine	Prevents re-uptake from synaptic cleft
Dopa	Antidepressant effect in some cases	Prevents sedation after reserpine	Greater supply of catecholamine precursors

Thus, a number of pharmacological and clinical findings can be interpreted to support both the catecholamine and the serotonin hypothesis of depression. Depressions do not represent a single uniform disease; there is evidence for catecholaminergic hypofunction in a proportion of depressive patients, whereas others have features of serotoninergic hypofunction. However, reliable relationships between biochemical alterations and clinical courses or states have not been found, and the hope that subgroups of depression could be defined by their biochemical features to optimize drug treatment (Maas, 1975; Asberg et al., 1976) was not fulfilled.

Numerous antidepressants were synthesized, developed and marketed on the basis of the serotonin hypothesis. The selective serotonin reuptake inhibitors (SSRIs) are similarly effective as the older tricyclic antidepressants, but have the advantage of being less toxic and not inducing anticholinergically mediated side effects (Chapter 1). From the scientific point of view they represent an example of mechanistic, hypothesis-driven research and development in psychopharmacology (Chapter 2).

Comment

As with the dopamine theory of schizophrenia, the monoamine hypotheses of depression emphasize one or more aspects of the actions of clinically effective drugs in well-described pharmacological tests. However, whereas dopamine antagonism seems to be a common element of action of all neuroleptics, antidepressants differ more widely with regard to their pharmacological spectrum of activities and a common 'core of action' has not been identified so far. This can be interpreted in various ways: firstly, one could assume that the actual mechanism of action of antidepressants is still unknown and that the pharmacological models used capture only epiphenomena of the actions relevant to the clinical effect. Another conclusion would be to interrogate critically the overemphasis on individual transmitter systems as postulated bases for depressions.

Because the various transmitter systems in the brain are directly and indirectly linked together, purely catecholaminergic or purely serotoninergic depressions are unlikely. Furthermore, the majority of antidepressants known today have multiple effects, especially after repeated administration, and thus affect a number of transmitter systems. This fact is taken into account by more recent hypotheses of depression in that a balance between several transmitter systems is postulated as a prerequisite for mental health, whereas affective psychoses are believed to be a reflection of an imbalance.

Outlook

Given that even the best and most recent antidepressants are clinically effective in only 60–70% of patients, cause many unpleasant (albeit less dangerous) adverse events and have a slow onset of action, it is a natural consequence that much preclinical and clinical research still aims at detecting and developing new principles of antidepressant therapy. Newer approaches have to come up with therapeutic agents that retain or improve the efficacy of the best currently available medications but are superior with regard to aspects mainly related to patient compliance and health economics, such as an improved side-effect profile, higher responder rates, earlier onset of action and lower rates of relapse or recurrence. Seen from the perspective of today, the most advanced and perhaps most promising new directions are the following:

Neurokinin Receptor Antagonists

Neurokinin-1 (NK1) receptor antagonists are considered to be the currently best validated and clinically most advanced novel approach for the treatment of depressive disorders (Rupniak and Kramer, 1999; Rupniak, 2002; for review see also Stout et al., 2001). It was in 1998 when Kramer et al. published that, by blocking the NK1 receptor, symptoms in patients with major depression could be alleviated. The compound used was MK-869, now also named aprepitant. In addition to its favorable effect on both anxiety and depression, the compound was described as being well tolerated and to have a more favorable side-effect profile than an SSRI. In the meantime this group and others have published evidence that selective and brain-penetrating NK1 receptor antagonists have anxiolytic and antidepressant effects also in several animal models (File 1997, 2000, Papp et al., 2000; Vassout et al., 2000; Cheeta et al., 2001; Gentsch et al., 2002). The race to develop and bring the first NK1 receptor antagonist to the market is ongoing and several major drug companies (Merck, Pfizer, Takeda and probably others) seem to be involved.

Corticotropin-releasing Factor-1 Receptor Antagonists

There are many preclinical and clinical observations indicating that abnormalities of corticotropin-releasing factor (CRF)-related mechanisms may underlie psychiatric disorders, especially states of anxiety and depression (reviews by Arborelius et al., 1999; O'Brien et al., 2001). Consequently, the concept of using selective, non-peptidic antagonists to block overactivity in these systems as a potential antidepressant mechanism has been put forward (Holsboer, 2000; Reul and Holsboer, 2002). A preliminary report on an antidepressant effect seen in patients treated with the experimental compound R121919 (Zobel et al., 2000) supports the concept that CRF-1 receptor antagonists will develop into a novel type of antidepressant. The compound R121919 had to be discontinued for toxicological reasons, but better tolerated molecules probably will be identified and eventually may represent an attractive new treatment principle for depression.

Multiple Uptake Inhibitors

The recent approach to consider compounds with a broad spectrum of pharmacological activities rather than being very specific with regard to one particular neurotransmitter or mechanism aims at generating therapeutic principles that would provoke fewer side effects linked to one single principle of action (such as serotonin-related sexual or gastrointestinal side effects) and become first-line treatments effective with different kinds of potential under-lying disturbances (i.e. be it deficits in noradrenergic, serotonergic or other transmitter pathways). Although these newer 'tailored' drugs have some similarity with the early, relatively unspecific tricyclic compounds, they are devoid of the additional activities – cholinergic or histaminergic – that are held responsible for many of the tolerability problems with the older drugs. Representatives of this new class of less-selective compounds are venlafaxine and reboxetine; a triple uptake inhibitor called duloxetine is close to approval by health authorities.

Sigma Ligands

As another new approach the sigma ligands should be mentioned. Although the detailed mechanism of their action remains unclear preclinically, selective sigma1 receptor agonists reduce the immobility time in the forced swim test and tail suspension test and are, in this respect, comparable to typical antidepressants (Noda et al., 1999). Igmesine, a selective sigma-1 ligand, was reported to exert an antidepressant action (Akunne et al., 2001) and, according to Sanchez and Papp (2000), the selective sigma-2 ligand Lu 28-179 has an antidepressant-like profile in the rat chronic mild stress model of depression. For this class of compounds the proof of beneficial effects in patients is expected to become available within the next few years. Interestingly opipramol, an old anxiolytic with pronounced antidepressant action, has been described recently as having one of the strongest interactions ever observed at the sigma-1 binding site (Möller and Müller, 2001).

Transcranial Magnetic Stimulation (TMS)

Although somewhat outside the scope of this text, a non-pharmacological treatment that may become an important therapeutic tool in the future deserves to be mentioned within this outlook section. Initial clinical data indicate that depressive patients are significantly improved after TMS treatment and the procedure is very well tolerated (Berman et al., 2000; McNamara et al., 2001). Interestingly for preclinical research, repeated TMS in rats has also been shown to have an antidepressant-like effect (Sachdev et al., 2002) in the forced swim test described later in this chapter. Whether or not there are psychopharmacological correlates of TMS is unknown at present.

Finally, newer technologies such as linkage studies or magnetic resonance imaging measures have started to be applied in an attempt to elucidate additional pathophysiological mechanisms in depression. These studies are expected to widen our view and to increase our understanding of depression in the years to come. One avenue currently being pursued is the proposed link between an altered neurogenesis in depressive illness and its restoration during treatment with antidepressants (Jacobs et al., 2000; Malberg et al., 2000). This is rationally linked with the notion that stress modulates neurogenesis and that chronic stress is very likely a causative factor for depression. Obviously this avenue is worth pursuing further and once initial progress is made, mainly on the preclinical side, it might lead to an entirely new treatment strategy for depression.

4.3.3 HYPOTHESES RELATING TO THE MECHANISM OF ACTION OF ANXIOLYTICS

Benzodiazepines

Benzodiazepines and a few closely related compounds are still in wide use as anxiolytics and their mechanism of action has been largely elucidated. These drugs interact with GABA-A receptors and reinforce the action of the neurotransmitter GABA. Because the action of GABA is inhibitory, the GABA-related inhibition within a neural circuit is intensified in the presence of a benzodiazepine. The particular localization of GABA neurons as interneurons throughout almost all regions of the CNS is considered to be the major reason why benzodiazepines are able to inhibit an excessive 'unphysiological' stimulation only, and why the inhibition will not exceed a given degree.

Recent data from molecular biology and knockout mice studies indicate that different benzodiazepines interact differentially with several GABA-A receptor subtypes and that a separation between sedative, muscle-relaxing and anxiolytic effects might, in principle, be achieved by the synthesis of subtype-specific molecules. If successful, this approach could help to overcome one major shortcoming of the benzodiazepines available today, namely the tight association of anxiolytic, general sedative and muscle-relaxant properties. This association is observed in clinical use with almost all known benzodiazepine derivatives, irrespective of whether they are direct agonists, partial agonists or inverse antagonists. On the other hand, benzodiazepines have one major clinical advantage: they relieve tension and anxiety immediately rather than following a lag phase of 2–3 weeks, as seen with other classes of anxiolytic compounds (such as SSRIs and buspirone; see Chapter 1). Thus, drugs with a fast onset of anxiolytic effect but without the known disadvantages of today's benzodiazepines, including the tendency to induce tolerance and dependence, would be highly desirable.

Beta-receptor Blockers

Some of these compounds are still in clinical use, typically to treat the fear of performing in public, such as giving a speech, acting on stage or passing an examination. Beta-blockers are primarily effective against the peripheral manifestations of stress and anxiety, such as increased heart rate, sweating and mild tremor, rather than having a major effect via the CNS. Their clinical effectiveness is usually explained by their ability to intercept the vicious circle developing between anxiety/stress → physiological manifestations of stress → perception of physiological stress reaction → increased anxiety/stress.

Outlook

Based on the available (essentially preclinical), evidence, NK1 and CRF-1 receptor antagonists might become alternative therapeutic approaches, not only as antidepressants but also as anxiolytics. Given the high comorbidity of anxiety and depression, drugs with combined anxiolytic and anti-depressant effect could be of great practical value. However, before becoming overenthusiastic about the two relatively new pharmacological approaches, clinical trials need to be performed and analyzed in order to evaluate properly the potential therapeutic benefit of the new concepts. Judging from preclinical observations, drugs interacting with some subtypes of the metabotropic glutamate receptor (mGluR) family (i.e. mGluR5 antagonists or mGluR2 agonists), as well as mitochondrial benzodiazepine receptor ligands, might also represent promising new therapeutic concepts. However, these newest classes of compounds are still at early stages of development.

4.4 INTRODUCTORY REMARKS REGARDING THE DEVELOPMENT OF NEW PSYCHOPHARMACEUTICALS

All processes involved in the 'life cycle' of a neurotransmitter, i.e. its synthesis, storage, release, reuptake, degradation and effects at the receptor, can be influenced and modulated by drugs. Depending on the assumed direction of the abnormality in a given disorder, the aim is to improve the function of the respective neurotransmitter system, i.e. to either increase or decrease its level of activity. Many of the conceivable possibilities at influencing neurotransmission are currently being used as powerful pharma-cotherapies.

4.4.1 DISORDERS DUE TO HYPOFUNCTIONALITY

Administration of a Precursor

In Parkinson's disease there is a degeneration of dopaminergic neurons in the substantia nigra, causing hypoactivity of dopaminergic neurotransmission due to a lack of dopamine in the respective synapses. Because orally administered dopamine will not reach the CNS, one of the successful therapeutic approaches in Parkinson's disease consists of substituting L-Dopa, the biological precursor of dopamine. This treatment, via a 'renormalization' of the dopaminergic neurotransmission, leads to functional recovery including amelioration of motor capacity in Parkinson patients.

Inhibition of a Degradating Enzyme

This approach is also applied successfully in Parkinson's disease. Drugs such as entacapone inhibit the activity of the enzyme catechol-*o*-methyltransferase (COMT), which is involved in degradation of the neurotransmitter dopamine, and thus increase and prolong the availability of dopamine in the synaptic cleft. Inhibition of COMT and substitution of L-Dopa are often combined in the therapy of Parkinson patients.

Alzheimer's disease is characterized by a degeneration of neurons producing and containing the neurotransmitter acetylcholine, leading to hypoactivity of this neurotransmitter system. Inhibition of the activity of acetylcholinesterase (AChE), the enzyme responsible for the degradation of acetylcholine, increases the availability of the failing transmitter at cholinergic synapses and leads to symptomatic improvement in many of these patients (Chapter 6). Donepezil, rivastigmine and galanthamine are drugs with this mode of action.

In depression, serotoninergic and/or noradrenergic neurotransmission is assumed to be deficient. One of the approaches to increase the availability of these neurotransmitters is to inhibit the activity of MAO, the enzyme involved in the degradation of serotonin and noradrenaline. Older drugs such as phenelzine and recently also moclobemide are representatives of this therapeutic approach used in some forms of depression.

Inhibition of Reuptake

Another approach to correct neurotransmission is to inhibit the reuptake of the neurotransmitters into their presynaptic endings. If the presynaptic reuptake mechanism of a neurotransmitter is blocked then more of the neurotransmitter will stay in the synaptic cleft and be functionally available. Many antidepressant drugs, called 'reuptake inhibitors', are thought to act via this mechanism. If selective for serotonin they are called selective serotonin reuptake inhibitors (SSRIs, Chapter 1), but if selective for both serotonin and noradrenaline they are called serotonin noradrenaline reuptake inhibitors (SNRIs). Most older antidepressants, such as the tricyclic compounds amitriptyline, imipramine and clomipramine, have little specificity for any of the neurotransmitters; fluoxetine, paroxetine, citalopram and a few others are specific for serotonin; venlafaxine is a representative of the SNRIs. A more recent mixed-uptake inhibitor is mirtazepine, and some similar compounds are about to be launched.

4.4.2 DISORDERS DUE TO HYPERFUNCTIONALITY

Blockade of the Receptor

In schizophrenia the dopaminergic neurotransmission is thought to be exaggerated. All known antipsychotic drugs are blockers of the dopamine

D2 receptor, albeit with different specificity. Older examples of dopamine antagonists are chlorpromazine, haloperidol and many derivatives of these prototype compounds. Newer antipsychotic drugs such as risperidone, olanzapine and quetiapine have retained this mechanism of action, although no longer exclusively.

4.4.3 SHOULD NEW COMPOUNDS BE VERY SPECIFIC OR HAVE A BROADBAND MODE OF ACTION?

When looking at the period between the early 1950s (the time when the first psychopharmaceuticals were discovered) and today, and trying to see what is ahead, some interesting observations can be made. The early psychopharmaceuticals, in particular the first antipsychotics and antidepressants, were not specific pharmacologically, i.e. they interacted with various targets at the same time. These multiple interactions were held responsible for the unfavorable side-effect profile of some early compounds. There followed a period, first with the antipsychotics (e.g. haloperidol and related compounds) and then with the antidepressants (e.g. SSRIs), when molecules with more selective mechanisms of action were put forward. These approaches had several merits and, at least in the case of antidepressants, reflected the increasing insight into the underlying neurochemical mechanisms of some mental disorders.

On the other hand, the first really novel antipsychotic drug after chlorpromazine – clozapine – had its origin in the late 1950s (Chapter 2) and was by no means a transmitter-selective or target-specific compound. Similarly, the more recent atypical antipsychotic drugs, especially olanzapine, have a multitude of pharmacological actions, and the same holds true for some of the newer antidepressants. Examples are the SNRIs and, more recently, the triple uptake inhibitor duloxetine, a compound that concomitantly interferes with the uptake sites for serotonin, dopamine and noradrenaline. As noted earlier, 'multi-functional' drugs may be expected to cause fewer transmitter system-specific side effects (such as the gastrointestinal upset and sexual dysfunction typical for SSRIs); in this respect, and given their potential to produce higher response rates, they might turn out to be superior first-line treatments. The entry into the market of these 'multifunctional' agents can be seen to reflect the notion that complex disturbances such as psychiatric disorders are more than just an aberration in one single neurotransmitter system and/or that disturbances in more than one neurotransmitter system may lead to similar clinical syndromes.

4.4.4 IS THERE A NEED FOR 'PURE' ANTIPSYCHOTIC, ANTIDEPRESSANT OR ANXIOLYTIC DRUGS?

Whereas some years ago a clear distinction was made between antipsychotic, antidepressant and anxiolytic drugs, the boundaries between these drug classes appear to have become less strict today. Thus, antidepressants – especially SSRIs – are now frequently and successfully prescribed to patients with anxiety disorders (Chapter 1) and atypical antipsychotics are used to treat mania in the course of bipolar disorder. From a diagnostic and psychopharmacological point of view, these therapeutic strategies would appear to break up the well-established distinction between psychotic, depressive and anxiety disorders and between antipsychotic, antidepressant and anxiolytic drugs. From a clinical viewpoint, however, these 'transgressions' reflect the fact that states of depression and anxiety have many symptoms in common and that a syndrome-orientated approach to therapy often may be more successful than one guided by strict adherence to diagnostic categories. This view is supported by the fact that the rate of comorbidity – the simultaneous occurrence of more than one disorder, e.g. depression and anxiety, in the same patient at the same time – is very high in psychiatry, which will support a 'broadband' therapeutic approach provided that effective and well-tolerated drugs with a broad spectrum of activities are available.

From a practical aspect, i.e. with regard to treatment compliance, convenience for the patient and drug safety, it is clearly preferable to use only one drug with a simple dosage schedule and without the risk of drug interactions rather than a combination of two or more drugs at the same time. Broadband psychopharmaceuticals, if available, would cover this need. Finally, one should consider an economic aspect. Drug companies invest many hundred millions of euros, dollars and Swiss francs in the development of each new drug and it is definitely in their interest that a new compound will be used in more than one indication. A strategy often used towards this goal is to have a new drug approved as quickly as possible for a well-defined, narrow indication and then to extend the range of indications based on the results of additional clinical trials (Chapter 5).

If these considerations are correct it is to be expected that more broad-band psychopharmaceuticals will enter the market in the years to come and that good tolerability and ease of practical use may become more important arguments than a specific and highly elaborate mechanism of action.

For additional reading, see Internet link:

http://kore.psy.du.edu/munakata/csh/neuron_minirvw_lewis&leiberman.pdf

4.5 ANIMAL MODELS FOR PSYCHIATRIC INDICATIONS

Mechanism-related pharmacological models, e.g. attenuation or reversal of an effect induced by an agonist by means of the respective antagonist or vice versa, as well as the so-called 'classical models' of psychopharmacology, i.e. interaction studies between a new compound and the effect caused by standard psychopharmacological agents, will not be described in the following paragraphs. It should be noted, however, that these models are still widely applied for the characterization of compounds in development.

4.5.1 SOME GENERAL COMMENTS AND PRINCIPLES REGARDING STUDIES WITH ANIMALS

Analogies and Homologies of Animal and Human Behavior

Behavioral pharmacology is a subdiscipline of psychopharmacology that deals with the behavior of animals and its modulation by drugs. In the context of biological psychiatry, behavioral studies are used because, in analogy to man, a behavioral pattern displayed by an animal reflects its current anxiety or its well-being, and because behavioral patterns can be quantified based on accurate observation. A distinction is made between pure ethological studies describing behavioral elements in a single animal (or representing interactions between animals) such as sit, push, crawl, etc. and the more applied studies describing an animal's behavior in terms of the number or duration of activities displayed when exposed to a specific experimental environment We will deal with the applied studies and use a few selected examples to explain some of the basic aspects.

One fundamental issue must be clarified from the beginning: there is no need to discuss whether or not a complex clinical picture of, say, depression can be found in experimental animals such as rats or mice because it cannot. However, some behavioral aspects of the multifaceted clinical picture that, following extensive verbal communication with and observation of a patient, allow a psychiatrist to make a specific diagnosis can be seen in animals. These common (analogous) behavioral elements are studied in experimental animals. This strategy also makes sense because many of our reaction patterns are, evolutionarily speaking, relatively archaic and therefore homologs or at least analogs to those present in species other than humans.

Two examples of this commonality may suffice. First, an increase in heart rate can be seen in both animals and humans when they are exposed to a threatening situation. The common underlying mechanism is the triggering of a stress reaction, which, following activation of the hypothalamic–pituitary–adrenal axis and excretion of cortisol, makes us ready for flight. Second, the avoidance of potentially dangerous situations or locations represents self-protection from being caught and occurs in both humans and animals. Observations of where people tend to walk on a pavement and where people tend to sit in restaurants when having a free choice will illustrate this point. Most people walk close to house walls rather than in the middle of a pavement and most single visitors of restaurants tend to take a seat close to a wall, probably in order to be maximally protected and to ensure an optimal scan on what is happening in their immediate, new environment. This phenomenon, called tigmotaxis, is also observed in animals: rats and mice avoid open areas and prefer close contact with walls.

Ethical Considerations Related to Animal Experiments

It is necessary continuously to ask questions about the ethical acceptability and usefulness of animal experimentation in general and, more specifically, also in biological psychiatry. However, anyone who has ever seen a patient suffering from severe mental disturbances will probably give a clear general answer: the burden of being mentally disturbed is so painful that every rational and promising attempt to come up with better therapeutics for these patients appears justified, even if this may entail some discomfort for experimental animals. Having said this, it is self-evident that animals should be treated optimally and used with the highest possible respect. Legislation regarding animal protection and other rules such as the famous '3Rs' (reduce, refine, replace) have to be fully respected and adequately applied. It should be added here that animals used for behavioral pharmacology experiments are among the best treated and all efforts are made in this discipline to minimize the animals' general level of anxiety and discomfort because it is exactly these dimensions that are the focus of many behavioral studies.

Individuality of Human Beings and Animals

Individuality is an accepted characteristic of human beings and it is accepted that each individual's repertoire of physiological and behavioral responses may be different and dependent upon his or her genetic background and previous experience. Who would dare to negate that some facets of the parents are mirrored in a child, and who will disagree that types of illnesses, be they somatic or mental, are seen with different incidences in various families ? For domestic animals such as cows, sheep or dogs the importance of both environmental and genetic priming is also accepted: one strain of dogs is more shy, another more aggressive, and another more social than the other, but also within a strain and even within a litter one individual dog is less shy, less aggressive or less social than other members.

When it comes to laboratory animals such as rats and mice, individuality is less widely appreciated, although influences of the genetic descent, age, gender and previous experiences cannot be disputed in these animals. If one accepts the concept and general impact of individuality in all creatures, discussions as to whether an individual's reactions are genetically or environmentally determined are no longer needed. Behavior is clearly determined by both, and then reflects individuality.

4.5.2 NON-GENETICALLY-BASED ANIMAL MODELS

Models of Schizophrenia

Among the animal models of schizophrenia a distinction can be made between pharmacological, lesion-induced and neurodevelopmental models. As is the case with models of depression and anxiety, it will be inappropriate to describe an animal with unusual behavior as suffering from schizophrenia; however, it is possible in animals to mirror at least some of the symptoms or parameters known to be predominant and aberrant, respectively, in schizophrenic patients.

A straightforward approach to generate an animal model bearing some analogy to schizophrenia is the administration of *psychostimulants*, i.e. compounds that can also induce psychosis-like states in healthy humans. Examples are high-dose amphetamine, ketamine and phencyclidine, i.e. compounds that in animals cause a kind of motor behavior that bears some resemblance to positive psychotic symptoms seen in patients. Thus, using stimulant-treated rodents as screening models, compounds that specifically counteract drug-induced hyperactivity will be identified. This is the case for most antipsychotic drugs that act primarily via blockade of dopamine D2 receptors. Following administration of phencyclidine, social contact and interaction between two treated rats is greatly disrupted. According to Sams-Dodd (1996) this may be seen as an analogy to some of the negative symptoms occurring in schizophrenic patients, and it is hypothesized that compounds that are able to re-establish social behavior in these animals (e.g. clozapine) have the potential to ameliorate negative symptoms in schizophrenic patients.

A characteristic disturbance in schizophrenic patients is thought to be their inability to distinguish between relevant and irrelevant stimuli due to inappropriate filtering (sensory gating) of information (Perry *et al.*, 1999). An experimental set-up to measure this capacity is the so-called *prepulse inhibition (PPI)* paradigm, which can be assessed in both human and animals. Prepulse inhibition describes the normal attenuation of a startle reflex that occurs when a reflex-eliciting stimulus is preceded by a weak stimulus (prepulse). Disruption of PPI as an indicator of disturbed sensory gating is consistently observed in symptomatic schizophrenic patients (Braff *et al.*, 1999; Cadenhead *et al.*, 2000) and has been proposed as an operational measure of these patients' inability to ignore or suppress irrelevant stimuli.

A disruption of PPI can be induced in normal animals with apomorphine or amphetamine, i.e. a direct and an indirect dopaminergic agonist. This induced disruption of PPI is reversed by dopamine antagonists, i.e. compounds known as clinically effective antipsychotics, and thus the paradigm can be used to identify novel compounds with potential antipsychotic activity. Interestingly, there is a strain of mouse – DBA/2 – that shows a PPI deficit even without being treated with dopaminergic agonists; this strain of mouse is now in wide use as an animal model to evaluate compounds for their potential to restore PPI disruption.

Another class of models is designated as *neurodevelopmental*. The rationale underlying these paradigms is that schizophrenic psychoses constitute a clinical consequence of wrong or suboptimal neuronal connections established during specific developmental stages within ontogeny. Animal models thus should mimic this developmental disorder. A typical approach is to administer toxic agents, e.g. the DNA-methylating agent methylazo-oxymethanol acetate (MAM), to pregnant animals (Talamini *et al.*, 2000): MAM interferes with cell division during development of the fetus and destroys populations of rapidly dividing neurons. The behavioral consequences of this drug-induced disturbance of neuronal pathways are particularly pronounced once the animals reach puberty or adulthood. Antipsychotic drugs are expected to normalize or attenuate abnormal behavior tested under standardized conditions. As for other models, it is hoped that novel types of antipsychotic drugs can be detected in this paradigm (for a review see Kilts, 2001).

Models of Depression

A popular model in behavioral psychopharmacology is the so-called *forced swim test*. A rat or a mouse is placed in a cylinder filled with water and left there, as described in the original protocol, for 15 min. The animal initially struggles and swims around trying to escape from the aversive situation, but it becomes more and more immobile during the later phase of the trial. The motor activity displayed in this later stage is restricted to the minimum necessary to keep the head above the water. The immobility posture acquired at this stage is thought to reflect a kind of 'giving up'. If removed from the water at the end of an initial trial and re-exposed later (after 24 h or after several days), an untreated (control) rat will remain in an immobility posture for a good part of the second trial. In contrast, animals treated with a clinically effective antidepressant between the two trials will be much more active (less immobile) throughout the second trial. Reduction of the overall immobility time displayed during the second exposure is considered an indication of a compound's potential antidepressant-like effect (Fig. 4.8).

The so-called *tail suspension test* applies a similar principle (Steru *et al.*, 1985; Fujishiro *et al.*, 2001). Instead of being immersed in water the animal (usually a mouse) is suspended by its tail. Following an initial period of struggling, untreated (control) animals remain predominantly in an immobile posture whereas animals treated immediately before the experiment with an antidepressant drug show a reduction in the time spent immobile.

Another, somewhat comparable paradigm is the so-called *learned help-lessness test*. Initially the rat is confronted with mild foot-shocks from which it cannot escape. Once it has learned that there is no way to avoid the unpleasant

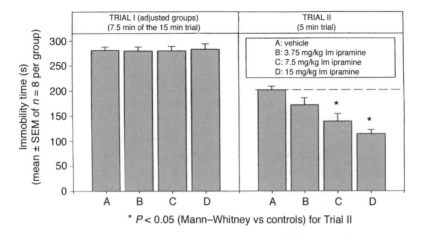

Figure 4.8 Effect of an antidepressant (imipramine) in the two-trial forced swim test in rats. Oral treatment between the initial (trial I) and second exposure (trial II) with imipramine at doses of 3.75, 7.5 or 15 mg/kg reduces the animal's immobility time dose dependently in the second trial

situation the animal will become immobile. On subsequent trials, the previously shocked animals remain immobile even when offered the possibility to avoid further shocks by moving to a safe, previously non-accessible compartment of the test box. In contrast, rats treated with clinically effective antidepressants will show a much higher number of escapes.

The last depression model to be mentioned is the *chronic mild stress model.* Normal rats show a clear preference for sweet liquids rather than water. In the current paradigm they are given a choice to drink, once or twice a week, either water or a sucrose solution. They are then exposed, according to an unpredictable random schedule, to various mild stressors such as 24-h continuous light, transient individual housing or crowding, partial food or water restriction, tilting of the cage, etc. Under these conditions the rats will drink less and less of the normally preferred sucrose solution. This change in behavior is thought to reflect *anhedonia,* an inability to enjoy pleasant stimuli, which is one of the core symptoms noted in depressed patients. If administered an antidepressant drug, and although still exposed to stress, the animals will slowly resume drinking more of the sucrose solution and the amount consumed will gradually regain the level seen previous to the stress period. It takes a few weeks until the stress-induced change in drinking preference is reversed, which, in view of the similarity in time scale with clinical use of antidepressants, makes this model attractive. Interestingly, most of the established antidepressants, irrespective of their mode of action – such as tricyclics, MAO inhibitors, SSRIs, electroconvulsive therapy and S-adenosyl-methionine or St John's wort – are effective in this model. It is assumed, therefore, that the chronic mild stress model has a high predictability for a compound's clinical antidepressant efficacy.

Models of Anxiety

Anxiety Based on a Conditioned Response

In this category of models the animal learns a performance, typically to abstain from a behavior that it would normally display according to its natural and current tendency. For example, in the so-called *Vogel test* a partly water-deprived and thirsty rat learns that, during a signaled period, every lick at the water spout will be followed by a mild electric foot-shock. This sequence induces anxiety and an untreated (control) animal will abstain from drinking. However, animals pretreated with anxiolytic drugs will overcome their inhibition and tolerate at least some of the shocks and drink even when punished.

Anxiety Based on an Unconditioned Response

Within this category two classes of paradigms can be distinguished – the so-called non-social and the social ones – depending on whether a single animal or a pair (or group) of animals is being tested. An example of an unconditioned, non-social model is the *elevated plus maze test,* used in mice and rats and recently also in gerbils. The test is based on the observation that rodents prefer enclosed over open environments, probably reflecting these animals' tendency to protect themselves from being caught by a predator.

In the elevated plus maze (EPM) a test naïve animal is given the opportunity to explore for a few minutes an environment made up of four identical arms (Fig. 4.9), two surrounded by walls (enclosed arms) and two without walls (open arms). Most rats or mice will preferentially explore the enclosed and only rarely enter the open arms. It is believed that in this set-up the animal is in conflict between its drive to explore the environment (there might be a potential partner or a preferred food source) and the avoidance of a potential threat (there might be a cat there).

Depending on the animal's level of anxiety, this conflict will be solved differently. An anxious animal will enter the more aversive open arms less frequently and for short periods only. As a measure of the animal's current level of anxiety, the ratio between the number of open arm entries over the number of total arm entries is calculated. A ratio of 0.15–0.30 will be found in untreated control rats but in animals pretreated with clinically effective anxiolytics, such as the benzodiazepines, the ratio is close to 0.50, indicating that they are no longer avoiding the more aversive part of the experimental

Elevated plus maze in mice

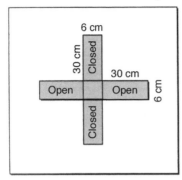

Experimental parameters:
Activity-related:
  • number of total arm entries
Anxiety-related:
  • ratio (% of open arm entries)
  • time spent on open arms
  • latency to leave closed arm

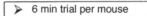

➤ 6 min trial per mouse

Figure 4.9 Schematic representation of the elevated plus maze used to evaluate the anxiety of a mouse based on its behavioral pattern displayed during an initial exposure

environment. Effective anxiolytics will also increase the duration of time that rats spend on the open arms. Note that the EPM test, due to its high practicability and ease of use, is also frequently applied to compare groups of rodents generated by both genetic engineering and selective breeding (see below).

There are other tests based on the same principles as those applied in the EPM, such as the light/dark box or the open-field test. In these experimental paradigms again it is the frequency and the duration that an animal stays in the more aversive and potentially more dangerous part of the test environment (such as the illuminated part of the light/dark box or the central part of the open field) that are recorded and, if low, reflect an animal's higher level of anxiety.

Another interesting model is the so-called *stress-induced hyperthermia test*. This is based on the observation that rodents, similar to humans, show a transient increase in body temperature when something unknown is going to happen (Lecci *et al.*, 1990; Zethof *et al.*, 1994). This reaction is mediated by the autonomic nervous sytem and reflects part of a stress reaction aiming at being alert and metabolically prepared to respond to a threat. Stress is induced in a group of mice housed in one cage by removing one animal after the other. Because the animals remaining in the cage do not know what is going to happen to them next, they become more alert and ready to react. The activation manifests itself as a mild increase in body temperature (up to 1.0°C) in the mice removed last compared with those removed initially (Fig. 4.10).

This difference in body temperature is called stress-induced hyperthermia (SIH) and is thought to reflect an anticipatory type of anxiety. Following pretreatment of all mice living in the same cage with an anxiolytic compound (chlordiazepoxide in the example given in Fig. 10), the body temperature of the

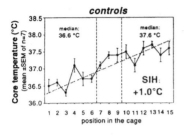

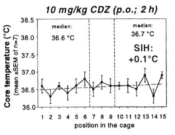

• **Design** (Lecci *et al.*, 1990)
• n=15 mice per cage, treated with compound (at 1 min intervals)
• 1 hour after treatment the rectal temperature is determined and mice are consecutively placed in another cage

• **Stress-induced hyperthermia**

defined as the delta of the median rectal temperature within the <u>six initially removed mice</u> and the median of the <u>six last removed mice</u> within a cage

Figure 4.10 Anxiolytic effect of chlordiazepoxide (CDZ) in the stress-induced hyperthermia paradigm in mice

mice removed last is increased less than in untreated animals and the temperature in those removed initially is unaffected. This results in a significantly attenuated SIH (0.1°C in the given example) following treatment with a benzodiazepine. A modified SIH test (Spooren *et al.*, 2002) that uses less animals is also well applicable and sensitive to benzodiazepines and other candidate anxiolytics.

An example of an unconditioned social paradigm is the so-called *social interaction test* in which two animals (rats or mice) unfamiliar with one another are placed together in a novel environment (File, 1980, 1985, 1997, 2000). In this situation the two animals follow two divergent drives: to explore the environment (there could be a cat around) and to enter into close contact with the unknown partner (for a male mouse it would be most attractive if the partner were a female mouse but potentially dangerous if it were an aggressive congener). During the initial confrontation, social contact between the two animals is usually minimal and this is thought to reflect the animals' situational inhibition or anxiety. If, however, two experimentally naïve rats, unknown to one another, are pretreated with an anxiolytic compound, the duration of time they spend in social contact increases significantly. Thus, the model allows quantification of the animals' current level of anxiety (or its degree of inhibition to engage in social activities) by measuring the duration of time spent in social contact. Furthermore, the level of environmental stress can be easily 'titrated' in this model by using, for example, different levels of illumination of the test arena or a difference in familiarity between the partners. Typical anxiolytics (most studies were performed with benzodiazepines) show the greatest efficacy under the most stressful condition (high light intensity and confrontation with an unfamiliar partner).

Another subset of models uses the confrontation with an *aversive stimulus coming from a natural enemy* to trigger and assess anxiety. The most popular stimuli are real cats or objects impregnated with the odor of a cat or an ingredient from fox urine (Dielenberg and McGregor, 2001). All these stimuli cause an attenuation of ongoing activities, and pretreatment with anxiolytic compounds causes rats or mice to react with less anxiety than untreated controls. In the case of mice as experimental animals, the presence of a rat is sufficiently stressful and produces significant behavioral inhibition.

4.5.3 MODELS USING GENETICALLY ALTERED ANIMALS

Genetically altered animals can, in principle, be obtained in two different ways: by *selective breeding*, i.e. by selection and subsequent breeding of (behaviorally or otherwise) extreme individuals within a population over several generations; and by genetic modification, i.e. by making use of recent molecular biological techniques to generate strains of animals characterized by specific properties or behaviors.

Studies in Strains Obtained through Selective Breeding

The following categories of strains can be distinguished:

(1) Strains showing relevance to psychiatric disturbances, although originally bred for some physical peculiarity. An example are Wistar Kyoto (WKY) rats, i.e. normotensive rats originally considered only as normotensive controls to spontaneously hypertensive rats. The WKY rats display low motor activity, increased immobility in the forced swim test and abnormal sleep patterns and, based on their behavior, are being used as an animal model of depression (Pare and Redei, 1993; Solberg *et al.*, 2001). An early study (Gentsch *et al.*, 1981) had also indicated that WKY rats have increased emotionality, i.e. attenuated activity in the open field and an increased defecation rate. Attempts are being made to breed behaviorally extreme WKY rats to increase further the potential of this model of depression.

(2) Strains originally bred for their differential sensitivity towards an experimental manipulation or a pharmacological agent, and subsequently recognized to be potential models of psychiatric disorders:

examples are the Flinders sensitive (FSL) and Flinders resistant (FRL) lines. The FSL rats show depression-like behavioral patterns, e.g. in the forced swim test (Overstreet *et al.*, 1995). Another example are rats more or less sensitive to the effects of apomorphine: when challenged with this dopamine agonist some rat strains display more severe alterations than others in a problem-solving test, with the more susceptible strains thought to be a partial model of schizophrenia (Coenders *et al.*, 1992; Ellenbroek *et al.*, 1995).

(3) Strains selected for differences in learning performance – Roman high avoidance (RHA) versus Roman low avoidance (RLA). In addition to the different performances displayed on the acquisition of an active avoidance task (RHA > RLA rats) these two strains have been described to differ in emotionality/level of anxiety (RHA < RLA) (e.g. Gentsch *et al.*, 1988).

(4) Strains selected and selectively bred for their behavior in the elevated plus maze, reflecting animals' anxiety upon being exposed to a novel environment. Two strains of rats, named the high anxiety line (HAL) and the low anxiety line (LAL), represent a very interesting example because it has been shown that the CRF-1 receptor antagonist R121919 was anxiolytic in rats with a high degree of innate anxiety, whereas the same compound was ineffective in rats with low anxiety (Keck *et al.*, 2001). This is reminiscent of experimental situations in humans where anxiolytic compounds are almost ineffective when taken by non-anxious persons (Janke and Debus, 1968).

Selective breeding often results in strains that drift bidirectionally from the original population. Any difference within such a pair of extremes needs to be interpreted with caution because at least in some of the available examples it is disputable which of the two sub-lines is more deviant from normality, i.e. from the original strain. With the inclusion of the appropriate control (normal) animals, selective breeding still remains an attractive approach because the individuals represent the extremes of the original (normal) population, this being quite analogous to some human psychopathologies.

Strains Derived from Direct Manipulations of the Genetic Background

General Considerations

(1) The emergence of gene technological methods during the last decade has extended the scope of animal experimentation dramatically. Older, time-consuming approaches to influence the characteristics of animal populations, which were based on spontaneous mutations (chance events) and subsequent selective breeding, are being superseded by newer technologies that allow direct and specific intervention with the genetic set-

up of living beings. Rather than criticizing and being worried about these novel technologies, one should consider that selection and subsequent breeding of special forms of individuals represents a strategy that has been applied for many centuries. More productive animals as well as many desired types and forms of plants and flowers were created in the past by means of selective breeding, i.e. a genetics-based but unfocussed approach.

(2) The possibility of studying the involvement of genetic factors in mental disorders directly has a major impact on preclinical investigations related to mental disorders. With the availability of newer technologies from molecular biology, genetic aspects can be studied in much more detail by using genetically modified experimental animals such as knockout strains (animals in which a gene has been removed) or overexpressing strains (in which replicates of a gene are present). Owing to practical reasons, genetically modified mice are used more frequently than transgenic or knockout rats. These studies are heuristically supported by the fact that the genomes (see Box 4.3 for explanation of terms used in genetics) of mice and humans are remarkably similar (Mural *et al.*, 2002): as an example, of the 731 genes contained in chromosome 16 of the mouse, only 14 could not be identified in the human genome. This similarity supports the concept that gene-targeting models in mice will produce valuable information about gene-mediated aspects of mental disturbances in humans.

Box 4.3 Definitions used in the Field of Genetics

Genetics: The field of science dealing with the molecular basis and underlying mechanisms of inherited characteristics and their transition to subsequent generations

Gene: A distinct sequence on the DNA strain that encodes for a peptide

DNA: Deoxyribonucleic acid is the repository of hereditary characteristics. The most commonly described form of DNA is the double-stranded form, arranged as a helix. Chromosomes are composed of double-stranded DNA. So called DNA fingerprinting offers a basis for evaluating the probability that blood, hair, semen or tissue samples originate from a given person, and thus offers a forensic tool as well as a means to determine lineages of humans and animals

RNA: Ribonucleic acids are macromolecules found in all cells in both the nucleus and the cytoplasm. Messenger RNA (mRNA) is an exact reflection of the genetically active DNA, carrying the message of the DNA to the cytoplasm where proteins are built up from amino acids as specified in the sequence of the RNA

Gene loci: Location of a segment of chromosomal DNA known or suspected to be linked with a heritable trait or a disease

Genotype: Characteristics of an individual reflected in its genetic 'lay-out'. Genotype is the counterpart of the phenotype that comprises the apparent characteristics of an individual, such as size, color of eyes, etc.

Genotyping: Determination of an individual's genetic background by using the so-called polymerase chain reaction (PCR), which permits the sequence of a gene to be replicated by using enzymes added *in vitro*. It is a diagnostic tool and is used also in criminology to identify individuals based on their genetic 'fingerprints'. It opens a new analytical and diagnostic avenue that is of great value beyond the basic sciences.

Gene technology: Methodologies to characterize and isolate genes of a living individual and transfer them to other living organisms. This transferred piece of genetic information may be modified or multiplied prior to its insertion.

Pharmacogenomics: Drugs are not equally effective in all patients and one of the reasons for this is thought to be the diversity of individuals' genetic repertoires at specific loci. It is estimated that there are some 3 million minimal variations, so-called single nucleotide polymorphisms, which may determine whether a patient is a responder or not to a drug or is less or more susceptible to drug side effects. Thus, in order to provide optimally effective treatment, it would be of value to know an individual's genetic pattern before initiating drug therapy. This possibility is still far from routine use, but genetic scanning of entire populations also has the aim to identify genetic markers that could be used as diagnostic tools to predict patients' reactions to a particular drug.

Genomic approach: Determination of alterations in the genetic make-up of patients, aimed at identifying altered gene sequences in order to predict the individual risk of contracting a specific illness.

Proteomic approach: Whereas the genomic approach focusses on the analysis of genetic material, the proteomic approach concentrates on the pattern of proteins present in patients.

(3) It has long been known that the risk for specific psychiatric disorders is much higher in some families than in others, indicating a genetic mediation of these disorders. Combined epidemiological and genetic studies might shed further light on the genetic predisposition for some disorders, and entire populations are currently being screened for the presence of indicator genes. A well-known example is a screening program for genetic indicators comprising the population of Iceland; according to preliminary information, 13 candidate genes for CNS disorders have been identified, among them also some genes associated with stroke and schizophrenia.

(4) The advances in large genetic screening studies are paralleled and supported by the dramatic increase in computer capacity and advances in semiconductor technology. So-called gene chips and microarrays make it possible to scrutinize, on a single glass slide of one square centimeter, details of the entire genome of an organism. Two chips are sufficient for the human genome! By comparing the pattern of activated genes between, for example, depressed patients and healthy persons, information on activated or inactivated genes in depressive disorder can be gathered. Existing and potential new therapeutic principles then can be tested for their potential to turn on or shut down the activity of selected genes. This approach is expected to generate relevant information on genetic correlates of mental disorders; it may also provide answers to currently unresolved questions, such as why some patients respond to treatment with a given drug whereas other patients do not. Once it is more developed and refined, this approach may lead to individually tailored treatments for mental illnesses. It may also help to shed new light on the trait versus state issue, i.e. whether a given genetic constellation (the activity pattern of certain genes) is present in a patient all the time ('trait marker'), or only at times when clinical symptoms are manifest ('state marker'). In the former, prophylactic treatment could be appropriate, but in the latter, a more interventive therapeutic procedure would probably be chosen.

Two typical gene-modified strains of mice that are currently used in pharmacological studies will now be described.

Corticotropin-releasing-factor (CRF)-over expressing Mice

Corticotropin releasing factor is a 41-amino-acid-containing peptide. Its physiological role is to trigger the release of adrenocorticotropin (ACTH), which in turn causes the release of cortisol – a stress hormone released in large quantities during any stress exposure. Once released, cortisol makes an organism ready to react by increasing the heart rate and turning on several metabolic processes; as a consequence of the stress reaction the individual becomes alert and, as evidenced in animals, ready to fight or flight.

Under normal conditions a stress reaction is shut off once the stimulus, e.g. an enemy or some other situation perceived as dangerous, has disappeared. If, however, due to any possible reason, the level of cortisol is not decreasing to its baseline level, one speaks of a hypercortisolemic state that, if chronified, can cause harm to an organism and ultimately may lead to physiological damage. Many chronically anxious or depressed patients are in a hypercortisolemic state.

The CRF-overexpressing mice are a genetically engineered strain with more than the normal number of copies of the CRF-encoding gene inserted in their genome. Compared with their wild-type counterpart, these animals show increased anxiety; they also have some of the abnormalities seen in hypercortisolemic patients, such as adrenal hypertrophy, marked thymus involution and increased abdominal fat (Beckmann et al., 2001). They have increased blood levels of cortisol and represent an animal model of hypercortisolemia (Stenzel-Poore et al., 1992, 1994; Holmes, 2001).

Neurokinin-1 Receptor Knockout Mice

Neurokinins are small peptides that participate in the modulation of many physiological processes. One neurokinin, called substance P, predominantly acts as an agonist at neurokinin-1 (NK1) receptors. The distribution of substance P and NK1 receptors in the organism suggests an involvement in physiological processes and subjective symptoms such as inflammation, emesis pain, migraine and gastrointestinal discomfort. Substance P is also located in brain regions involved in the regulation of emotions, such as the amygdala and the septum, and newer studies with specific NK1 receptor antagonists in rats, mice and gerbils indicate that this class of compounds may have anxiolytic potential (File, 2000; Vassout et al., 2000; Cheeta et al., 2001; Gentsch et al., 2002). Based on these findings it was anticipated that studies in animals lacking NK1 receptors (so-called NK1 receptor knockout mice) would provide additional information about the relevance of this receptor. Such animals have now been generated and are reported to be less anxious than control animals (Santarelli et al., 2001). These and other experimental findings suggest that the physiological consequence of shutting down the NK1 receptors by either knocking out this receptor or completely blocking it by means of a potent, selective and centrally active NK1 receptor antagonist will be identical. It is anticipated that NK1 receptor antagonists will turn out to be of clinical use in anxiety syndromes.

A Possible Limitation of Genetically Engineered Experimental Animals

It is thought that CNS receptors in man have normal function most of the time but may lose some of their normal function transiently, a loss that will translate clinically into symptoms of anxiety, depression, etc. In contrast, knockout animals do not have the respective receptor at any time in their life, including the various developmental stages. This permanent deficiency is likely to affect all functions normally controlled by the receptor during ontogenesis. Thus, in an attempt to come closer to the (hypothetical) clinical situation, more recent preclinical approaches aim at generating so-called conditional knockouts, i.e. animals with transiently inactivated receptors during a specific developmental period or at a certain age only.

To conclude this paragraph it should be stated that modifications in any creature's genetic background must be made with respect and should always include ethical considerations, because scientifically interesting but physiologically harmful mutations can be created by these interventions. Close evaluation of vital functions and observation of the behavior of any new type of animal created by genetic engineering will help to avoid unnecessary or inappropriate suffering of any newly established population. Interested readers are referred to a recent article by Cryan *et al.* (2002), which summarizes genetically modified strains of mice currently used as models in anxiety- and depression-directed experimental research.

4.6 FINAL COMMENT

There will be many new challenges ahead of those working in the field of psychopharmacology. However, the development of new ideas and concepts in the future should not be guided exclusively by scientific interest, aiming solely at understanding the complex mechanisms involved in our normal and pathological feelings and emotions. The dedication to come up with better drugs for patients suffering from mental disorders should remain the prime goal of all our efforts. Thereby – and note that this is mentioned here by a behavioral pharmacologist – clinicians and particularly the patients might tell us best which directions psychopharmacology should take in its efforts to try to alleviate the burden of mental disorders. Needless to say that tight interdisciplinary contact, as it traditionally exists in neuropsychopharmacology, will ultimately decide whether we succeed together in our mission to help suffering patients to overcome their disturbance and attain full remission.

Acknowledgment:

I am grateful to Albert Enz for having created Fig. 4.2 and for his critical reading of the manuscript.

Additional Information on Topics in this Chapter

- Glossary of concise definitions of terms covering the various aspects of medicinal chemistry:
  http://www.chem.qmul.ac.uk/iupac/medchem/cont.html
- References and further reading on depression, antidepressants and mood-brighteners:
  http://www.biopsychiatry.com/refs/index.html
- References and further reading on anxiety, anxiety medications, anxiolytics:
  http://www.fpnotebook.com/PSY15.htm
- Internet Mental Health, a free encyclopedia of mental health information created by a Canadian psychiatrist, Dr Phillip Long:
  http://www.mentalhealth.com/
- Information from the National Institute of Mental Health (USA)
  http://www.nimh.nih.gov/publicat/index.cfm
- Daily updated information on health aspects provided by news channels:
  http://www.cnn.com/HEALTH/
  http://www.abcnews.go.com/sections/living/

Periodicals Reporting on Original Contributions within the Field (in Alphabetical Order)

- *Behavioral Brain Research*
- *Brain Research*
- *European Journal of Pharmacology*
- *Journal of Affective Disorders*
- *Journal of Pharmacology and Experimental Therapeutics*
- *Pharmacogenomics*
- *Pharmacology, Biochemistry and Behavior*
- *Proceedings of the National Academy of Sciences, USA*
- *Psychopharmacology*
- *Psychiatry Research*
- *Schizophrenia Research*
- *Science*

5

Clinical Research in Psychopharmacology

By
FERENC MARTENYI

5.1 INTRODUCTORY CONSIDERATIONS

Clinical research involves sick persons and aims ultimately at improving existing treatments and discovering new and better ones. Questions of diagnosis and classification of diseases, as well as parts of basic medical research, also come under the heading of clinical research insofar as they concern the study of causes and mechanisms of diseases and their symptoms in humans. In psychiatry, clinical research in the sense of therapy research includes pharmacotherapeutic and non-pharmacological therapeutic approaches. This chapter deals exclusively with research on drug treatments.

The search for new psychopharmaceuticals lies largely in the hands of pharmaceutical companies and is thus strongly influenced by commercial interests. During the development of new compounds, these companies work closely with universities and other research institutes, and later with doctors and psychologists in clinics, hospitals and private practices. This cooperation is supervised to different degrees by the state or regional authorities in different countries.

As a rule, drug companies have a *research and development (R&D) portfolio*, i.e. a more or less well-defined collection of short- and long-term scientific projects. With the progress of medicinal sciences and changes in the pharmaceutical markets, the R&D portfolio undergoes regular revisions. Typical questions at the time of portfolio revision may be:

Psychopharmacology, Fourth Edition. By R. Spiegel
© 2003 John Wiley & Sons, Ltd: ISBN 0 471 56039 1: 0 470 84691 7 (PB)

- What are the urgent unsolved therapeutic problems in an area of medicine such as psychiatry?
- What is the ratio between the estimated prevalence of a disease and the number of adequately diagnosed patients? How many of the diagnosed patients are receiving adequate treatment?
- What are the health-economic consequences of a disease, in terms of healthcare utilization (number and duration of hospitalizations, frequency of use of healthcare resources, direct and indirect cost of treatment, lost productivity and activity, the overall burden of a disease on the environment and society)?
- Is the company already present in this segment of the health market? With which products? How are the company's products and those of its competitors developing in terms of market shares? What changes can be forecast for the market in question?
- What are the prospects for resolving other therapeutic problems in this area? On what time scale? With how many resources? Do the company's R&D departments have experience in the therapeutic field in question? Are there cooperations with other research groups?
- What impact will there be on the rest of the organization if the field considered to be of interest is developed further (or newly taken up)?

Some of these questions are of a qualitative type and cannot be answered with precise figures, so that entrepreneurial decisions are required. Because decisions concerning the R&D portfolio will tie up personnel and financial resources for years, they are of highest relevance to the company as a whole. In order to limit the risk, most companies compile a portfolio of R&D projects that includes a mixture of long-term and short-term, partly conservative and partly high-risk R&D areas.

Once the R&D portfolio is determined, questions regarding a specific *research strategy* need to be approached, such as:

- How is a specific objective within the R&D portfolio, e.g. the search for anxiolytic drugs with a fast onset of action (like benzodiazepines) but lacking cognitive side effects and addictive potential (unlike benzodiazepines), to be partitioned and sequenced so that individual groups within R&D, with their different approaches and methods, can be integrated sensibly into the project?
- Which areas are preferably dealt with inside the company, with its own R&D know-how, and which sub-projects should be farmed out to external organizations such as other research companies, biotech companies or university institutes?
- How many compounds from a given chemical class, with a given pharmacological profile and starting from a given hypothesis should be developed and taken up to clinical testing?

Unlike the R&D portfolio, which forms part of business policy, questions of this type are usually discussed and decided upon not by the company top management but within the specialist divisions.

When an interesting compound or series of compounds is identified in preclinical R&D, a clinical development strategy needs to be agreed upon. A key element of this process is the definition of a *target product profile* (TPP). The TPP contains a comprehensive product description of the new drug, which reflects its potential therapeutic uses (indications) based on information regarding the preclinical pharmacokinetic profile, the expected route of administration, the receptor-affinity profile, data from animal models, etc. The TPP needs to consider the potential advantages and disadvantages of the new drug based on preclinical efficacy and safety findings. Positioning of the new drug in relation to existing treatment and differentiation from other molecules with the same or similar indication are essential elements of the TPP. The TPP follows the structure of the package insert; it is an evolving and dynamic version of the expected drug labeling that is used and modified during the entire drug development process. The TPP drives the development plan: it determines the orientation, size and other specifics of clinical trials to support the predicted profile of the drug. The TPP, together with the clinical development strategy, represents a flexible learning-by-results system: the results of clinical trials confirm or challenge the TPP.

At this level a number of *methodological issues* concerning clinical research need to be addressed:

- Stratification of targeted indication and patient population.
- Objectives and hypotheses for sequences of individual experimental and clinical studies.
- Statistical planning of individual studies and *a priori* determination of statistical methods.
- Selection of patient samples: definition of inclusion and exclusion criteria.
- Definition of the levels of assessment, evaluation criteria and measurement instruments.
- Duration of treatment and dosage of the experimental product and reference substances.

A challenging situation arises when a substance possessing a 'high degree of innovation' is to be tested clinically. Such compounds would be derived from as yet relatively unknown chemical classes, with the mechanism of action not established so far; they would have shown a qualitatively novel profile of action during animal experiments or would have been tested using methods about which little was known to date. In circumstances such as these, the pharmacological hypothesis must be tested in specifically designed proof-of-concept (PoC) trials before large efficacy and safety trials are undertaken in Phases II and III.

Regulatory requirements predefine in many ways the preclinical and clinical development of new compounds. The US Food and Drug Administration (FDA) requires primarily two positive, independent, adequately powered, placebo-controlled clinical trials supporting the indications of a new antidepressant, antipsychotic or antimanic compound. In this special regard the European regulations are different: the European Medicines Evaluation Agency (EMEA) primarily requires data about the non-inferiority of a new potential psychotropic drug compared with an existing standard treatment. European regulations are asking for maintenance data as well, even in the case of a short-term treatment claim.

The clinical study of a new substance proceeds in several steps or phases. The purpose of this subdivision is to minimize the risk to the participating subjects and patients at each point in time and to allow each individual part of the study to flow one from the other so that a maximum of information from one trial can be obtained for the following studies.

5.2 ETHICAL ASPECTS OF CLINICAL RESEARCH IN PSYCHOPHARMACOLOGY

5.2.1 GENERAL REMARKS

The mission of clinical research is to provide scientifically appropriate and accurate information about new treatments in patients, keeping the safety of the patient as absolute priority; referring to the law of Hippocrates: "Nil nocere" (Not to harm). An additional ethical aspect of clinical research is the demand of high scientific standards. Therefore " ... at the start of the trial, there must be a state of clinical equipoise regarding the merits of the regimens to be tested, and the trial must be designed in such a way as to make it reasonable to expect that, if it is successfully conducted, clinical equipoise will be disturbed" (Freedman, 1987).

Research in the field of mental illnesses raises specific ethical challenges that derive from the unique aspect of psychiatric disorders and from the personal and social consequences of often stigmatizing, chronic, debilitating and many times life-threatening diseases. It is difficult to estimate the impact of mental diseases on the socio-economic dimension (Chapter 9). One in four people worldwide will suffer from a mental or neurological disorder at some point during their lifetime. It is estimated that more than 120 million people worldwide suffer from major depression and some 24 million from schizophrenia at any time. Unipolar major depression is now the leading cause of disability globally and ranks fourth in the causes of global burden of disease; it is forecasted to be the second disease in 2020 in terms of socio-economic burden, expressed by disability adjusted life years (DALY; World Health Organization, 2001).

As in other domains of medicine, there is an unabated demand for new, more efficacious psychiatric drug treatment with a better tolerability and side-effect profile. But is it really desirable to add further to the long list of psychopharmaceuticals with their often similar properties of actions? This question certainly must be answered in the affirmative for several psychiatric indications because there is a perceived lack of:

- Antipsychotic drugs without extrapyramidal action and not causing other medical or tolerability problems after short- and long-term use.
- Antidepressants with fast onset of action and a broader spectrum of efficacy in both unipolar and bipolar depression.
- Anxiolytics with fast onset of action but not causing sedation or leading to drug dependency.
- Mood stabilizers with antimanic and antidepressive efficacy, preventing affective episodes in different types of bipolar disorder from occurring, with considerably better tolerability than lithium.
- More effective drugs for the treatment of cognitive and behavioral disorders occurring in the elderly.

Given the need for development and clinical testing of novel drugs in patients, and the right of each patient to benefit from optimal treatment, there is obviously a conflict of purposes in clinical research that has been and still is evaluated differently at different times and under different circumstances. Opinion today is that a patient should, whenever possible, be the master of his own fate and not be delivered defenseless to the doctor – an opinion that has been reflected in laws and guidelines.

5.2.2 PROTECTING THE PATIENT

Medical activity is covered, on the one hand, by national civil and criminal law and, on the other hand, by what are known as medical ethics. These are standards of behavior that govern the doctor's dealings with his patients and by which every doctor should feel himself bound. The Hippocratic oath is part of the medical code of ethics that has been extended further over the past 30 years, particularly in view of clinical research. The 18th World Medical Association Conference in 1964 passed the Declaration of Helsinki, containing recommendations intended to guide physicians engaged in biomedical research on human subjects. This Declaration was revised in 1975 in Tokyo, in 1989 in Hong Kong, in 1996 in South Africa and in 2000 in Edinburgh (see p. 325 ff., and the homepage of the World Medical Association: www.wma.net/e/policy/17-c_e.html).

Four major elements act as a safeguard for patients participating in clinical trials:

(1) *The knowledge, expertise and integrity of the investigators.* Only highly qualified, experienced experts are able to generate high-quality data with scientific impact. Beyond scientific and clinical experience, a professional commitment related to regulations and basic ethical principles of biomedical research is required. Knowledge of Good Clinical Practice guidelines (see Box 5.1) is requested from investigators.

Box 5.1 Principles of Good Clinical Practice (GCP)

"Good Clinical Practice is an international ethical and scientific quality standard for designing, conducting, recording, and reporting trials that involve the participation of human subjects. Compliance with the standard provides public assurance that the rights, safety, and well-being of the trial subject are protected.... The objective ... is to provide a unified standard for the European Union (EU), Japan, and the United States to facilitate the mutual acceptance of clinical data by the regulatory authorities in these jurisdictions."

Detailed information on GCP is available under www.fda.gov/cder/guidance/index.htm.

Overall Principles of GCP

- Protection of the rights, safety and well-being of the human subjects participating in clinical trials are the most important considerations
- Clinical trials should be described in a clear, detailed protocol
- The protocol should be approved by an independent ethics committee/institutional review board prior to study start
- Freely given informed consent should be obtained from every subject prior to the subject's participation in the study
- All study information should be recorded, handled and stored in such a way that it allows accurate reporting, interpretation and verification
- The confidentiality of records that could identify subjects should be protected
- Investigational products should be manufactured, handled and stored in accordance with applicable good manufacturing practice (GMP) and should be used only in accordance with the protocol

(2) *Full disclosure of financial liaisons and relationships of investigators.* An important aspect is to exclude any conflict of interest between the study participants and the investigator's self-interest (financial, scientific, carrier, etc.). Only voluntary participation in a study is acceptable, and patients (participants) must have the right to withdraw from a study at any time.

(3) *Accurate information of study participants resulting in 'informed consent'.* This process is intended to provide comprehensive information to study participants (or their legal representative), allowing them to make an informed decision about participation or non-participation in a clinical trial. The details of the investigational procedures must be explained: e.g. the randomization and allocation of treatments, placebo lead-in, washout, frequency of visits, experimental paradigms, challenge maneuvers, restrictions related to concomitant medication, the nature of medications, potential side effect(s) of the active treatment(s) and the potential hazard of placebo treatment. All explanations must be transparent, written in an easy-to-understand language. In the case of additional questions related to the trial protocol, an additional independent expert has to give the detailed explanation.

(4) *Institutional Review Boards.* In university clinics and other hospitals engaged in research, ethics committees (also called Institutional Review Boards, IRBs) have been formed over the last three decades to monitor clinical research activities from scientific, legal, ethical and social viewpoints. All protocols relating to clinical trials must be submitted to these committees, which are generally made up of one or several doctors, a lawyer, a representative of the nursing staff and also community representatives such as priests. This composition forces clinical researchers to set out their intentions in such a way as to be clear enough for a lay person to understand and to assess whether the inconvenience and risks involved for the patient are in a reasonable relationship to the possible benefit of the planned trial.

A basic ethical issue in several areas of psychiatric research is whether participants are able to provide informed consent, particularly for protocols entailing medication washout and/or placebo treatment. The majority of psychiatric patients who are asked to participate in clinical trials have adequate capacity to provide consent. Thus, in a study specifically designed to examine the capacity of schizophrenic patients to give informed consent, cognitive dysfunction and negative symptoms (apathy and avolition), but not psychotic symptoms (hallucinations, delusions), were found to be associated with impaired decisional capacity (Moser *et al.*, 2002). These features are probably not unique to schizophrenia but are likely to apply to many other forms of illness.

When a clinical trial involving placebo or no-treatment control (see Box 5.2) is undertaken, the researcher and the IRB are obliged to ensure that patients or authorized third parties are fully informed about any therapy withdrawn or withheld for purposes of the research project, about the anticipated consequences of withdrawing or withholding the therapy and about the reasons why investigators deem a placebo-controlled trial to be necessary.

Box 5.2 Issues of Placebo Control in Clinical Trials

Use of *placebo controls* in clinical trials is judged differently by the health authorities of different countries. Most Institutional Review Boards in Europe are reluctant or even negative about allowing placebo-controlled trials in cases where accepted and established treatment is available for the respective disease – which is obviously the case for major depression, schizophrenia or bipolar disorder. The US point of view differs (Laughren, 2001). A major concern with regard to placebo-controlled trials is the potential increase of suicidality, which represents a high risk both in major depression and in schizophrenia. However, analysis of suicidality data from eight placebo-controlled trials in depressive patients and four studies in schizophrenic patients failed to support the hypothesis of increased risk of suicide in patients on placebo compared with the standard treatments or the investigational new compounds used in these studies. On the other hand the failure rate (about 50%) of placebo-controlled trials in depression, even for established compounds, would argue in favor of placebo-controlled studies to provide scientifically valid data about efficacy. The ratio of failed trials in placebo-controlled studies with established antipsychotic treatment is lower (about 25%), providing a reason to consider the possible validity of a non-inferiority design in this condition (Laughren, 2001).

Ethically motivated opponents consider trials with placebo control unacceptable if and when standard therapies or interventions are available for a particular patient population. Accordingly, placebo-controlled trials would be permitted only in the following circumstances:

- If there is no standard treatment or if standard therapy has been shown to be no better than placebo.
- If evidence has arisen creating substantial doubt regarding the net therapeutic advantage of standard therapy (e.g. due to side effects).

- If effective treatment is not available to patients due to cost constraints or short supply (however, a placebo-controlled trial is not permissible when effective but costly treatment is made available to the rich but remains unavailable to the poor or uninsured).

Placebo-controlled trials also can be considered in the following circumstances:
- In a population of patients who are refractory to standard treatment and for whom no standard second-line treatment exists.
- When testing add-on treatment to standard therapy, assuming that all subjects in the trial receive all treatments that would normally be prescribed.
- If patients have provided an informed renunciation of standard therapy for a minor condition for which patients commonly refuse treatment, and when withholding such therapy will not lead to undue suffering or the possibility of irreversible harm of any magnitude.

5.3   BASICS OF CLINICAL PSYCHOPHARMACOLOGY

5.3.1   THE BASIC OF BASICS: CORRECT DIAGNOSIS AND PATIENT SELECTION

A fundamental aspect in clinical psychopharmacological research is the precision (*reliability*) and accuracy (*validity*) of a particular diagnosis given to a patient. Validity in this context is the ability of a diagnosis to allow accurate decisions during a study (inclusion or exclusion of patients according to the criteria specified in the protocol; judgments as to the onset of the disease, of improvement or remission; differentiation of the symptoms of the disorder from potential adverse events of the treatment). Reliability is the ability of a diagnostic procedure to provide consistent results. It depends on the skills of the investigator how patient interviews are being performed, under what conditions the patients are interviewed and how the answers given by the patient are interpreted (interrater reliability). The validity and reliability of diagnosis affect all aspects of a clinical study in psychopharmacology. Invalid diagnoses will lead to inappropriate inclusion or exclusion of patients in a trial, and the findings may simply be wrong, possibly biasing all conclusions from a study. On the other hand, if diagnoses are valid but not reliable (precise), signals coming from a study are blurred (Kraemer, 1994). Thus, low diagnostic reliability decreases the power of a trial and larger sample sizes will be needed to detect differences between treatments.

Making a diagnosis is a more complex task than just the detection of a disorder. A disorder represents a pathophysiological abnormality, manifested in mental and/or physical symptoms. Diagnosis considers patients within a more complex, multiaxial system that is the essential concept of the DSM-IV system. The DSM-IV provides a comprehensive approach to evaluate patients according to: pathological mental conditions (clinical disorder) = Axis I; personality disorders/mental retardation = Axis II; general medical condition = Axis III; psychosocial and environmental problems = Axis IV; global assessment of functioning = Axis V (APA, 1994). A diagnosis in this regard is a composite of the disorder of the patient (A), characteristics of the patient irrespective of the current disorder, i.e. possible contaminants such as education, rural or non-rural status, civil status, employed or not employed (B), and random error (C). Sources of random error are inconsistencies in patient reports, diurnal variation of symptoms, observational errors of the investigator, etc. The diagnosis of a patient represents the sum of all these factors: diagnosis = A + B + C. The validity or accuracy of diagnoses in a sample of patients can be defined as:

$$\frac{A}{A + B + C}$$

The reliability or precision of the diagnosis for a group of patients represents:

$$\frac{A + B}{A + B + C}$$

In this sense one can speak only about the validity and reliability of diagnoses in a population of patients. Reliability is always greater than validity. A reliable diagnosis can be invalid but an unreliable diagnosis cannot be valid.

In clinical trials patients are selected according to a number of inclusion and exclusion criteria. Selection criteria in a clinical trial consist of:

- The specific diagnosis according to a diagnostic system (DSM-IV, ICD-10 or other established classification instrument).
- Patient selection based on symptom severity. This can be defined directly by a minimal acceptable severity score as measured by a rating instrument (e.g. the Hamilton Rating Scale for Depression, the Positive and Negative Symptom Scale or other established assessment instruments; see Section 5.6). An indirect definition of symptom severity may be a consequence of the status of a patient population: a clinical trial designed for inpatients generally implies a more severe symptom profile than a study with

outpatients. Involvement of outpatients in a study usually excludes the upper range of severity of the patient population.

- The previous course of a disorder and its resolution with treatment can be a key element of patient selection. Investigation of the effects of a drug in *de novo* diagnosed, first-episode patients will lead to different conclusions than a trial in mainly chronic, multitreatment-exposed patients. Some key inclusion criteria can be defined according to the treatment response history of patients; a study with clozapine in "treatment resistant schizophrenic patients" (Kane *et al.*, 1988; see Chapter 2) is an example for this.
- Exclusion criteria limit the sample of the trial by the segregation of patients: those who may contribute undue risk to a trial, such as potential high-risk patients (due, for example to suicidality) or patients with severe somatic comorbidity or special Axis II comorbidity (e.g. antisocial personality disorder); and those who are affecting the potential effect size of the investigated compound (e.g. treatment-resistant patients, patients exposed to adequate treatment within a predefined time frame or patients suffering from drug abuse).

Although narrow inclusion and extensive exclusion criteria may increase the internal validity of a study, results of a very 'clean' trial become less generalizable. Thus, at the very beginning of a clinical development, highly controlled PoC trials strive for high levels of homogeneity mainly by extensive exclusion criteria. In contrast, an important goal of so-called naturalistic studies (which are characteristic of late stages of clinical drug development) is to collect information about the efficacy and safety aspects of pharmacological interventions in a broader patient population not limited by overly strict exclusion criteria.

5.3.2 PHARMACOKINETIC–PHARMACODYNAMIC ASPECTS OF CLINICAL TRIALS

This section deals with the question of whether there are quantitatively detectable and interpretable correlations between the dose of an administered drug, or the concentration of a drug and its metabolites measured in the blood or plasma (blood or plasma level), and the therapeutic action or side effects observed. Investigations relating to questions of this type are called PK–PD (pharmacokinetic–pharmacodynamic) studies. The PK–PD analysis is a bidirectional approach: pharmacokinetics represent what the body does with a drug, and pharmacodynamics describes what a drug does to the body. The PK–PD analyses are key elements of early drug development, and PK–PD trials are able to answer specific disease-related efficacy and safety questions.

Basic Pharmacokinetic terms and models

Pharmacokinetics is a discipline that uses mathematical models to describe and predict the time course of drug concentrations in body fluids. Methods for quantitative analysis of drug concentrations in plasma and tissues are nowadays highly sensitive and specific. For some psychotropic drugs, the ranges of therapeutic and potentially toxic plasma concentrations are reasonably well established; for others, such ranges are tentatively established or postulated. Owing to the different blood–brain penetration parameters, pharmacokinetic data of molecules measured in blood do not necessarily reflect the psychotropic (central nervous system) effects. *Pharmacodynamics* – the study of the quality, intensity and time course of drug effects on the organism – has also undergone major changes, largely due to technological advances in our capacity to measure drug effects. So-called kinetic–dynamic modeling uses mathematical methods to link drug concentrations directly to clinical effects (Fig. 5.1).

The most important processes assessed in pharmacokinetic studies are *absorption* (uptake of a drug from the digestive tract), *distribution* (compartmentalization in the body), *metabolism* (conversion or breakdown, especially in the liver) and *elimination* (excretion), summarized by the abbreviation ADME.

The time elapsed from ingestion of a drug until peak concentrations (C_{max}) are reached in the blood or plasma is called t_{max}. The elimination half-life ($t_{1/2}$) is the interval between t_{max} and the time at which the remaining concentration amounts to 50% of the previously achieved C_{max}. In the case of drugs that produce their intended effect after a single dose, such as hypnotics, the relevant pharmacokinetic properties differ from those of medication that has to be taken repeatedly over a longer time (such as antipsychotics, mood stabilizers and antidepressants). Thus, assuming that the pharmacokinetic features coincide in time with the pharmacodynamic properties of a drug, an optimal hypnotic should have a short t_{max} and a short $t_{1/2}$, i.e. a fast onset of action and a fast decline. In the case of antipsychotics and antidepressants, t_{max} is less important and $t_{1/2}$ should be 12 or more hours so that no more than one or two drug doses are required each day. Typical $t_{1/2}$ values for antidepressants are 12–50 h, and it takes about four to five half-lives to reach a stable concentration or 'steady-state' concentration (C_{ss}) after repeated administration. Therapeutic plasma level monitoring, e.g. for compliance control, is sensible only under steady-state conditions (Fig. 5.2).

Drug *absorption* is influenced by many biological and physiological factors within an organism. The membrane of the gastrointestinal epithelial cells is composed of a phospholipid bilayer interspersed with proteins. The transcellular passage of a drug depends on its *solubility* in water and its permeability characteristics to penetrate the lipid bilayer of the epithelial cell membrane, which in turn is dependent on the *lipophilicity* of the drug

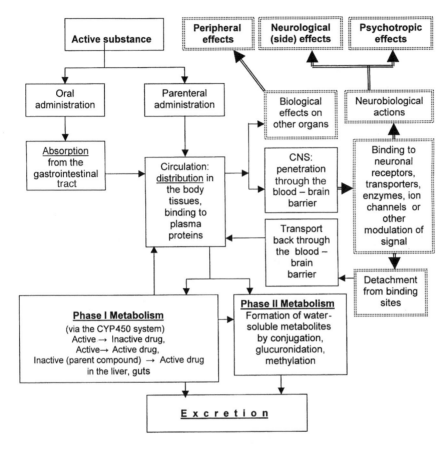

Figure 5.1 Pharmacokinetics and pharmacodynamics of the psychotropic drugs in the body. Pharmacokinetic routes of absorption, distribution, metabolism and excretion are represented by single lines. Pharmacodynamic effects such as biological and neurobiological effects, receptor binding, modulation of signal transudation, etc. are represented by double-dotted lines

molecules. As an example, absorption of barbiturates increases with higher lipophilicity as a result of better membrane penetration. The lipophilic character of the central nervous system (CNS)-acting drugs has an additional aspect: it is a critical feature in the penetration of the *blood–brain barrier* because all psychotropic drugs must be able to diffuse passively from the blood to the brain.

Because the entire blood supply of the upper gastrointestinal tract passes through the liver before reaching the systemic circulation, a drug may be metabolized by the gut wall and the liver during its first passage of drug

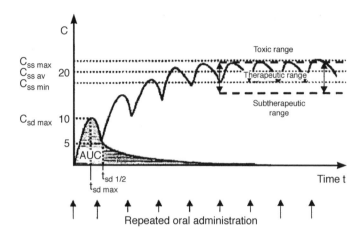

Figure 5.2 Plasma concentration curve of drug after single and repeated administration: $C_{ss\ max}$, maximal steady-state plasma concentration after repeated administration; $C_{ss\ av}$, average steady-state concentration after repeated administration; $C_{ss\ min}$, minimal steady-state concentration after repeated administration; $C_{sd\ max}$, maximal plasma concentration after single oral dose; $t_{sd\ max}$, time to maximal concentration after single oral dose; $t_{sd\ 1/2}$, plasma half-life after single oral dose; AUC, area under the concentration vs. time curve

absorption: the *first-pass effect*. In general, the higher the lipophilicity of a drug, the better its permeability and the greater its first-pass metabolism and hence its metabolic clearance.

Pharmacokinetic Metabolic Studies

There is no specificity for CNS compounds in the design of pharmacokinetic and metabolic studies, which should provide information about the ADME characteristics of a new drug (see Box 5.3). An important part of pharmacokinetic investigations is the exploration of drug metabolism. Biotransformation is a critical step during the metabolism of endogenous ligands (e.g. hormones, neurosteroids) and drugs. Cytochrome P-450 (CYP450) enzymes are heme-containing proteins that occur predominantly in the liver and to a lesser extent in the small intestine, kidney and adrenals. The CYP450 enzymes are responsible for the deactivation of active compounds or the transformation of psychopharmacologically inactive molecules (so-called parent compounds) into active molecules. A classification system has been developed in which each P-450 is assigned a family, subfamily and number. For example, CYP2D6 stands for family 2, subfamily D and gene 6. The importance of the P-450 enzymes to psychopharmacology follows from the fact that they mediate most of Phase I drug metabolism.

Box 5.3 Pharmacokinetic Studies Conducted During the Development of Psychotropic Drugs

- Basic *ADME* characteristics (absorption, C_{max}, plasma half-life, area under the curve, terminal half-life, volume of distribution, protein binding, clearance)
- *Dose proportionality* characterizes the relationship between the dose administered and the plasma concentration of a drug. The ideal dose–concentration curve is linear, i.e. the plasma concentration of the drug correlates linearly with an orally administered dose of the drug. Over-proportionality means a positive alteration from linear dose–concentration kinetics, i.e. a pronounced concentration increase with increasing drug dose (e.g. in the case of fluoxetine), whereas under-proportionality means a negative alteration from linear kinetics (e.g. in the case of carbamazepine). An over-proportional pharmacokinetic profile of a drug usually implies a more pronounced efficacy and adverse event profile at higher dose ranges, whereas in cases of under-proportionality the opposite should be expected
- *Food effect*: absorption of most psychotropic drugs is not significantly affected by concomitant intake of food. An exception is buspirone, with a twofold increase of absorption with food intake
- *Absolute bioavailability*: this implies a comparison of plasma levels after oral and i.v. administration of the drug. Most psychotropic drugs have a good bioavailability, i.e. values between 30 and 100%. Low bioavailability, as seen with buspirone, is associated with highly variable drug plasma concentrations and is not a desirable feature of a drug
- The *relative bioavailability* of different formulations needs to be studied if different galenical forms, e.g. capsules, tablets and liquid formulations, are used during the development of a compound
- *Inter- and intrasubject variability* of pharmacokinetic parameters: there are many sources of variability (age, gender, pharmaco-genetic factors, hepatic impairment, renal impairment, smoking vs. non-smoking, pregnancy, concomitant use of other drugs) that need to be investigated during drug development. In addition to the generally required program, the specific pharmacokinetic studies depend on the intended clinical use of a new medication

Phase I (presystemic or first-pass) metabolism can occur during drug absorption either in the gut wall or in the liver, i.e. before a drug reaches the systemic circulation. Typical phase I pathways are oxidation, reduction and hydrolysis of molecules; these reactions are responsible for the transformation of compounds into more polar, i.e. more water- and less lipid-soluble, molecules that can be eliminated by the kidneys and the biliary system. First-pass metabolism determines the fraction of an oral drug dose that will reach the systemic circulation (i.e. the fraction of the drug that is bioavailable and has a chance to get into the CNS). Drug that reaches the systemic circulation is redistributed to the liver via hepatic arterial blood. The unspecified term 'clearance' refers to the rate at which a drug is cleared from the systemic circulation. Thus, presystemic and systemic clearance together determine the concentration achieved after a given dose of a given drug in a given patient.

The importance of the P450 enzymes extends beyond determining the concentration of a parent drug. These enzymes also determine the concentration of drug metabolites that may or may not be pharmacologically active. Active metabolites of a drug can have pharmacological profiles different from those of the parent compound. For example, carbamazepine is a well-known anticonvulsant drug with antimanic properties; however its epoxy-metabolite, although inactive in terms of CNS effects, is responsible for the significant enzyme-inductive effect of carbamazepine. Nefazodone is an antidepressant with anxiolytic properties, whereas its active metabolite, meta-chlorophenyl-piperazine (mCPP), is anxiogenic. The concentration of mCPP is generally only a fraction of that of the parent drug: however, mCPP is dependent on the enzyme CYP2D6 for its biotransformation prior to elimination. Thus, concentrations of the anxiogenic metabolite can be appreciably higher than usual (and thus induce anxiety) in individuals who are deficient in CYP2D6. More generally, the activity of P-450 enzymes can be an important determinant of atypical responses to medication if the usual ratio of parent drug to active metabolite is altered.

Both CYP2C19 and CYP2D6 are P-450 enzymes known to be genetically polymorphic, meaning that there are, within a population, several groups of individuals with different abilities to metabolize a given type of drug. For example, Caucasian populations comprise a large percentage of individuals who are genetically deficient in CYP2D6 – some 5–10% of the population are so-called 'slow metabolizers'. Conversely, about 20% of Orientals are genetically deficient in CYP2C19, leading to different metabolizing capacities for certain drugs.

The activity of CYP enzymes is also influenced by external factors such as food and other drugs taken concomitantly:

- Grapefruit juice contains a substance called naringine that inhibits CYP3A4; thus, if grapefruit juice in large quantities is taken together with drugs that are metabolized by this CYP450 subtype, a higher than normal drug exposure will result (Greenblatt *et al.*, 2001; Ho and Saville, 2001) and side effects may occur that are normally seen at higher doses of the respective medication.

- Drugs such as barbiturates and carbamazepine induce certain enzymes and will then trigger faster breakdown of some concomitantly used antipsychotics and antidepressants. In contrast, paroxetine, fluoxetine and fluvoxamine, acting by different mechanisms, inhibit the breakdown of other concomitantly administered drugs such as benzodiazepines, antidepressants, antiepileptics and neuroleptics (Table 5.1).

Phase I reactions are followed by *Phase II metabolic pathways*: chemical reactions such as conjugation, glucuronidation, methylation and acetylation are responsible for the formation of more water-soluble products by binding the compound with endogenous glucuronide, sulfate or glycine. Pharmacokinetic interactions with other drugs may also occur at this level. Thus, valproic acid blocks the glucuronidation of compounds such as lorazepam and

Table 5.1 Compounds interacting with CYP enzymes

Compound	CYP enzyme	Action
Antipsychotics		
Haloperidol	1A2	Substrate
Olanzapine	1A2	Substrate
Risperidone	2D6	Substrate
Antidepressants		
Paroxetine	2D6	Inhibitor
Desipramine	2D6	Substrate
Fluoxetine/Norfluoxetine	2C19, 2C9, 2D6, 3A4	Inhibitor
Fluvoxamine	1A2	Inhibitor
Nefazodone	3A4	Inhibitor
Paroxetine	2D6	Inhibitor
St. John's Wort	3A4	Inhibitor
Clomipramine	2D6	Substrate
Anxiolytics		
Diazepam	2C19	Substrate
Midazolam	3A4	Substrate
Others		
Carbamazepine	3A4	Inducer
Phenobarbital	2D6, 2C9	Inducer
Donepezil	2D6	Substrate
Estrogen	3A4	Substrate
Grapefruit juice	3A4	Inhibitor
Tobacco	1A2	Inducer

carbamazepine, leading to accumulation and possibly stronger clinical action of these drugs. Tricyclic antidepressants and all benzodiazepines are potent inhibitors of glucuronidation of morphine; as a consequence, they increase the plasma concentration of morphine, resulting in an additive effect beyond the pharmacodynamic interaction (Pacifici *et al.*, 1986; Wahlstrom *et al.*, 1994).

In summary, both Phase I and Phase II metabolic drug interactions are of clinical relevance because they alter the steady-state concentrations of drugs and thereby attenuate or enhance their pharmacological effects; in extreme cases this can either lead to a lack of therapeutic efficacy of a drug or to drug intoxication. The purpose of drug plasma level measurements here is to adjust the dose to suit the new situation.

Pharmacodynamic and PK–PD studies

The objectives of pharmacodynamic studies early in development are to delineate and confirm the range of pharmacologically active doses in humans, together with the maximum tolerated dose (MTD), and to describe the time-course of pharmacodynamic activity of a new compound. A variety of methodological approaches are used in pharmcodynamic studies, ranging from simple questioning of subjects and behavioral observations to the more recent brain imaging and functional procedures (more detail in Chapter 3). For putative CNS-active drugs, studies usually focus on:

- Effects on psychomotor performance and cognitive function (in young and older subjects, males and females) after single and multiple doses (Patat, 2000).
- Effects on electrophysiological parameters (pharmaco-electroencephalo-gram, evoked potentials); polygraphic sleep studies.
- Driving tests; interactions with alcohol.
- Effect on brain metabolic and perfusion parameters measured by functional brain imaging (SPECT, PET, fMRI: see Chapter 6).
- Habituation and tolerance phenomena; withdrawal effects, rebound phenomena.
- Neuroendocrine changes.

Dose-escalation studies performed in an early phase of drug development provide preliminary information to explore pharmacodynamic parameters at different dose levels up to the MTD. If the focus of a study is on the relation-ship between the pharmacokinetic and pharmacodynamic parameters (rather than on dose–response relationships), then the term PK–PD studies is used.

5.3.3 ENDPOINTS AND MARKERS IN CLINICAL TRIALS

A *biological marker* is a physical sign or laboratory measurement that occurs in association with the pathology of a given disease and has a potential diagnostic or prognostic utility. Biological markers can reflect efficacy as well as safety aspects of a drug, e.g.:

- Atrophy of the *substantia innominata* on magnetic resonance imaging (MRI), reflecting degeneration of cholinergic neurons in the *nucleus basalis* of Meynert, may be an *in vivo* marker of cholinergic deficiency typical of Alzheimer's disease. The thickness of the substantia innominata shows a significant positive correlation with the Mini Mental State Examination (MMSE) and thus may be useful as a predictive biological marker for the efficacy of cholinesterase inhibitors (Hanyu *et al.*, 2002).
- A prolongation of the QT interval seen in the electrocardiogram (ECG) serves as a *safety biological marker* for heart function. Several psychotropic drugs (chlorpromazine, imipramine, maprotiline, pimozide, thioridazine, sertindole, ziprasidone) prolong the QT interval and this has been associated with the occurrence of arrhythmias, in several cases with potentially fatal ventricular arrhythmia, known as torsade de pointes; QTc is the QT interval corrected by the square root of the heart rate interval; and prolongation of QTc represents a major safety concern for drug regulatory authorities because it was responsible for about half of the safety-related withdrawals of new drug applications at the FDA since 1998.

A *surrogate endpoint* of a clinical trial is a biological marker used to substitute for a clinically meaningful endpoint that directly measures feelings, functions or events that are difficult to assess, or survival. Changes induced by pharmacological intervention on a surrogate endpoint are expected to reflect changes in a clinically meaningful endpoint (Fleming and DeMets 1996; Temple, 1999). A surrogate endpoint for 'survival' needs to be supported by epidemiological evidence that the marker is indeed a risk factor, i.e.:

- The marker must be consistent with pathophysiology.
- The marker must be correlated with a true clinical outcome and fully capture the net effect of treatment on the clinical outcome.
- It must be on the pathway of the pharmacological intervention.
- It must not be confounded with adverse drug reactions.

Strictly speaking, no generally accepted, valid surrogate efficacy marker has been established in psychopharmacology so far. Several authors declare biological markers as surrogate endpoints, e.g. some specific patterns of receptor occupancy seen in positron emission tomography (PET) trials (see Chapter 6). As an example, D2 receptor occupancy trials may predict the outcome of treatments with antipsychotics because they indicate the pathway of the pharmacological intervention, show correlation with extrapyramidal side effects but are not fully consistent with the pathophysiology of schizophrenia. Early reports of elevated postsynaptic D2 dopamine receptors in schizophrenic brain post mortem have not been consistently confirmed by brain imaging studies of young neuroleptic naïve patients with schizophrenia (Farde, 1997). Furthermore, the psychotogenic effect of ketamine is not mediated by any significant changes in the dopamine release in the dorsal caudate, dorsal putamen or ventral striatum as measured by ^{11}C-raclopride in a PET study of healthy volunteers (Kegeles *et al.*, 2002).

On the other hand, there are some biological markers in the cerebrospinal fluid (CSF) of patients with Alzheimer's disease showing a correlation with the severity of the disease, the extent of neurodegeneration, oxidative stress or neuroinflammation (see Chapter 7).

The clinical endpoint is a clinically meaningful measure of how patients feel, function or survive. Investigator-rated or self-assessed rating instruments are the most frequently used clinical endpoints. A *primary endpoint* is the main outcome that a study protocol is designed to evaluate. The statistical power and the sample size calculation of a particular trial are determined by the primary endpoint. Depending on the purpose of a study the primary endpoint can be

- An efficacy outcome measure (e.g. change from baseline in a symptom assessment instrument, response rate according to a predefined response criterion, remission rate, time to response, time to relapse according to predefined relapse criteria, etc.). For Phase III trials the primary endpoint should be a clinical event (such as full recovery) or clinical improvement relevant to the patient (e.g. disappearance of specific symptoms).
- A safety parameter: examples are drop-out rate due to adverse effects, adverse effects measured by a (side-effect-specific) rating instrument, biological markers, etc.
- Bioequivalence (e.g. equivalence of efficacy) of two different galenical formulations of the same compound as measured by maintained remission rates in schizophrenic patients after an oral or depot antipsychotic formulation.
- Other relevant pharmacokinetic or pharmacodynamic parameters.

An *intermediate endpoint* is a clinical endpoint assessed at some stage of a study but not at its very end. *Ultimate outcome* is a clinical endpoint such as survival, onset of serious morbidity or symptomatic response that captures the benefits and risks of a treatment. Admission to a nursing home could serve as an ultimate outcome in the case of a drug intended to treat outpatients with Alzheimer's disease.

5.4 STUDY DESIGNS

5.4.1 THE NEED FOR CONTROLLED STUDIES

Studies in psychopharmacology have some specific features differentiating them from other disciplines of clinical research:

- There is a significant degree of experimental variability across studies.
- Diagnostic categories are phenomenological constructs rather than biologically homogenous entities (no specific biomarkers are established for psychiatric disorders to differentiate mental illness from 'normality'). Criteria for diagnosis are based on behavioral disturbances observed by the diagnostician or reported by the patient (possibly people in his environment).
- Effect size of most treatments with psychotropic drugs tends to be modest.

For these reasons, hypothesis-testing studies in psychopharmacology must be well controlled, i.e. employ one or more control groups (Leber, 1991). Because of the duration of treatment required to demonstrate a therapeutic effect (weeks or months in the case of antipsychotics, antidepressants, antipanic, etc. compounds), as well as the highly variable course of psychiatric disorders, double-blind, placebo-controlled studies with parallel-group design are recommended in most situations. A clinical trial design that involves more than one control treatment, typically a standard drug used in the same indication and a placebo, represents one of the most informative designs, for several reasons:

- A trial that demonstrates superiority of the new drug over placebo, plus superiority of the standard drug over placebo, has demonstrated its assay sensitivity and may be considered a valid experiment.
- A trial of this kind provides a useful efficacy and safety standard to quantify the treatment effects of a new drug against both an established drug and placebo.
- Because two active drugs (causing effects and side effects) are involved, the double-blind character of the study is better protected throughout the trial.
- The study design increases the chances that a patient will receive an active treatment rather than placebo.

5.4.2 PARALLEL-GROUP DESIGNS

This design is generally preferred for large clinical trials. Parallel groups, i.e. statistically equivalent and concomitantly treated groups, are achieved by assigning patients randomly to one of two or more groups ('treatment arms'). A clear advantage of the parallel-group design is its simplicity; its major downside is the large variance due to individual differences between patients included in the parallel groups. To decrease the variance it is recommended that patients are randomized according to one of the treatment groups by treatment blocks.

There is no completely satisfactory alternative to a parallel placebo control group when seeking to establish the efficacy of psychopharmacological agents.

However, if the use of a placebo is impractical, or inappropriate for ethical or technical reasons, a multiple fixed-dose study without a placebo arm may be an acceptable option. This approach involves comparison of responses to a range of doses of the test drug in comparison with a standard compound. When significant differences between treatment groups are observed, some positive conclusions regarding efficacy can be derived from the data. However, a multiple fixed-dose study design also has some disadvantages:

- There is a risk of false negative judgment if the wrong doses are selected because of uncertainty about the therapeutic dose range of a drug.
- If significant differences between doses are not detected, no inference can be drawn about drug efficacy.
- Purposely selecting a low dose outside the therapeutic range, or even a dose that is thought to be marginally effective, raises the same ethical concerns as use of a placebo.

5.4.3   PLACEBO-CONTROLLED STUDY DESIGNS

The parallel-group, double-blind, placebo-controlled study design represents the golden standard of acute treatment trials of depression, mania and anxiety disorders. This design is intended to limit bias, in particular selection and measurement bias. Trials based on this design are expected to provide information about the effect size of a new compound and its side-effect profile.

There appears to be an emerging trend for rising placebo response rates during the past two decades in almost all pharmacotherapy trials of psychiatric diseases. The reported placebo response rates were around 10% in placebo-controlled trials of lithium treatment of bipolar mania (Pope *et al.*, 1991); however, the proportion of placebo responders exceeded 40% in a trial of olanzapine by the end of the 1990s (Tohen *et al.*, 2000). In early efficacy trials of obsessive–compulsive disorder (OCD) the placebo response rates used to be around 5%, whereas the rates reported in studies published in the 1990s have risen to more than 25%. A meta-analysis of clinical trial data from 9 antidepressants and 13 anxiolytics approved by the FDA between 1985 and 2000 pointed at the consequences of placebo response rates in depression trials (Khan *et al.*, 2002). These studies comprised a total of 18 370 patients suffering from depression or anxiety disorders who participated in 93 treatment arms of a new or established antidepressant in 52 different antidepressant studies, or in 75 treatment arms of 40 different anxiolytic trials. Less than half of the antidepressant or anxiolytic treatment arms showed superiority over placebo (48% in both indications: 45 of 93 for the antidepressant; 36 of 75 for the anxiolytics). Elimination of placebo controls in favour of non-inferiority designs (Section 5.4.4) would have resulted in a high likelihood that ineffective antidepressants or anxiolytics had been approved, and potentially effective compounds would have been missed (Khan *et al.*, 2002).

Another meta-analysis of placebo-controlled trials in depression published between 1980 and 2000 showed an increase in the response rates in the placebo arms of trials with a variety of antidepressants (Walsh *et al.*, 2002). Responses to placebo increased significantly in recent years, as shown by the high positive correlation with the year of publication. The association between response rate and year of publication was more statistically robust for placebo than for active medication. The change in placebo response rate did not appear to be explained directly by changes in study characteristics such as patient age, placebo lead-in or minimum required Hamilton Rating Scale for Depression score. A potential explanation could be the changing awareness of patients and the fact that many patients in recent clinical trials had been exposed to several previous treatments and thus expected to improve (see Box 5.4).

A large response in the placebo group of an antidepressant trial clearly reduces the power of the study. One-third of all published trials of antidepressants fail to demonstrate efficacy, therefore new strategies are required for the reduction of variance. Meta-analysis of baseline characteristics of more than 2000 depressed patients included in the development program of an antidepressant showed remarkable differences between study participants in the USA and Europe (Niklson and Reimitz, 2001): European patients had significantly higher average baseline scores on several depression scales, particularly on items indicative of anxiety/agitation, somatization and sleep disturbance. Overall their depression appeared more severe, with more melancholic features than seen in the US patients. Such differences are probably relevant because observations made in other studies indicate that inclusion of patients with mild depression increases the risk of non-discrimination between drug and placebo. Thus, a meta-analysis of studies with four antidepressant medications showed that 41% of patients with scores of 18–20 on the Hamilton Rating Scale for Depression (HRSD) responded to placebo, whereas patients with scores of 21–24 and 25–29 had considerably lower (23 and 22%, respectively) placebo response rates (Wilcox *et al.*, 1992). Similarly in a number of studies with selective serotonin reuptake inhibitors (SSRIs), less severely depressed patients, i.e. those with HRSD baseline scores of less than 28, had higher placebo response rates than patients with higher scores (Schatzberg and Kraemer, 2000). On the other hand, a severity of illness above 'moderately severe' is not a major factor predictive of significant active-versus-placebo treatment differences (Montgomery, 1999).

Another important factor that may favor placebo responses in clinical studies is probably the *patient recruitment* strategy, as suggested by the following observation: two almost identically designed studies with fluoxetine vs. placebo in the treatment of post-traumatic stress disorder (PTSD) were performed, but only one of them resulted in a significant difference between

Box 5.4   Factors Responsible for Placebo Effects

(1) *Natural course of the disorder*. Some apparent placebo effects
    may be due to spontaneous remissions whereas others are
    clearly not. Spontaneous remissions are only partly predictable
    for a given time interval. Patients on waiting lists show clearly
    the natural course of the disease, spontaneous remission and
    worsening (see Fig. 5.3).

(2) *Conditioning*. A Pavlovian explanation of placebo effects has
    been based on the traditional model of classical conditioning:
    active ingredients serve as unconditional stimuli and the
    vehicles in which they are delivered (pills, injections), particu-
    larly the elements of therapeutic procedures, function as
    conditional stimuli. After repeated pairing of unconditioned
    and conditioned stimuli, the conditional stimulus elicits a
    conditional response even if the conditioned stimulus (e.g. the
    pill) is presented alone (without active ingredient).

(3) *Expectancy*. The aim of placebo control is to challenge and
    avoid the perception of clinical changes (improvement or
    worsening) caused by expectations on the part of both patients
    and physicians. The expectancy effect is "the tendency for
    experimenters to obtain results they expect, not simply because
    they have correctly anticipated nature's response but rather
    because they have helped to shape that response through their
    expectation" (Rosenthal and Rubin, 1978). Expectancy is
    different from distortion: "The distortion effect comes from
    seeing what you want to see, even if it's not there. The
    expectancy effect involves creating the objective results that we
    want to see. We don't distort results to conform to our
    expectations as much as we make the expectations come true.
    Strictly speaking: the expectancy effect is not a response effect
    at all" (Bernard, 1995).

active drug and placebo (Martényi, 2002). Inclusion criteria according to the
protocol were the same in both studies, but a possible explanation for the
differential outcomes could be the different sources of patients in Europe and in
the USA. All patients recruited in Europe, South Africa and Israel were
spontaneous arrivals in the study with positive outcome, whereas the patients
in the negative US study had been recruited by newspaper and similar
advertisements. These and other findings suggest that the power of studies with

antidepressants and anxiolytics is increased if placebo responses are reduced by recruitment of moderately to severely depressed or anxious patients (Thase, 1999; see Box 5.5).

In contrast to experience with depression, placebo response rates of trials in social phobia show a rather constant pattern during the past decade: between 9 and 29% of patients were characterized as placebo responders as measured by the Liebowitz Social Anxiety Scale (Kobak *et al.*, 2002).

Owing to the variable nature of most mental disorders, the preferred design for studying acute treatment of depression, mania, generalized anxiety disorder (GAD), social phobia, panic disorder, PTSD, OCD, several psychotic disorders, agitation in the elderly, etc. is the randomized, double-blind, placebo-controlled parallel-group trial, using patient samples of adequate size. As noted earlier, there are differences between the USA and Europe with regard to registration requirements: the FDA requires two independent, adequately powered, placebo-controlled trials to support an acute indication claim (depression, schizophrenia, mania, panic disorder, OCD, PTSD, etc.). The EMEA-CPMP guidelines require comparison of a new compound with established active treatment, and in many cases with placebo as well, preferably in three-arm designs.

Specific Placebo-controlled Trial Designs

Depending on the purpose of a study there are several subtypes of placebo-controlled trials (see Fig. 5.3). One design makes use of a single-blind *placebo lead-in period*. The purposes of this pretrial period of up to 4 weeks are:

- To allow time for washout of previously taken psychotropic medication.
- To allow time for medical assessments and evaluation of laboratory tests.
- To permit patients to change their minds regarding participation in the trial.
- To assess the patients during a prospectively monitored drug-free interval for substance use (drug screen, blood and/or urine level measurement).
- To allow for repeated assessment of symptom severity and stability, i.e. to identify and take out patients with clear placebo response or early spontaneous improvements.

This design may help to screen out placebo responders as well as bipolar depressed patients with transient exacerbations of symptoms, or subjects suffering from anxiety disorders in response to environmental psychological stressors. However, the value of this design is limited because it will not reduce potential investigator bias, i.e. the expectation of pharmacological effects after a given time.

An interesting approach to deal with this specific issue and to reduce further the placebo response rates is the use of a *blinded lead-in as well as a blinded lead-out period*. The purpose of the procedure is to mask the timing of

Box 5.5   Reducing placebo responses in clinical trials

Numerous factors influence placebo response rates in clinical trials. The following is a non-exclusive list of techniques that potentially are able to minimize placebo response rates in psychiatric indications, particularly in major depression and anxiety disorders.

Factors Related to Investigators
- Invitation of investigators who have previously demonstrated drug–placebo differences in other trials

Factors Related to Patient Recruitment
- Exaggerated pressure to recruit rapidly may lead to inclusion of patients in whom the response to placebo is unusually high
- Patients recruited by advertisement may cause higher placebo response rates than the 'spontaneously' incoming patients of out- or inpatient departments

Factors Related to Trial Design
- Double-blind placebo lead-in
- Blinded randomization
- Lead-in phase of several weeks during which subjects receive psychoeducation about handling disease

Factors Related to Frequency and/or Duration of Assessments, Visits
- Minimize the frequency and duration of assessment visits
- Use short investigator-rated instruments

Factors Related to Inclusion/Exclusion Criteria
- Increase the homogeneity of the population (use standard diagnostic tools; maximum feasible reduction of comorbidities with other Axis I disorders)
- Recruit patients with moderate to severe psychopathology. Exclude Axis II comorbidities
- Shift inclusion criteria to an acute/subchronic rather than a very chronic population. But patients in the acute phase of an episode may show spontaneous recovery.
- Exclude patients with drug or alcohol abuse and/or dependence
- Minimize participation of patients recruited by means of advertisement
- Limit recruitment of patients suffering from dissociative symptoms, histrionic features

Parallel placebo control (2 arms)
Patients are randomized into placebo or
investigational treatment arm.

Placebo lead-in followed by 3-arm active- and placebo-controlled treatment phase design
Patients are randomized into placebo, investigational
treatment or active control treatment arms after a placebo
lead-in period. Responders of the placebo lead-in period
should be excluded.

Crossover design
Patients are randomized into a placebo or active treatment arm
at baseline and switched into the other arm in the middle of
the trial. All patients are treated by both placebo and active
drug during the trial, with two different sequences: active
treatment followed by placebo or placebo followed by active
treatment.

Blinded randomization
Patients are randomized into a placebo and one or more
treatment arms. The treatment phase is preceded by different
lengths of placebo lead-in phases; the time of switch to the
active treatment(s) remains blinded. The treatment phase is
followed by a placebo lead-out period; the timing of switch
from the active treatment to placebo is blinded.

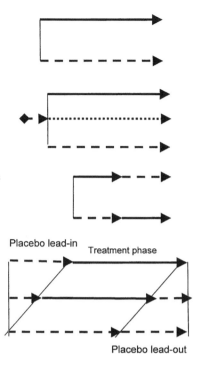

Relapse prevention design. Comparison of placebo with 3 different lengths of treatment
Patients responding in open-label acute
treatment to the investigational drug qualify to
enter the placebo-controlled double-blind
relapse prevention phase. Patients are
randomized into different lengths of active
treatment followed by placebo administration.

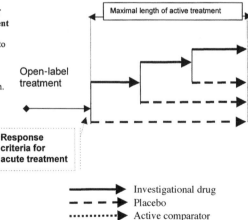

Figure 5.3 Placebo-controlled designs

transition to potential active treatment: the patients will be allocated to active or placebo treatment arms after different durations of placebo lead-in. All patients will be treated with active compound or placebo for the same length of time, and therefore the study will also end with a blinded placebo lead-out phase of variable duration. This design was used in a placebo-controlled trial with duloxetine (a norepinephrine and serotonin reuptake inhibitor) in the treatment of major depression. The study showed a significant difference between the active treatments and placebo as early as after 4 weeks, i.e. with a delay similar to that seen in conventional studies, and therefore the additional value of the blinded lead-in and lead-out approach remains doubtful (Faries *et al.*, 2002; Goldstein *et al.*, 2002).

A design intended specifically to investigate the effect of discontinuation or withdrawal symptoms of a particular compound, or comparing different compounds with regard to withdrawal symptoms, is the *placebo-controlled discontinuation or cessation design*. Insertion of a placebo treatment phase within the course of active treatment for several days allows the observation of discontinuation and withdrawal symptoms. The design requires frequent sampling during the entire length of study. A placebo-controlled trial was designed to differentiate fluoxetine, paroxetine and sertraline from each other based on discontinuation symptoms. The 5–8 day placebo substitution interrupting the antidepressive treatment provoked detectable differences between the drugs, favoring fluoxetine (Rosenbaum *et al.*, 1998).

Several trials have been performed with antidepressants in the prevention of recurrence of major depression. In an exemplary trial of this kind, Reimherr *et al.* (1998) explored the optimal length of therapy in a long-term, *placebo-controlled continuation study* of patients who had responded to 12–14 weeks of open-label fluoxetine treatment (20 mg/day) for major depression. Different maintenance schedules were represented by four treatment arms:

- Group A: 50 weeks of treatment with placebo.
- Group B: 14 weeks on fluoxetine, followed by 36 weeks on placebo.
- Group C: 38 weeks on fluoxetine, then 12 weeks on placebo.
- Group D: 50 weeks on fluoxetine.

Relapse rates were significantly reduced among the patients on continued fluoxetine treatment (group D) compared with those who were switched to placebo after the open 12–14 week period of active drug treatment (group A). Group B also showed significantly higher relapse rates than group D, whereas the difference in relapse rates between groups C and D was smaller and not statistically significant. The authors concluded that patients "treated with fluoxetine for 12 weeks whose depressive symptoms remit should continue treatment with fluoxetine for at least an additional 26 weeks to minimize the risk of relapse" (Reimherr *et al.*, 1998).

Placebo-controlled long-term trials can also produce additional clinically relevant information. Thus, in a trial of 18 months of treatment with recently hypomanic or manic bipolar patients, both lamotrigine and lithium were superior to placebo at prolonging the time to further mood episodes, i.e. both drugs prevented relapse or recurrence. However, the study also showed that lamotrigine was superior to placebo regarding the prolongation of the time to the next depressive episode, whereas lithium was superior to placebo in prolonging the time to the next manic episode (Calabrese *et al.*, 2002).

Generally speaking, success of placebo-controlled *relapse prevention trials* depends on:

- The duration of a trial: the longer the study, the higher the chances of differentiation between active drug and placebo.
- The homogeneity of the patient population studied.
- The probability of relapse: the previous pattern of relapses is the best predictor for further relapses.

A much discussed approach to the study of disease-modifying treatment effects, e.g. in degenerative disorders such as Alzheimer's disease, is the *randomized placebo-phase lead-in* design. This design is intended to address the question of whether subjects who begin active treatment earlier in the course of their disease have a stronger (or more sustained) response to a pharmacological intervention than those who start treatment later. Patients enter the active treatment phase after being assigned randomly to a period of time (from several months up to a year) on placebo treatment. Groups of patients are then switched blindly from placebo to active drug (Feldman *et al.*, 2001). A stronger and better sustained therapeutic response seen in patients switched to active medication earlier in time would suggest an effect on the progression of the disorder, i.e. a potential disease-modifying drug action. However, the randomized placebo phase needed for this design raises some ethical questions: it is certainly not acceptable to delay treatment in cases of potentially life-threatening diseases, although this design may be able to provide relevant information about the optimal onset of treatment in a chronic, progressive disease.

5.4.4 *ALTERNATIVES TO PLACEBO-CONTROLLED DESIGNS*

Given the ethical concerns about placebo-controlled study designs, several alternative procedures to reduce bias in clinical trials have been proposed:

- Use of historical (placebo) data.
- Comparison of current treatment with waiting list.
- Comparison of the new with an established standard treatment.

Use of Historical (Placebo) Data

This option assumes a comparable or even standard placebo response rate for historical data and the current trial. The historical improvement rate (on placebo or without any treatment) is then used for purposes of comparison with results of subsequent non-placebo-controlled studies involving the same investigator and protocol design but different drugs. For historical placebo response data it is recommended that a small placebo treatment arm is used for safety data purposes and to avoid observer bias – although this proposal may resolve or diminish some ethical concerns, it raises a number of scientific problems:

- The approach neglects the fact that placebo or no-drug treatment responses are dependent on a number of factors that are likely to change over time.
- Expectations on the part of doctors and patients regarding treatment effects change over time.
- The clinical and/or comorbidity profile of the same disease can change within a limited period, increasing or decreasing the chances of a new treatment.

In summary, and as supported by the shifting placebo response rates quoted earlier, use of historical placebo or no-treatment data does not appear to be a reliable alternative to the use of concurrent placebo.

Comparison of Current Treatment with Waiting List

Instead of using a placebo treatment arm, this approach compares a treated patient population with subjects receiving no treatment at all (see Fig. 5.4). Assuming that the status of patients remains unchanged or does not deteriorate during the waiting period, this approach may be permissible in cases of less severe diseases. However, there are several significant downsides of so-called waiting list comparisons:

- From a therapeutic aspect the 'no treatment' condition provides much less attention to patients' problems than participation in a placebo treatment arm.
- Spontaneous fluctuations of symptoms are not usually assessed during the waiting list period.
- Living longer with the prevailing symptoms may have a negative 'disease-modifying effect' and demoralize a patient, hence contributing to a self-down-rating bias.

5.4.5   COMPARISONS WITH ACTIVE COMPARATOR DRUGS

Direct comparison of a new compound with an active drug used in the same indication can provide the following information:

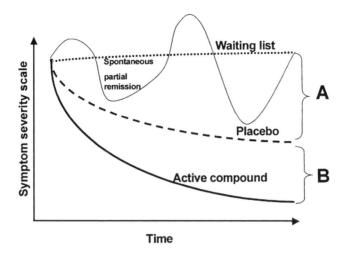

Figure 5.4 Theoretical comparison of results of a placebo-controlled trial compared with the 'waiting list' or no-treatment approach: A, placebo effect; B, effect size of treatment; A+B, clinical effect

- Equivalence of the new drug with standard (established) treatment.
- Superiority of the new drug over standard (established) comparator treatment.
- Non-inferiority of the new drug compared with established treatment.

Equivalence trials aim to show that the effects of two treatments differ by no more than a specific amount. To show the equivalence, two one-sided statistical tests are performed to ascertain that the new treatment is not inferior to the established active treatment and that the established treatment is not inferior to the new drug. The allowed tolerance is known as the equivalence margin (δ). In an equivalence trial, if the effects of the two treatments differ by more than the equivalence margin in either direction, the assumption of equivalence does not hold. When comparing a new psychotropic treatment with an active comparator, the hypothesis usually being tested is the assumption of *non-inferiority* of the new drug (predefined as an a priory equivalence margin) in one-sided statistical tests: the aim is to show that the experimental treatment is not inferior to the active control by more than the equivalence margin. Demonstration of equivalence is not requested by health authorities, except in some specific indications outside of psychiatry.

A finding of no significant difference in outcome between two treatments is ambiguous unless a non-inferiority design is used. Two-arm non-inferiority designs require much larger sample sizes to test adequately the statistical hypothesis of no true difference in efficacy between a test and reference drug.

Small differences in efficacy are very hard to detect using a two-arm study design because of the inherently large variance of psychopharmacological studies.

The results of a non-inferiority design trial can lead to one of the following conclusions:

- The new drug is non-inferior to the standard treatment (see Box 5.6).
- The new drug failed to show the non-inferiority criterion to the standard treatment.
- The new drug is superior to the standard treatment.

An adequately powered trial initially designed to demonstrate the non-inferiority of a new compound compared with a standard treatment can also demonstrate the superiority of the new compound provided that a statistically significant difference in favor of the new treatment was detected. However, trials intended to show the superiority of one of the treatments cannot be interpreted, in the case of a statistically non-significant difference, as showing non-inferiority of the new chemical entity compared with the standard treatment.

Box 5.6   Amisulpride vs. Paroxetine: a Non-inferiority Trial

A non-inferiority trial was designed to show that amisulpride is not clinically less efficacious than a widely used antidepressant. Paroxetine was chosen as the reference compound because of its recognized efficacy in major depression. A 15% difference in response rates was predefined as clinically acceptable and methodologically justifiable because it is smaller than the average difference in response rates between paroxetine and placebo reported in the literature. A total of 277 so-called double-depressed patients (major depression with comorbidity of dysphoria) were randomized to paroxetine (20 mg/day) or to amisulpride (50 mg/day). A high response rate was achieved in both groups: there were 76% responders in the amisulpride group and 84% in the paroxetine group by week 8, the difference being 8% and the 95% upper limit being 15.7%. Because the upper limit of the confidence interval included the predefined non-inferiority margin, the null hypothesis of a clinically relevant difference was rejected and amisulpride was considered to be non-inferior to paroxetine in the treatment of double depression (Cassano *et al.*, 2002).

Selecting the Dose of an Active Comparator

Active comparators are used in placebo-controlled trials primarily to validate the study results. In addition, the effect size seen with an active comparator provides guidance concerning the effect size of the new treatment in comparison with an established treatment. In studies without a placebo arm and not demonstrating a significant difference, it is often not possible to determine whether the lack of difference was due to equal effectiveness of the treatments or the result of a type II error, i.e., the erroneous assumption that there was no difference between treatments (although in fact there was a difference).

A crucial issue in comparative trials is to choose the appropriate dose range of the comparator drug. Inappropriate doses of the standard drug, e.g. doses outside the recommended range, will lead to inconclusive results or to biased competitive advantages (Safer, 2002). A trial with hypericum perforatum compared with placebo and sertraline in the treatment of major depressive disorder provides an example: this outpatient study in moderately-severe depressed patients failed to show significant differences between hypericum and placebo treatment on the HRSD but also failed to demonstrate significant differences between sertraline and placebo. Response rates were 38.1%, 50% and 48.6% for hypericum, placebo and sertraline, respectively. The dosage schedule allowed a maximum daily dose of 1800 mg of hypericum, whereas the dose of sertraline was restricted to 100 mg/day (although the recommended dose range is 50–200 mg/day). Given the unwarranted dose limitation for sertraline and the non-significant differences between the three treatments, the study results are inconclusive and much time, effort and money was essentially wasted (Hypericum Depression Trial Study Group, 2002).

Safety and partly efficacy outcomes of several comparative antipsychotic drug trials were biased by the implementation of unnecessarily high doses of haloperidol (20 mg/day or more). Meta-analysis of data from more than 12 000 patients included in 52 randomized trials comparing atypical antipsychotics (amisulpride, clozapine, olanzapine, quetiapine, risperidone and sertindole) with conventional compounds (usually haloperidol or chlorpromazine) led to the conclusion that doses of haloperidol of greater than 12 mg/day produced fewer favorable symptom changes than doses of less than 12 mg/day (Geddes et al., 2000). If the doses of haloperidol were restricted to a maximum of 12 mg/day, atypical antipsychotics had no more clear-cut advantages in terms of efficacy or overall tolerability but still caused fewer extrapyramidal side effects. Doses of haloperidol above 10 mg/day produce no better clinical response than the dose range of 4–10 mg/day (Baldessarini et al., 1988; Rifkin et al., 1991).

Some published examples illustrating the use of (biasing) high doses of standard drug are trials with risperidone in the treatment of schizophrenia, with haloperidol used as a comparator (Chouinard et al., 1993; Marder and

Meibach, 1994). In these comparisons the high doses of haloperidol ensured that the investigational new atypical antipsychotic had a better extrapyramidal side-effect profile than the conventional antipsychotic.

5.4.6   WITHIN-PATIENT DESIGNS

Single-case Design

The purpose of within-patient designs is to reduce variability between patients by using the study subjects as their own controls. This design can be used only in diseases having a chronic course, or in cases of recurrence of disease episodes within a reasonable period of time. Intensive and systematic tracking of a small number of patients who are put, for example, on active drug and placebo at variable and randomized intervals can provide valuable information about the efficacy and safety profile of a new drug. An example is the treatment of chronic primary or secondary sleep disturbance, where the episodic improvement due to a hypnotic drug will not solve the sleep disorder for a longer period. Results of single-case studies can be useful for early hypothesis testing; however, the strong impact of each individual's response and of the very specific experimental conditions on the results need to be considered.

Crossover Designs

A randomized crossover design has theoretical appeal because it eliminates the largest source of experimental variance: interindividual variability. This could significantly enhance statistical power and permit much smaller samples sizes to detect a treatment effect. Unfortunately, a crossover design is appropriate only in rare cases in psychopharmacology, namely in studies:

- dealing with chronic stable conditions
- where within-subject variability is expected to be less than between-subject variability
- if patients return to the baseline condition after each therapeutic intervention

However, if the response to the first treatment is likely to affect the second one ('carryover effect'), the results of a trial may be jeopardized. Carryover effects from earlier to subsequent treatment can be corrected partially by random assignment of patients to the sequence of treatments used. Nevertheless, in the case of a significant degree of carryover effect (as is the case in therapeutic trials leading to definite symptom resolution or remission), a parallel-group design is clearly preferable for a reliable estimation of treatment effects (Willam and Pater, 1986). Pharmacological carryover effects between two active compounds can be reduced by inserting a placebo period after the first treatment. The

Group I	Drug A	Drug B	Placebo
Group II	Drug B	Placebo	Drug A
Group III	Placebo	Drug A	Drug B

Figure 5.5 Illustration of a 3×3 Latin Square design: trial of two different drugs and placebo

duration of the placebo period then has to be justified based on the pharmacokinetic properties of the compounds involved (Senn, 1994).

Latin Square Design

This is an extension of the crossover design that applies in situations where more than two treatment conditions are being evaluated. Each subject receives each treatment successively but in a different sequence. This design can be used in the case of single-dose experimental trials, such as studies of cognitive function, psychomotor performance, psychophysiological responses, etc. in healthy volunteers (Chapter 3) but also in therapeutic short-term trials of hypnotics or anxiolytics.

5.4.7 METHODOLOGY TO MINIMIZE BIAS IN OPEN-LABEL TRIALS

In some situations double-blind placebo-controlled trials are not acceptable from an ethical standpoint; examples are studies on patients in life-threatening conditions such as severe withdrawal symptoms (e.g. delirium tremens) or diseases with a high risk of suicide. To keep double-blind conditions in long-term treatment may also be difficult or even impossible, e.g. if one of the drugs used needs special safety monitoring or if the side-effect profile requires special treatment considerations.

In this situation the use of trial-independent, blinded raters assessing the primary endpoints of a study can ensure unbiased ratings, although it will not eliminate other confounding factors operating during a trial.

Independent blinded raters are health professionals from a different department or from outside, with no information about details of the treatment studied. Their involvement in the trial is limited to providing ratings for the primary study endpoint(s).

Independent endpoint committees are groups of experts who, based on blinded and standardized reports, decide whether specific event(s) reported for a patient meet the criteria of a defined primary endpoint. Examples of endpoints are imminent need of hospitalization, suicide attempt, etc. (see Box 5.7).

5.4.8 LONGITUDINAL STUDY DESIGNS

In principle three different types of questions require long-term studies:

(1) Does a given treatment provide benefit in terms of *prevention of relapse*? This question can be approached with a design of open-label acute (symptomatic) treatment followed by a double-blind, placebo-controlled period, randomizing responders to acute treatment into a maintenance treatment or into a placebo arm. An *'enrichment design'* (enriching the sample for responders) of this kind has inherent limitations regarding the generalizability of results, because only responders in the open treatment phase are included in the long-term continuation, and attrition during the open-label treatment phase may reach 50% or more. An alternative to the enrichment design is to randomize patients to active drug or placebo maintenance treatment arms in an inter-episode period, i.e. at a time when they are remitted from the disorder.

(2) What is the *minimum duration of maintenance treatment* providing clinical benefit, e.g. to prevent relapse or recurrence of a depressive episode (see p. 277 f.; Reimherr *et al.*, 1998)? The design addressing this issue is similar to the previous one but with different durations of active-maintenance treatment arms compared with a full-time placebo treatment arm.

(3) In cases of chronic disease, does early treatment initiation provide benefit for the long-term outcome of the disease, i.e. does the treatment have a *disease-modifying effect*? Questions of this type are often asked with regard to the drug treatment of attention deficit hyperactivity disorder (Rappaport *et al.*, 1998) or early drug treatment of high-risk children from parents with affective disorders (Duffy, 2000) and schizophrenia (Cornblatt, 2002; McGorry *et al.*, 2002). Evidence from both retrospective and prospective studies suggests that a longer duration of untreated psychosis in the early stages of schizophrenia is associated with a prolonged time to remission, with lower levels of recovery, a greater likelihood of relapse and poorer overall outcome. Early intervention and optimal maintenance treatment are thought to improve the long-term course of schizophrenia (Sheitman and Lieberman, 1998).

The ethical and methodological issues of long-term placebo-controlled designs are basically the same as in shorter trials. However, long-term studies pose

Box 5.7   An Open-label Comparative Trial with Blinded Assessments

A recent example of how rater bias can be reduced in an open-label comparative trial is given in a comparative study between clozapine and olanzapine with regard to their effect on suicidality in patients with schizophrenia and schizoaffective disorder with a high risk of suicide (Meltzer *et al.*, 2003). Because one of the medications used in this prospective, randomized parallel-group trial requires regular blood monitoring for safety reasons, the study was open-label. Its duration was 2 years in order to provide time to obtain a sufficient number of endpoints to differentiate between the two treatments. Two approaches were used to minimize the bias of the open-label treatment conditions upon assessments: blinded ratings of clinical status by specifically trained, study-independent assessors; and determination of whether certain actions and events met the criteria for a suicide attempt or hospitalization to prevent suicide. The second assessment was performed by an independent expert Suicide Monitoring Board (SMB) who had no contact with the participating sites, i.e. neither with the patients nor the medical staff involved.

Significant differences were observed with regard to all primary outcome measures:

(1) A hazard ratio of 0.76 was established for suicide attempts or hospitalizations as determined by the SMB for the clozapine-treated patients, i.e. suicide events were reduced by 24% ($P = 0.03$) compared with olanzapine.
(2) The cumulative probability of a suicide attempt or hospitalization to prevent a suicide was significantly different by Kaplan–Meier estimates ($P < 0.02$) in favor of clozapine.
(3) Actual suicide attempts were made by 6.9% of clozapine- and 11.2% of olanzapine-treated patients ($P < 0.05$), and 16.7% of patients on clozapine vs. 21.8% on olanzapine ($P < 0.05$) required hospitalization to prevent suicide as determined by the SMB.

In the total sample of 609 patients the mean (SD) prescribed dosages of study drugs were 16.8 (7.4) mg for olanzapine and 306 (166) mg for clozapine.

added complexities, some of which remain unresolved despite growing emphasis on continuation and maintenance treatment in several areas of psychopharmacology. Because long-term placebo administration is not feasible in a number of conditions, several types of single-blind designs have been proposed, none of them able to provide fully satisfactory answers. An often used procedure is periodically to discontinue and/or replace active drug treatment with placebo. Another type of longitudinal study is the 'mirrored image' trial, in which the course of illness during the study treatment is compared with the course of illness during an equivalent period of prior treatment with another drug or no treatment at all. These designs can provide some useful information about a drug's long-term efficacy but are not regarded as being conclusive due to the lack of a concurrent control group (Wyatt, 1991).

Longitudinal, non-blinded observation studies are a practical way to accrue much valuable safety data during chronic use of a new drug. In the case of bipolar disorder, or more generally in the case of cyclic mental diseases, a life-charting methodology can provide relevant data concerning the influence on the course of disease of the introduction of a new drug as monotherapy or in an add-on manner (Leverich and Post, 1993).

5.4.9 CASE–CONTROL STUDIES

In contrast to the previously discussed prospective trial designs, case–control studies are retrospective in nature. Clinically defined *cases*, e.g. patients treated with a specific drug for a given time, are compared with matched *controls*, i.e. patients with the same diagnosis, age, gender, etc. but treated with another drug or not treated at all. Control subjects are selected from existing databases containing information on patients from the same population observed at the same time as the cases. Case–control studies can provide evidence about treatment effects as well as information on whether a particular intervention was effective to prevent serious or fatal outcomes. Two published examples illustrate the importance of case–control studies in psychopharmacology:

- In the 1970s a strong association had been suggested between *in utero* exposition to lithium treatment of pregnant women and a particular damage (Ebstein's anomaly) to the heart in the offspring. The relative risk for Ebstein's anomaly among such children was estimated to be 400 (i.e. 400 times higher!) on the basis of data collected in a registry of spontaneously reported cases. However, subsequent controlled (case–control) epidemiological studies consistently showed a lower risk. In four independent case–control studies of Ebstein's anomaly involving more than 200 affected children, no mothers who had taken lithium during pregnancy were found. Thus, although initial information regarding the teratogenic risk of lithium treatment was derived from spontaneous, uncontrolled reports,

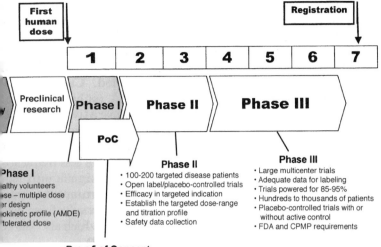

First human dose

Registration

| 1 | 2 | 3 | 4 | 5 | 6 | 7 |

Preclinical research

Phase I

PoC

Phase II

Phase III

Phase I
- Healthy volunteers
- Se – multiple dose
- er design
- okinetic profile (AMDE)
- tolerated dose

Phase II
- 100-200 targeted disease patients
- Open label/placebo-controlled trials
- Efficacy in targeted indication
- Establish the targeted dose-range and titration profile
- Safety data collection

Phase III
- Large multicenter trials
- Adequate data for labeling
- Trials powered for 85-95%
- Hundreds to thousands of patients
- Placebo-controlled trials with or without active control
- FDA and CPMP requirements

Proof of Concept
- 40-80 Patients
- Biological/clinical markers
- Efficacy/safety measures
- Statistically not highly powered trials
- Adaptive or other innovative designs

Phases of clinical drug development: from drug discovery to Phase III pivotal

Required duration of toxicology studies to support clinical Phase I, II and III

f human trial	Rodent study	Non-rodent study
inical Phase I and II Trials		
	2–4 weeks	2 weeks
eks	2–4 weeks	2 weeks
onth	1 month	1 month
onths	3 months	3 months
onths	6 months	6 months
n 6 months	6 months	Chronic
inical Phase III Trials		
eks	4 weeks	4 weeks
onth	3 months	3 months
onths	6 months	6 months
n 3 months	6 months	Chronic

Industry. M3 Non-clinical Safety Studies for the Conduct of Human Clinical Trials for icals (www.fda.gov/cder.guidance).

systematically collected data from case–contr
that the teratogenic risk of first-trimester lithiu
than previously suggested (Cohen *et al.*, 1994

- The potential impact on suicidality of diffe
analyzed in a study of 61 suicide victims with
than 27 000 admissions during a 20-year peri
were matched for age, gender and diagnosis
disorder) at the time of discharge. This comp
significant differences between the treatment
with the non-suicidal patients: lorazepam witho
more frequent and the use of mood-stabilizers
schizophrenic suicide victims. Lithium was give
non-suicidal patients than to patients who then
et al., 2002). These findings are consonant with
of prospective, placebo-controlled lithium trials
suicidal effect of lithium (Baldessarini *et al.*, 19

5.5 PHASES OF DRUG DEVELOPMENT

5.5.1 PHASE I CLINICAL TRIALS: TOLERABILITY,
PHARMACOKINETICS, HUMAN PHARMA(

Tolerability and Pharmacokinetic Trials

The testing of a new psychotropic substance in
investigations into its tolerability. These are usu
subjects who are informed about the aims and po
who then volunteer to participate in the trial for so
Tolerability trials call for close medical supervision
any emergencies, even though the first doses of the r
in man, based as they are on the results of animal ex
they generally have no effect at all. The dosage is in
to keep the risk for the volunteers as low as possibl

A human single-dose exposition trial must be prec
and 2-week non-rodent toxicity studies. The animal
incremental by exposition: for up to 1 month the Ph
1-month rodent and 1-month non-rodent toxicity stu

Because this is the first time the new drug is bein
beings, only a small number of individuals will be
persons may be involved. First tolerability trials co
without placebo control until dosages are reached
become apparent. However, owing to the nature of

possible expectancies on the part of subjects and investigators (*nocebo effect*), only placebo-controlled conditions will provide a reliable impression about the pharmacological activity of the new compound. At this very early stage of clinical development, tolerability problems will serve as a clear no-go decision criterion. It should be noted, however, that the tolerability profile of psychotropic drugs given as single doses to healthy volunteers is likely to vary from what is seen in psychiatric patients on repeated-dose administration; as a rule, antipsychotics and antimanic compounds are usually better tolerated by patients than by healthy subjects.

Although it is not normally feasible to include comprehensive psychological or psychophysiological testing during the first tolerability trials, because medical aspects have to be paramount at this stage, it is possible to determine with considerable reliability any pronounced central actions of a substance as well as the approximate duration of such effects. Examples are effects on vigilance, attention, concentration and potential side effects such as sedation, stimulation, euphoric effects, etc. Further data also will be available as to the effects of the preparation on vital functions such as ECG, respiration and circulation, as well as on biochemical laboratory tests, liver enzyme and renal functions.

Within the context of initial tolerability testing, blood samples should be taken from the subjects at predetermined intervals of time. Tests are then conducted to determine if, when and in what concentrations the substance and its metabolites are detectable in the blood, when peak blood levels are reached and the way in which they decrease (Section 5.3.2). These data make it possible to establish more precisely the intervals that should elapse between doses during later studies involving repeated administration of the substance.

Initial Dose and Dose Escalation in Early Human Studies

The first dose administered to man is a fraction of the 'no-effect' dose or no adverse event level (NOAEL) determined in animal toxicology studies. Typically the first human dose is 1/25 to 1/100 of the NOAEL in mg/kg. So-called allometric scales are used by clinical pharmacologists to estimate human doses from toxicology findings. *Allometric scaling* is expected to optimise predictions from one species to another; it takes into account body weight, clearance, volume of distribution and elimination half-life (Mahmood and Balian, 1999). Several methods are then available to determine the increments during dose escalation. Depending on the pharmacological profile and toxicological findings in animal studies, three different schemes are recommended: doubling the dose at each step; increasing the dose in a logarithmic manner; and using the Fibonacci scheme (1, 2, 3, 5, 8, etc.). A pharmacologically guided dose escalation is based on PK–PD considerations: when comparing the animal and human doses, equal toxicity is expected for equal drug exposure. The doses are adjusted based on unbound ('free') plasma concentrations of the molecule.

Early Multiple-dose Studies

The aim of these trials is to establish the tolerability and pharmacokinetic profile of a new drug on a small number of healthy volunteers after multiple doses. The administration scheme of the drug is driven by the previous animal and single-dose human pharmacokinetic data. In the case of a plasma half-life of less than 10 h the administration should be twice daily (b.i.d.), for a shorter plasma half-life it should be three times daily (t.i.d.). This approach has importance only in drugs used potentially for chronic administration (depression, anxiety, psychosis, etc.); hypnotics with typical episodic use do not require this approach. Additional PK–PD information can be obtained during early multiple-dose trials by combining blood sampling with pharmacodynamic parameters such as pharmaco-EEG, evoked potentials, endocrine parameters, reaction time, cognitive tests, etc.

The Bridging Approach: Phase I Trials in Patients

In some instances, patients may respond differently to healthy young or older volunteers. Separate studies are then needed to determine the maximum tolerated dose (MTD) in the target patient population with '*bridging studies*' prior to designing Phase II efficacy trials. Well-controlled safety/tolerability trials with a small number of patients on an inpatient basis are performed to establish the population- and disease-specific MTD and to characterize the most frequent adverse events. Early studies in patients can be used also to investigate PK–PD relationships, to optimize the dosing regimen for subsequent trials, to confirm that the drug is affecting the targeted receptor and to measure correlations between drug activity and potential surrogate markers.

5.5.2   PROOF-OF-CONCEPT (PoC) TRIALS (PHASE IIa TRIALS)

A *proof-of-concept* (*PoC*) *study* is a "human clinical trial that provides scientifically sound evidence supporting the postulated effect(s) of a new therapeutic product in human, where effects may be relevant pharmacological or disease biomarkers, surrogate endpoints, or clinical assessments, and may be beneficial and/or toxic in nature" (Lesko *et al.*, 2000). The terms *proof of principle* and *proof of concept* are sometimes used interchangeably, although PoC occurs generally earlier in drug development than proof of principle. The PoC trials are designed to provide evidence that a pharmacological model is reliable and predictive and that a pharmacological treatment paradigm may be feasible. The PoC trials comprise:

- *Proof-of-mechanism* (PoM) trials: the objective is to demonstrate the mechanism of action of a new compound using biological markers. A frequent question in early drug development is whether the new compound penetrates the blood–brain barrier. Targeted radiotracer displacement studies (with isotope-labeled receptor agonists or antagonists), changes in brain glucose metabolism measured by single-photon-emission computed tomography (SPECT) methods (Chapter 6) or general non-specific changes detected by functional MRI or pharmaco-EEG methods can provide early information about the blood–brain barrier penetration and basic mechanisms of action of a molecule. The sample size of PoM studies is usually limited to 10–20 persons.
- *Proof-of-efficacy* trials: these studies should provide, within a limited time frame and with a low-cost program, sufficient information for a go/no-go decision concerning efficacy and safety aspects of a new compound. The traditional approaches are Phase IIb trials based on placebo-controlled dose-finding designs. These studies need relatively high power, which means the inclusion of several dozen to several hundred patients.

Challenge Paradigms in PoC Trials

The aim of challenge paradigms is to evoke specific, transient mental alterations or symptoms in healthy volunteers or patients under controlled experimental conditions, allowing the effect of treatment on the symptoms provoked to be investigated. As an example, challenge paradigms to investigate the antipanic effect of anxiolytics have good predictive validity. Thus, antipanic drugs (imipramine, clomipramine, several SSRIs) show significant action on CO_2-*induced panic hyperreactivity* (Perna *et al.*, 2002). Relatively small groups (20 patients per treatment arm) are sufficient to provide satisfactory predictive results. Some more challenge tests used in anxiety disorder are shown in Table 5.3.

The CO_2 *inhalation challenge* and *sodium lactate infusion challenge* paradigms show high specificity for panic disorder but less sensitivity than the *cholecystokinin* (*CCK*) or *methyl-chlorophenylpiperazine* (*mCPP*) *challenge* tests, which are also able to provoke panic symptoms and anxiety in healthy volunteers. *Flumazenil* – a benzodiazepine antagonist – can provoke panic attacks in some panic disorder patients but with lower sensitivity than sodium lactate infusion, CO_2 or CCK.

The alpha-2-adrenoreceptor antagonist *yohimbine* increases adrenergic activity and may provoke anxiety and panic symptoms in patients but no or only mild symptoms in healthy volunteers. Yohimbine infusions evoke intrusive symptoms, i.e. flashbacks together with significant increase of

Table 5.3 Challenge tests in anxiety disorders

	Panic	Social phobia	Generalized anxiety disorder	Post-traumatic stress disorder	Obsessive–compulsive disorder
CCK-4, CCK-8, pentagastrin	+ + +	+ +	+		
Sodium lactate	+ + +	+/–	–/+	–	
CO_2	+ + +	+ +	–	–	
Flumazenil	+	–/+	?	?	
mCPP	+ + +		+ +	+ + prolactin and cortisol response	+ + +
Fenfluramine	+/–	+		+ + prolactin response	
Yohimbine	+ +	+ +	–	+ + +	

Data from: Charney *et al.*, 1989; Targum, 1990; Tancer *et al.*, 1994; Potts *et al.*, 1996; vanVliet *et al.*, 1997; Strohle *et al.*, 1998; Goddard *et al.*, 1999; Southwick *et al.*, 1999; Coupland *et al.*, 2000; Rinne *et al.*, 2000; Jetty *et al.*, 2001; Bell *et al.*, 2002.
+ + +, strong predictive value, challenge-paradigm-provoked panic/anxiety symptoms are attenuated by different compunds; + +, modest predictive value, data suggest attenuation of challenge-paradigm-provoked panic/anxiety symptoms by a few compunds; +, weak predictive value, data suggest weak attenuation of challenge-paradigm-provoked panic/anxiety symptoms; –, no predictive value; +/–, inconclusive data; ?, no data available.

anxiety symptoms in patients with post-traumatic stress disorder (PTSD). *Fenfluramine*, a serotonin-releasing compound, evokes anxiety similar to generalized anxiety in panic disorder patients.

Selective serotonin reuptake inhibitors (SSRIs), clonazepam and alprazolam attenuate the panic attacks occurring in CO_2 and CCK challenge paradigms and thus support the predictive validity of these tests. Only limited data are available about potential antipanic compounds with mechanisms of action different from those of SSRIs and benzodiazepines, such as the GABAergic anticonvulsant including vigabatrin (Zwanzger *et al.*, 2001). A comprehensive hypothesis suggests that both CO_2 and lactate induce panic states by triggering a suffocation false-alarm in individuals with a hypersensitive 'suffocation detector'. An advantage of the CO_2 and the CCK challenge paradigms is their relatively good tolerability: both methods provoke a panic attack for 1–2 min (which is dose-dependent in the case of CCK), i.e. much shorter than a 'real' panic attack. The discomfort caused by mCPP or lactate extends much longer, leading to higher dropout rates among both patients or healthy volunteers after the first and before the second challenge test in a crossover study design.

The *scopolamine challenge* paradigm is a frequently used model for the investigation of impairment of attention and memory, and for modeling some aspects of Alzheimer's disease. Effects of oxiracetam in this paradigm were demonstrated in a placebo-controlled crossover study: this nootropic drug attenuated the negative effects of scopolamine on cognitive performance, with a statistically significant difference from placebo at a dose of 1600 mg on delayed recall of word lists; it also showed dose-related antagonism of scopolamine-induced impairments on semantic memory and attention (Preda *et al.*, 1993).

A promising approach is to study the effects of a scopolamine challenge on performance in a face-name-associative encoding paradigm, with functional MRI brain scanning providing a direct signal of the activity of the anatomic regions involved. In a crossover placebo-controlled trial with 0.4 mg of scopolamine and 1.0 mg of lorazepam in healthy volunteers, significant decreases were seen in both the extent and magnitude of activation within the hippocampal, fusiform and inferior prefrontal brain regions (Sperling *et al.*, 2002), which may mimic some of the alterations typical of Alzheimer's disease.

General Remarks on PoC Studies

Proof-of-concept studies with a new compound are recommended provided that:

(1) The scientific basis of a compound is sound and its basic pharmacokinetic parameters look promising.
(2) The compound is novel and may lead to a truly innovative treatment.
(3) Early exploratory data are required and sufficient for a go/no-go decision.

Pharmacological and methodological requirements to launch PoC trials are as follows:

- The modeling of a new – hypothetical – pharmacological action can be based on a well-defined homogeneous population representing a highly homogeneous diagnostic category, possibly characterized by well-defined biomarker(s).
- There are well-defined, valid endpoints (biomarkers and/or clinical measures) to assess the hypothetical action of the investigated compound. Although biomarkers are preferred in PoC trials, the number of these markers is limited in psychopharmacology; for this reason clinical outcomes are often used as endpoints in PoC trials.
- The detectable signal provides sufficient qualitative or quantitative information about the effect of the new compound to allow reliable go/no-go decisions about further development.
- In view of the limited sample size of PoC trials, minimization of bias and control of unspecific effects are essential; double-blind, randomized, placebo-controlled studies are the rule.

- Approachable methodology is required for PoC studies. Close collaboration between the study sponsor and the research institutes providing the research methodology is mandatory.

The combination of sophisticated challenge paradigms with biomarker detection provides new and technically advanced quantitative opportunities for PoC trials. However, objective and balanced evaluation of PoC and PoM paradigms sometimes may be hindered by publication bias: trials with negative or inconclusive outcome tend to be published less frequently than studies with positive outcome, a fact that can mislead readers with regard to the predictive validity of certain models.

5.5.3   LATER PHASE II (IIb) AND III TRIALS

Overview

Late Phase II (sometimes called IIb) trials are aimed at identifying the optimal dose to be used in Phase III trials and, ideally, to identify those compounds that will not make it through the next phase of development. Typically, these trials are double-blind and have placebo controls. Compared with Phase I trials, where the primary objective is to establish the tolerability limits of a new compound, Phase II type trials are dedicated to establish efficacy data in patients. This includes clarifying the effective and safe dosage range for single and repeated administration, defining the precise pattern of action, including side effects under hospital and outpatient conditions, and the question as to whether the new substance possesses sufficient advantages over existing drugs to make its introduction on the market medically and commercially advisable.

Phase III studies represent the confirmatory phase of drug development, which takes several years and usually involves several thousand patients at multiple trial centers. Large patient numbers are required in these trials to provide convincing documentation of clinical efficacy and safety, a more complete adverse event profile and covariates and estimates of variability in dose–response relationship due to individual differences in pharmacokinetics and pharmacodynamics. They are aimed at definitively determining a drug's effectiveness and side-effect profile. Most of these studies are double-blind and placebo-controlled, sometimes with the option of open-label long-term extensions.

Dose–Response Trials

A typical feature of Phase IIb are dose–response trials regarding a drug's safety, efficacy and side effects. No single study design can address all aspects of dose–response relationships for a new drug, and so a number of different trials are needed, each supplying complementary information. Multiple-dose randomized clinical trials (RCTs) can be particularly rich sources of information because they compare different dosages of the test drug concurrently in the same study. In addition, optimal dosage schedules and therapeutic dose ranges for a new drug must be determined in different patient populations. Study designs that compare either different fixed doses or different dose ranges of a drug are used to obtain this information.

Fixed-dose (Dose-finding) Designs

Fixed-dose studies using multiple dose arms have gained popularity for evaluating dose–response relationships. A fixed-dose design can be implemented if the patients to be studied are diagnostically homogeneous and if their therapeutic responses are expected to be similar. Multiple fixed-dose trials are often used to establish optimal 'effectiveness', i.e. an optimal balance between efficacy and safety of a drug. Fixed-dose study designs have some obvious advantages over flexible-dose approaches:

• It is not necessary to determine or assume milligram equivalence between the experimental and the reference drugs used.
• Dosage and time factors are independent of each other so that time to response can be assessed better.
• It is possible to determine, within the range of the doses studied, an optimal fixed dose for the new drug, allowing the study of the relationship of plasma drug concentrations to both clinical response and side effects.

On the other hand, multiple fixed-dose designs have one definite drawback: because the doses cannot be adjusted to the individual patients' needs, the risk of patients dropping out of a study, due to insufficient efficacy or significant adverse events, particularly in the first few weeks of treatment, is relatively high.

Some typical, published examples of multiple fixed-dose studies are:

(1) A trial comparing 10, 20, 40 and 60 mg/day of citalopram and placebo in the treatment of moderate-to-severe major depression. This study showed that the 40 and 60 mg dose arms had significantly superior efficacy in comparison with placebo (Feighner and Overo, 1999).
(2) A trial comparing daily doses of 50, 100 and 200 mg sertraline with placebo for 12 weeks in patients with panic disorder. No consistent evidence of a dose–response effect was found because all three doses of sertraline produced significant efficacy compared with placebo and, surprisingly, there was no significant between-dose difference with regard to discontinuations due to adverse events (Asheikh *et al.*, 2000).

(3) A four-arm trial of fluoxetine in the treatment of OCD designed to compare 20, 40 and 60 mg/day of fluoxetine and placebo during a 13-week period. The results indicated greater efficacy of the 60 mg/day dose, suggesting that the optimal dose of fluoxetine is higher in the treatment of OCD than in depression (Tollefson *et al.*, 1994).
(4) A three-arm trial during six menstrual cycles evaluating the efficacy and safety of fluoxetine treatment of premenstrual dysphoria. Both 20 and 60 mg/day were significantly more effective than placebo, without any salient benefit of the higher dose; however, the women on 60 mg/day of fluoxetine reported significantly more side effects than those at the lower dose or placebo. Based on the results of this three-arm fixed-dose and similar trials, the recommended dose in this indication is 20 mg of fluoxetine (Steiner *et al.*, 1995).

These examples demonstrate the heuristic value of fixed-dose comparative studies, which admittedly do not reproduce clinical reality, characterized by individual dose adjustment according to patient response.

Dose-titration Designs

Dose-titration studies, i.e. trials with adaptation of doses to the needs of individual patients, are a closer approximation to actual clinical practice and arguably can provide a better assessment of dosage and therapeutic benefit of a drug for patient populations treated in usual practice settings. This approach is preferable if the homogeneity of a patient population cannot be assumed *a priori* (e.g. inclusion of patients with rapid cycling, non-rapid cycling, euphoria or mixed states in a study of bipolar mania), or if the severity of symptomatology varies within a very wide range. Advantages of a dose-titration design are as follows:

• Individual dose titration to a desired clinical effect, or until side effects occur, mirrors the actual clinical management of patients.
• Use of both a placebo and individually optimized reference control treatment allows an estimation of what has been termed 'assay sensitivity'.
• The design provides a more realistic answer to the question of whether the new medication is comparable to or better than a currently available one in terms of its therapeutic effect and side effects.

Limitations of dose-titration designs are:

• Dose titration makes it impossible to determine, within a single study, whether there is one optimal dosage within the range studied;
• Differences that are attributed to dose may be a function of time. Time and dose factors are 'confounded', therefore flexible-dose designs do not allow

CLINICAL RESEARCH IN PSYCHOPHARMACOLOGY

reliable assessment of the relationship of plasma drug concentrations and clinical response.

- Correlation of dose and response may well show that those patients who received the highest dose of a drug showed the poorest response (inverted dose–response relationship) because the doses are likely to be increased if patients do not respond at lower doses.

To overcome some of these limitations, a fixed dose-titration schedule can be implemented in the beginning of a flexible-dose trial in order to reach a minimum effective dose for each patient, followed by a flexible dose-titration schedule. Use of titration points, anchored to a clinical assessment (e.g. forced titration to the next level in the case of Clinical Global Impression severity scores of $\geqslant 3$), makes the titration schedule and the results more homogeneous and tends to unify investigators' judgments (for details see Martényi et al., 2002).

Concentration-controlled Studies

Concentration-controlled study designs (Peck, 1990) have been advocated as a more cost-effective and efficient alternative to standard clinical trials to investigate the clinical pharmacology, safety and efficacy of an investigational drug, especially during early stages of development. This approach is based on the assumption that the plasma concentrations of a drug correlate more meaningfully with clinical responses than do dosages. There are, however, a number of limitations to a concentration-controlled study approach in psychopharmacology. Psychotropic drugs are lipophilic and show high brain/plasma concentration ratios; as a consequence, the pharmacokinetic profile measured in peripheral compartments (i.e. plasma drug levels) is less informative than in the case of drugs with primarily peripheral action. Concentration-controlled approaches are recognized to be clinically relevant in the case of some anticonvulsants and lithium used in affective disorders. In the case of antipsychotics and antidepressants, drug plasma level determinations are relevant if compliance needs to be checked but are not generally considered helpful to determine optimal dosage ranges.

5.5.4 PHASE IV TRIALS

After a new drug has been approved by health authorities and launched in national markets, pharmaceutical companies usually conduct numerous further studies of its therapeutic performance in more extended patient populations. Some typical clinical and scientific goals pursued in Phase IV trials are:

- Dosing strategies different from the administration schedules established in pre-registration trials (e.g. use of high doses of antipsychotics in treatment-resistant patients).
- Combination strategies to assess the benefits and risks of treatment with a new drug if added on to an established administration regimen (e.g. in treatment-resistant patients, bipolar disorder, etc.).
- Treatment of patient groups with specific sociodemographic or medical characteristics (geriatric populations, patients suffering from comorbidity, e.g. HIV, renal or hepatic impairment, diabetes).
- Treatment of patients suffering from psychiatric and similar comorbidity, especially alcohol or drug dependence, who are usually excluded from Phase I, II and III trials.
- Treatment of patients with high suicidal risk who are excluded from Phase I, II and III trials, especially from placebo-controlled studies.
- Treatment of female patients during pregnancy or lactation because both conditions are primary exclusion criteria in Phase I–III trials.

Furthermore, clinical trials are performed in various cultural and geographical settings. Transcultural differences may play a significant role in drug efficacy: e.g. oriental populations require much lower doses of antipsychotic drugs compared with Caucasian patient populations. Phase IV trials also may be performed to explore possible novel uses for compounds approved and marketed in other indications (e.g. treatment of anxiety disorders with antidepressants, treatment of bipolar disorder with anti-convulsants, etc.).

Another important topic for Phase IV are *predictor studies* (see Spiegel, 1996, pp. 143–153). Because prescribing clinicians are highly interested in knowing which particular patient population or subpopulation is most likely to benefit from a treatment, retrospective analyses of large data sets typically collected in Phase III and prospective Phase IV trials provide opportunities to characterize the most likely responders and non-responders to a given medication. Finally, the *long-term safety* of a new drug is another topic usually studied in Phase IV. Large-scale trials, with simple designs adapted to real-life conditions, are key contributors to post-marketing surveillance (PMS) programs. If needed, randomized controlled clinical trials or case–control studies (Section 5.4.9) can provide comparative data about predefined specific adverse events of drugs (e.g. sexual dysfunction evoked by SSRIs; weight gain and/or diabetes induced by atypical antipsychotics).

Phase IV trials must be conducted according to the same ethical, scientific and Good Clinical Practice standards as those required in Phase I–III studies. A more detailed account on PMS studies can be found in a chapter by Hollister *et al.* (1994).

5.6 SYMPTOM ASSESSMENT

The therapeutic effects of psychopharmaceuticals are expressed as changes in well-being and behavior. The clinical testing of new substances therefore involves the reliable determination of these modifications in a form that can subsequently undergo statistical analysis. Three basic types of methods are available for this purpose: questioning of the patients themselves (or other procedures to determine subjective effects); behavioral observations of various degrees of complexity; and test procedures for specific mental functions.

5.6.1 QUESTIONING OF PATIENTS

Whenever possible, the treated patients should be the first source of information about a drug effect. Depending on the nature of a psychiatric disorder, questioning a patient can be difficult or even impossible but it is essential in the case of depressive patients, neurotics and many schizophrenics. Only the patients themselves can give information on how they feel, their anxieties, hopes, etc., and in addition many side effects of psychopharmaceuticals are exclusively of a subjective nature. In addition, some rating scales focusing on behavior also include items that have to be scored on the basis of the patient's own statements. Scales of various types are available for the quantification of statements made by patients (see *ECDEU Asessment Manual*, 1976; CIPS, 1986). Further methods are referenced in a book edited by Sartorius and Ban (1986). A detailed source of the standard rating instruments used across psychopharmacology is available in the book by Sajatovic and Ramirez 2002.

5.6.2 OBSERVATION OF BEHAVIOR

The behavior of a patient under hospital conditions can be observed by nursing staff, doctors or observers specially engaged for this purpose. In particular, nursing staff who see patients in their own environment for days and weeks can reliably determine if and to what extent they engage in activities, whether they make contacts with other patients or tend to keep to themselves, and how they react to questions, requests and other contacts. These are all features that make it possible to evaluate and, to some extent, quantify the need for nursing and the patient's social behavior and mood, although it must be borne in mind that personal likes and dislikes play a direct role even in apparently objective observations. Difficult, quarrelsome, withdrawn patients are generally less favorably assessed and contaminations may occur between various assessment levels. Moreover, times of observation and the conditions under which a patient is observed fluctuate from day to day. It is therefore possible to engage independent observers, uninvolved in the day-to-day nursing schedule, to rate the patients under conditions that are as standardized as possible and at predetermined times. In the case of outpatient treatment, relatives and other contact persons can observe the behavior of patients. Relatives are understandably often by no means neutral observers and therefore cannot always make reliable observations. In many instances it would also endanger the doctor–patient relationship if a system of communication were to be set up with the relatives behind the patient's back. Nevertheless, standardized behavioral observations in the habitual environment have great value in the case of children, e.g. in the documentation of drug therapy of attention deficit hyperactivity disorder (Whalen *et al.*, 1979; MTA Cooperative Group, 1999), and should also play an important role in the psychopharmacology of elderly patients with age-associated cognitive deficits (Crook *et al.*, 1983; Coper *et al.*, 1987).

5.6.3 *RATING SCALES*

Owing to the lack of well-defined, broadly established and valid biological markers in psychiatric diseases, the clinical assessment of patients is routinely based on different rating scales. When selecting a scale for use in the investigation of the effect of a drug on a particular disorder, some potential sources of error should be kept in mind:

- Most psychiatric rating scales only cover pathologically orientated items and, in the event of clinical improvement, merely indicate reduction in pathology or, in the best case, normalization. What they do not record are positive, desirable forms of behavior that are also present or can supplant pathological characteristics in the course of therapy.
- The individual items within a scale are not independent of one another and, for this reason, it is unlikely that one characteristic will change in isolation. However, by dividing up the observed behaviors into several differently formulated questionnaire items, one may create the wrong impression of independence and the equal significance of symptoms.
- Adding up the scores of several items to form sum scores can give misleading figures as estimates of the severity of an illness. Because the individual items are not independent of each other and not equivalent, caution must be adopted when arriving at and interpreting sum scores. Similar sum scores in different patients do not necessarily indicate comparable psychopathological conditions.
- Rating scales can flatten out the clinical situation. An event that would stand out as a dramatic situation in a case history may be leveled out when rating scales are used.

- Individual behavior that is part of a sensible whole is artificially broken down and looked at in isolation, at the risk of becoming incomprehensible.

Despite these limitations, rating scales today are the preferred clinical recording instrument in most areas of psychopharmacology. In order to cancel out the disadvantages, they are often combined with brief case histories or occasionally with symptom lists, which can be prepared individually for each patient.

Psychiatric Diagnostic Scales

These are instruments developed to identify specific psychiatric disorders. Most of these scales are based on a structured or semi-structured interview lasting some 60–90 min. Structured interviews contain a mix of open-ended and closed questions. Open-ended questions are essential for the validity of a diagnostic procedure; closed questions support the reliability and the standardization of diagnostic tools. The primary goal for the use of diagnostic scales is to reduce the variance within samples caused by diagnostic differences, i.e. to create homogeneous patient populations included in clinical trials.

General Diagnostic Instruments

The most commonly used semi-structured diagnostic scale is the *Structured Clinical Interview for DSM-IV Axis I Disorders* (SCID; First *et al.*, 1997). A clinical version of the SCID (SCID-CV) is designed for use in clinical settings and covers the most commonly seen diagnoses according to DSM-IV. The research version of the SCID includes ratings for different subtypes, severity and course specifiers of mental disorders. The SCID-CV contains six modules: (A) Mood Episodes; (B) Psychotic Symptoms; (C) Psychotic Disorders; (D) Mood Disorders; (E) Substance Use Disorders; (F) Anxiety and Other Disorders.

The *Mini-International Neuropsychiatric Interview* (MINI) is a short structured diagnostic interview for DSM-IV and ICD-10 psychiatric disorders. With an administration time of approximately 15 min, it was designed to meet the need for a short but accurate structured psychiatric interview for multicenter clinical trials and epidemiology studies, and to be used as a first step in outcome tracking in non-research clinical settings (Sheehan *et al.*, 1998).

5.6.4 DIAGNOSIS-SPECIFIC RATING INSTRUMENTS

Depression Scales

The two most widely used scales for the measurement of severity of depression are the *Hamilton Rating Scale for Depression* (HRSD) and the

Montgomery–Asberg Depression Rating Scale (MADRS) (Hamilton, 1959; Montgomery and Asberg, 1979).

The HRSD is an observer-rated scale that consists of 17 items (21 items in a more recent version). The instrument was originally developed for diagnostic purposes, specifically in depression, but its main use was and still is in clinical trials of all kinds, including drug studies in patients with schizophrenia, bipolar disorder and other disorders. Use of a standardized, semi-structured interview guide for the HRSD (e.g. Williams, 1988) is recommended to improve the accuracy of ratings in large multicenter trials. Three different subscales (see Table 5.4) have been developed based on HRSD items (Bech *et al.*, 1984; Maier *et al.*, 1988; Gibbons *et al.*, 1993) and they are claimed to be more sensitive to therapeutic changes than the full scale.

The MADRS is a ten-item investigator-rated instrument for the assessment of depressive symptoms. It focuses on symptoms of sadness, lassitude, pessimistic thoughts and suicidality; in contrast to the HRSD, no items are dedicated to the somatic aspects of depression.

The *Raskin Depression Rating Scale* (Raskin *et al.*, 1969) is a very simple clinician-rated three-item instrument for non-psychotic, non-bipolar depression. The source of information may include a patient interview, nursing reports and observations made during the interview. Administration of the Raskin Scale is very quick but, owing to a lack of specificity, it is recommended that it be combined with other, more specific instruments, e.g. some self-administered scales. The structure of the Raskin scale is similar to that of the Covi Anxiety Scale (Lipman, 1982) and parallel use of the two scales allows the primary pathology to be delineated in cases of comorbidity of depression and anxiety: a higher score on the Covi Anxiety Scale argues for an anxiety indication and a higher Raskin score indicates depressive symptoms.

The *Beck Depression Inventory* is a 21-item self-rating scale to assess key symptoms of depression such as mood deterioration, pessimism, guilt, self-punishment, self-dislike, self-accusations, suicidality, crying, irritability, social

Table 5.4 The three subscales of HRSD

Gibbons (HRSD8)	Bech (HRSD6)	Maier (HRSD6)
Depressed mood	Depressed mood	Depressed mood
Feelings of guilt	Feelings of guilt	Feelings of guilt
Work and activity	Work and activity	Work and activity
Psychic anxiety	Psychic anxiety	Psychic anxiety
Agitation	Retardation	Retardation
Somatic anxiety	Somatic symptoms	Agitation
Suicide		
Genital symptoms		

withdrawal, indecisiveness, change in body image, work difficulty, insomnia, fatigue, change of appetite, weight loss, somatic preoccupation, loss of libido (Beck *et al.*, 1988). The cognitive performance subscale may be particularly useful in the case of trials among elderly patients, or as a screening tool in the case of comorbid depression and somatic diseases (e.g. to detect cognitive decline in cases of hypertensive or diabetic encephalopathy, HIV, etc.).

The *Zung Depression Scale* (Zung, 1972) has a patient-rated version and an identical investigator-rated version. The instrument is heavily focused on somatic symptoms such as sleep disturbance, weight loss, constipation, tachycardia, fatigue and decreased appetite.

The *Center of Epidemiologic Studies Depression* scale (CES-D) was originally developed for the Community Mental Health Assessment, a population-based study of depressive symptoms. The 20-question survey contains items chosen from other validated mental health instruments designed to measure depressive symptoms. The questions assess symptoms experienced in the past week using a scale from zero to three, with the highest possible score of 60 (representing more depressive symptoms). The original four-factor structure included 16 of the 20 CES-D items: depressed affect (blues, depressed, lonely, cry, sad), positive affect (good, hopeful, happy, enjoy), somatic and retarded activity (bothered, appetite, effort, sleep, get going) and interpersonal feelings (unfriendly, dislike) (Radloff, 1977).

The *Inventory of Depressive Symptomatology – Self Report* (IDS-SR) is a 29-item self-rating scale for the evaluation of depressive symptom severity. Each item is rated on a defined four-step scale (0–3). Analysis of sensitivity to change in symptom severity in an open-label trial showed that the IDS-SR was highly correlated with the 17-item HRSD (Rush *et al.*, 1996).

A specific depressed population was originally targeted with the development of the *Edinburgh Postnatal Depression Scale*. This was designed as a screening tool to be used in women during the postnatal period. The scale can be completed in 5 min. The ten-item self-rating scale showed sensitivity and reliability among non-postpartum females and in males as well (Cox *et al.*, 1987). Another specific depressed population was addressed with the development of the *Calgary Depression Scale for Schizophrenia* (CDSS; Addington *et al.*, 1993). The CDSS comprises nine items selected from the HRSD) and the Present State Examination (PSE), and assesses symptoms of depression at any stage of schizophrenia.

Anxiety Scale

The *Hamilton Rating Scale for Anxiety* (HRSA) is the most widely used instrument for the assessment of anxiety symptoms in patients suffering from diagnosed anxiety disorders. The HRSA consists of 14 items and focuses to a great extent (7/14 items) on somatic symptoms (Hamilton, 1959).

The *Covi Anxiety Scale* is a simple three-item scale for the assessment of severity of anxiety symptoms. The scale measures three dimensions: verbal report, behavior and somatic symptoms of anxiety. Administration of the Covi Scale is very easy but, owing to a lack of specificity, it is recommended that it be combined with other, more specific instruments (e.g. some self-administered scale or the HRSA; see Lipman, 1982).

The *Liebowitz Social Anxiety Scale* (LSAS) measures fear, anxiety and avoidant behavior in 24 commonly feared social situations and performances. There are 13 performance-related items and 11 items that rate the social situations (Heimberg *et al.*, 1999). The LSAS is the standard established outcome measure in most of the pivotal trials for social anxiety. Cut-offs of 30 for social anxiety disorder and 60 for its generalized subtype on the LSAS total scores represent a balance of specificity and sensitivity. There are two valid versions of the LSAS: a clinician-administered version and a self-rating version (Fresco *et al.*, 2001).

The *Panic Disorder Severity Scale* (PDSS) is an investigator-rated instrument, that contains items assessing the severity of seven dimensions of panic disorder and associated symptoms: frequency of panic attacks, distress during panic attacks, anticipatory anxiety, agoraphobic fear and avoidance, interoceptive fear and avoidance, impairment of work functioning, impairment of social functioning. The PDSS is a simple, sensitive instrument for clinicians to rate the severity in patients with established diagnoses of panic disorder (Shear *et al.*, 1997).

The *Spielberger State–Trait Anxiety Inventory* (SSTAI) is a self-rating assessment that differentiates the state anxiety experienced during specific situations from chronic, situation-independent anxiety symptoms (trait anxiety). The SSTAI has 20 items covering statements on feelings "right now" and 20 items with statements related to feelings "in general" (Spielberger, 1984). The SSTAI is a useful screening tool, as well as in clinical trials of anxiety disorders or comorbid anxiety accompanying somatic disorders.

The *Fear Questionnaire* (FQ) is a 24-item self-rated scale used mainly for assessments in phobias. One component of the scale evaluates phobic behavior associated with a number of situations, whereas another component assesses symptoms of anxiety, depression and general distress caused by phobia (Marks and Mathews, 1979). The social phobia, strongly related to social anxiety, and most of the subscales are significantly related to neuroticism. The FQ has been utilized in several trials of social anxiety disorder.

The *Hospital Anxiety and Depression Scale* (HADS) is a 14-item self-report scale that was developed originally to indicate the possible presence of anxiety and depressive states in the setting of medical outpatients between 16 and 65 years (Zigmond and Snaith, 1983). The HADS is widely utilized in clinical trials of treatment of comorbid depression and/or anxiety symptoms in somatic disorders (stroke, cardiac disease, cancer, etc.).

Post-traumatic Stress Disorder (PTSD) Scales

The *Treatment Outcome PTSD Scale* (TOP-8) is a clinician-rated instrument that measures the presence and severity of eight PTSD symptoms that occur frequently in PTSD patients and are sensitive to treatment. The scale was developed from the Structured Interview for PTSD (SI-PTSD; Davidson *et al.*, 1997), an alternative to the SCID. The TOP-8 questions are representative of the three major PTSD symptom dimensions (intrusive, avoidant and hyperarousal symptoms). Each symptom is rated on a defined step scale (0–4), with a high numeric rating indicating greater symptom severity (Davidson and Colket, 1997). The TOP-8 has proved sensitive to changes of PTSD symptoms in studies with antidepressants.

The *Clinician-Administered PTSD Scale* (CAPS) for DSM-IV is a lengthy structured interview based on DSM-IV that assesses the presence and severity of PTSD and associated symptoms. The CAPS is available in two versions: the CAPS-DX (also known as the CAPS-1), which is used as a diagnostic instrument as well as a measure of current severity of PTSD; and the CAPS-SX (also known as the CAPS-2), which provides a rating of the severity of current symptoms during the past week. A CAPS total score can be drawn from either version and is based on the patient's response to 25 questions that assess the frequency and severity of current PTSD symptoms on a scale of 0–4. A high numeric rating reflects a greater degree of symptom severity (Blake *et al.*, 1990, 1995).

The *Davidson Trauma Scale* (DTS) is a 17-item self-rated instrument that allows the patient to assess the level of distress caused by various symptoms. Patients are asked to rate both the frequency and severity of each item on a scale of 0–4, with a higher numeric rating reflecting a greater degree of distress (Davidson *et al.*, 1997).

Additional trauma-related rating instruments are discussed in detail in Briere (1997).

Obsessive–Compulsive Disorder Scales

The *Yale–Brown Obsessive–Compulsive Scale* (YBOCS) is an OCD-specific instrument in which ratings are based mainly on patients' self-report in a semi-structured interview. Five items are addressed to rate the severity of obsessive symptoms and five items to assess the compulsive symptoms (Goodmann *et al.*, 1989). The YBOCS is the best-established and standard instrument to diagnose OCD; it has been used in most of the clinical trials in this area.

Psychosis Scales

The *Brief Psychiatric Rating Scale* (BPRS; Overall and Gorham, 1962) is an 18-item rating instrument covering a wide range of psychopathology. Ratings are partly based on observation of the patient (for symptoms such as tension, emotional withdrawal, mannerism and posturing) and partly on verbal answers given during the interview (items such as conceptual disorganization, unusual thought content, anxiety, guilt feelings, grandiosity, depressive mood, hostility, somatic concern, hallucinatory behavior, suspiciousness and blunted affect). The BPRS was designed primarily for inpatients, but it may be utilized also for outpatients; it has been used in hundreds of drug trials.

The *Positive and Negative Symptom Scale* (PANSS) is a 30-item rating instrument specifically designed to assess the psychopathology of schizophrenic patients. Ratings are based on a semi-structured clinical interview and any supporting available clinical information. Subscores of the PANSS are Positive, Negative, General Psychopathology and Affective Symptoms composite scores (Kay and Opler, 1986). Positive and negative syndromes, together with depression and excitement, comprise the fundamental symptomatic components of schizophrenic patients as described by Kraepelin (Kay and Sandyk, 1991). The PANSS is almost routinely used today in clinical trials with antipsychotic drugs.

The *Krawiecka–Goldberg Scale* (or Manchester Scale) is a brief ten-item scale for assessment of changes in the clinical status of patients suffering from psychosis. The items include depression, anxiety, delusions and hallucinations, incoherence, flattened affect, poverty of speech and psychomotor retardation. The absence of items typical of schizoaffective and manic psychoses limits the use of this instrument. It is, however, useful for follow-up of inpatients and outpatients for longer periods of time (Krawiecka *et al.*, 1977).

Mania Scales

The *Young Mania Rating Scale* (YMRS) comprises 11 items corresponding to the published core symptoms of mania. Four items are graded on a scale of 0–8 (irritability, speech, thought content, disruptive/aggressive behavior) and have double weight; the remaining seven items are graded on a scale of 0–4 (elevated mood, increased motor activity, sexual interest, sleep, language thought disorder, appearance and insight). The scale is easy to use and suitable for serial ratings, even every second day (Young *et al.*, 1978).

The *Bech–Rafelson Mania Scale* also comprises 11 items. It was originally developed to cover the whole affective spectrum in combination with the HRSD. All items are rated on a scale of 0–4. The last item is dedicated to the work/activity ability, with a separate first rating and follow-up assessment part (Bech *et al.*, 1979).

The *Manic State Rating Scale* is a clinician-rated 26-item instrument. All items measure the intensity (0–5) as well as the frequency (0–5) of symptoms (Beigel *et al.*, 1971).

Bipolar-disorder-specific *life charting methodology* (LCM) allows the collection of detailed information about changes of symptoms over longer periods of time. Prospective and retrospective LCMs have been developed (Leverich and Post, 1973). The retrospective LCM is constructed from recollections of the patient with the help of a trained clinician and measures mood, social and professional functioning and medication dosage by months. The prospective LCM is a self-report instrument used to collect daily prospective data relating to bipolar disorder; it can be completed alone at home or with assistance by a clinician. Prospective LCM charts are more detailed and include sleep, comorbid symptoms and menstrual cycle data, for example, in addition to mood and functioning. Both charts include space to record significant life events and rate their impact on the patient. Life charting methodology allows the bipolar nature of bipolar disorder to be approached over time rather than just the changes measured by other instruments specified for mania or depression (HRSD, YMRS, etc.).

Dementia Scales

The *Alzheimer's Disease Assessment Scale* (ADAS) is a 21-item scale with 11 items assessing cognitive–behavioral performances (spoken language ability, comprehension of spoken language, recall of test instructions, difficulties in word-finding, following commands, naming objects and figures, constructive capabilities, ideational praxis, orientation, word recall and word recognition) and 10 items for non-cognitive–behavioral disturbances (tearful, depressed mood, concentration/distractibility, uncooperativeness, delusions, hallucinations, pacing, increased motor activity, tremor and change in appetite). Rating of the individual items varies: several cognitive items require active participation of the patient, e.g. drawing or copying geometric forms on a sheet of paper, whereas other items require assessment by the person administering the test. The ADAS is not a diagnostic scale but an instrument applicable to patients already diagnosed as suffering from Alzheimer's dementia (Rosen *et al.*, 1984).

The *Mini-Mental State Evaluation* (MMSE) is a very popular instrument and includes components of orientation, calculation, registration, memory and praxis. It required active participation by patients who have to perform a number of simple tasks. The MMSE provides a rough estimate of cognitive decline; it is useful for screening purposes because it takes a very short time to perform (Folstein *et al.*, 1975).

The *Behavioral Pathology in Alzheimer's Disease* (BEHAVE-AD) scale comprises 25 items rated on a scale of 0–3. The part on paranoid and delusional ideations contains seven items typical in Alzheimer's disease, such as delusions of stealing, "one's house is not one's home" and "spouse is an impostor" type delusions; five items assess hallucinations in different modalities and three items refer to activity disturbances such as wandering, purposeless and inappropriate activities. Aggressive behavior, which is quite frequent in advanced dementia, is covered by three items, followed by one item on diurnal rhythm disturbances. Six items rate general affective and anxiety symptoms such as tearfulness, depression, anxiety regarding upcoming events, other anxieties, fears and phobias. The second part of the BEHAVE-AD is a global rating of severity of symptoms on a scale of 0–3. The BEHAVE-AD is a sensitive instrument to assess the effects of, for example, antipsychotics on the behavioral symptoms of Alzheimer's disease (Reisberg *et al.*, 1987).

Substance Use Scales

Among patients with bipolar disorder, schizophrenia and major depression the prevalence of comorbid substance use disorders may be as high as 50%. Substance use disorders are usually associated with Axis II (personality) disorders, poor treatment compliance and poorer response to pharmacotherapy; exclusion or at least adequate diagnosis of these patients is therefore essential for clinical trials.

The *Addiction Severity Index* (ASI) is a structured clinical interview developed to fill the need for a reliable, valid and standardized diagnostic and evaluative instrument in the areas of alcohol and drug abuse. The ASI may be administered by a technician in 20–30 min, producing ten-point problem severity ratings in each of the following six areas commonly affected by addiction: medical complications, psychological difficulties, legal issues, family and social disruption and employment status (McLellan *et al.*, 1980).

The *Clinical Institute Withdrawal Assessment for Alcohol Scale* (CIWA-Ar) is a short and practical ten-item instrument for clinical quantitation of the severity of an alcohol withdrawal syndrome. It can be incorporated into the usual clinical care of patients undergoing alcohol withdrawal and into clinical drug trials of alcohol withdrawal (Sullivan *et al.*, 1989).

5.6.5 GENERAL SCALES

The Hopkins 90-item *Symptoms Checklist – Revised* (SCL-90-R) is a patient-rated multidimensional instrument that measures how bothersome each of 90 symptoms is to a patient. Symptoms are rated on a scale of 0–4 ('not at all bothersome' to 'extremely bothersome'), with a higher numeric rating reflecting a greater degree of distress (Derogatis, 1983; Rief and Fichter, 1992). Answering 90 questions requires considerable patient compliance that cannot always be assumed in, for example, patients suffering from high levels of anxiety. Not being a disease-specific scale, the SCL-90-R is often used together with other, more specific investigator- or self-rated instruments.

The *SF-36* is a widely used self-rating general health survey used as a general indicator of functional health, well-being and perception of general health (Ware *et al.*, 1994). The questions comprise the following dimensions: physical functioning, role limitations due to physical health problems, bodily pain, social functioning, general mental health, psychological distress and well-being, role limitations due to emotional problems, vitality, energy or fatigue, general health perception. The SF-36 can be used for assessment in a variety of somatic and psychiatric diseases. It also provides valuable information about the quality of life of patients in clinical trials of psychotropic drugs and has been used, in combination with other, more specific instruments, as a secondary outcome measure in clinical trials of depressive and anxiety disorders.

The *Sheehan Disability Scale* (Sheehan *et al.*, 1996) measures subjects' evaluation of the extent to which their symptoms have disrupted work, social and/or home life. Each item is rated on an 11-point semi-analog continuum. This scale is utilized as a secondary outcome measure, combined with other more disease- or symptom-specific scales.

6

Neuroimaging Studies in Psychopharmacology

By
MARK E. SCHMIDT

6.1 INTRODUCTION

The last two decades have seen the introduction of several distinct 'functional' imaging techniques that can be used to investigate centrally active compounds working in the brain *in vivo*. These techniques provide windows through which to observe phenomena in the intact and fully functional central nervous system. When applied to studies with human volunteers or patients one can obtain information that cannot be extrapolated from animal models, and from areas such as the brain and neurotransmitter systems that would otherwise be inaccessible *in vivo*. When combined with peripheral measurements and objective and subjective assessments of behavior, these methods can be used to explore how psychopharmaceuticals influence central nervous sytem activity and behavior. Moreover, compounds with a known mechanism of action can be employed as tools to understand how different elements of the central nervous system work.

The imaging techniques that will be discussed are emerging from developments in radiochemistry, imaging physics and computer science. These methods detect signals that depend on the metabolic and physicochemical state of tissues and tissue components and can be sensitive to change in these signals over short time intervals. As a consequence, they are sensitive to a much larger range of physiological conditions, tissue properties and elements

Psychopharmacology, Fourth Edition. By R. Spiegel
© 2003 John Wiley & Sons, Ltd: ISBN 0 471 56039 1: 0 470 84691 7 (PB)

than radiographic imaging, which relies only on the degree to which tissues absorb x-rays. It is this greater sensitivity to change and the wide range of biological phenomena that can be explored that has given rise to the term 'functional' imaging. As a class, these methods can detect signals reflecting drug disposition and/or activity throughout the brain and therefore offer superior spatial information and resolution relative to electroencephalography, another principal method of assessing the effect of psychoactive compounds on brain function (Chapter 3). The temporal resolution of these techniques depends on the detection method chosen and experimental design; however, all currently available methods require integration of information over time époques one or more orders of magnitude greater than that achieved with electroencephalography.

Although many reports are being published with these methods, it is important to realize that technical execution of these studies, data acquisition and image processing are complex and functional imaging methods are still very much evolving. Reasonable interpretation of the data depends on knowledge of the performance characteristics of the methods, skilful experimental design and realizing that there are significant gaps in our understanding of the path from drug action to image signal.

6.2 NEUROIMAGING TECHNIQUES

6.2.1 FUNCTIONAL IMAGING WITH RADIOISOTOPES

The types of signals measured in functional imaging studies fall into two broad categories: compounds labeled with radioisotopes and compounds that generate a paramagnetic signal. The compounds may be biologically active molecules such as glucose derivatives, water or hemoglobin; small synthetic molecules such as benzamides; or larger synthetic molecules such as technetium (^{99}Tc) chelates. This section will introduce some of the concepts involved in the application of radiolabeled compounds to the study of psychopharmaceuticals.

Radioisotope-labeled biomolecules have been used for decades to dissect and measure metabolic pathways at the molecular, cellular and tissue level. Radiolabeled pharmaceuticals permit quantitation of signals expressed as low as the nanomolar range and, as such, are particularly useful for drug distribution and receptor occupancy studies. The isotopes that are used for *in vivo* brain imaging are of two types: single-photon emitting and positron emitting. These two types of isotopes require different signal detection systems and selection of the type of isotope depends on the compound being labeled and the intended use. The isotopes used in these studies are a select group of radionuclides that can be readily synthesized and then incorporated into a carrier molecule that can be used safely for *in vivo* studies in humans. These

Table 6.1 Isotopes used in central nervous system studies

	Radioisotope	Half-life
Single-photon Emitters	^{99}Tc	6 h
	^{123}I	13 h
Positron Emitters	^{15}O	2.01 min
	^{11}C	20.5 min
	^{18}F	109.8 min
	^{76}Br	16.2 h

isotopes decay, and this process generates gamma photons of sufficient energy that they project outside the body where the photons can be detected by a scintillation camera. In some cases the rapid decay or 'half-life' of the isotope permits serial studies to be obtained within a subject on a given day while the total radiation exposure is limited. Table 6.1 lists the most frequently used isotopes for psychopharmaceutical studies.

For studies of psychotropic drugs, the metal ^{99}Tc has most commonly been chelated with hexamethylpropyleneamine oxime (HMPAO). Following injection, 70% of this substance is transported across the intact blood–brain barrier and 'trapped'. As a consequence, images of the distribution of the tracer can be used to estimate relative cerebral blood flow. The heavier halides of iodine (^{123}I) and bromine (^{76}Br), can be substituted for their stable isotope counterparts in pharmaceuticals or derivatives that include iodine or bromine in their structure. Fluorine-18 (^{18}F) can be substituted for ^{19}F or, in selected cases (such as 2-deoxyglucose), for a hydrogen atom. Carbon is ubiquitous in endogenous compounds and drugs, therefore the carbon isotope ^{11}C is a very commonly used label following an isotopic substitution for ^{12}C in either naturally occurring molecules (such as amino acids, fatty acids, or sugars) or pharmaceuticals. The very short-lived oxygen isotope ^{15}O is incorporated in water, butanol or carbon monoxide to measure blood flow.

When single-photon-emitting isotopes decay they generate a gamma photon signal that can be detected using an Anger scintillation camera. The location or source of the signal is determined by attaching a collimator to the camera: a lead shield or septum with a geometric array of holes. These holes permit the detection of only those photons traveling along a line within some angle of the axis of the hole (the angle being a function of the location and geometry of the hole). The collimator therefore discriminates among photons based on their line of travel, defining one axis of the volume of tissue from which the signal was generated. The source of the signal is determined by back-projecting this line when a scintillation event is detected. For imaging the brain, the camera is rotated around the head and the intersection of back-projected lines is mapped

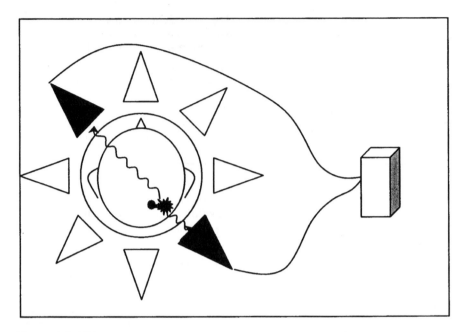

Figure 6.1 A ^{11}C atom emitting a positron is depicted (small star) somewhere in the head of a subject of a PET scan. These particles travel some distance from the nucleus (generally 2 mm or less, depending on the energy associated with the decay of the isotope, which depends on the atomic weight of the isotope). If the positron meets an electron somewhere in the surroundings, mutual annihilation occurs (large star), producing two gamma rays that project at an angle of 180° from each other. These gamma photons can be sensed by the detectors (triangles) arrayed in pairs around the bore of the camera. Multiple rings of these paired detectors constitute the camera. When a pair of detectors senses photons simultaneously, this is recorded in the computer as a 'true' coincidence event that occurred along the line between the detectors. If annihilation occurs outside the volume of space between two detectors, only one of the photons can be detected and the event is rejected. Many millions of such events are recorded during a PET scan and used to create an image of isotope distribution

to create the two-dimensional distribution or image of the signal, as with navigation by triangulation.

Positron-emitting radionuclides differ from single-photon emitters in that a positron is emitted as part of the radioactive decay process. A positron is an anti-matter electron and when these particles meet electrons in the surrounding tissue a mutual annihilation occurs. This produces two high-energy gamma photons that travel in opposite directions. Positron emission tomography (PET) cameras are constructed of rings of multiple scintillation detectors that are paired diametrically. When two such opposing detectors simultaneously detect an event, this determines the line in space on which the annihilation occurred, depicted in cartoon form in Fig. 6.1. Back-projection of the source of

Cerebral metabolic effects of the
α2-adrenoceptor antagonist ethoxyidazoxan

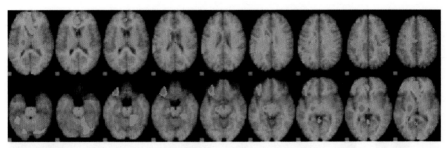

9 μg/kg i.v.

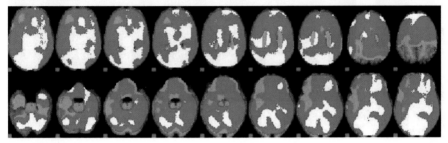

12 μg/kg i.v.

Plate 6.1 In this experiment, healthy adult male volunteers were assigned to intravenous infusions with either 9 (*n*=8) or 12 (*n*=8) μg/kg of ethoxyidazoxan, a selective α2-adrenoceptor antagonist. Presynaptic α2-adrenoceptors are located on monoamine terminals, where they provide feedback inhibition of neurotransmitter release. Postsynaptic receptors have been identified on a variety of neurons (Raiteri *et al.*, 1990, Aoki *et al.*, 1994). In the periphery, these compounds result in an increase of norepinephrine release through blocking the presynaptic receptors on noradrenergic neurons. The FDG-PET scans were obtained before and after the infusion. The individual image files of glucose metabolic rate were warped into the Talairach atlas. The post-drug metabolic rate was compared to the pre-drug metabolic rate voxel by voxel within subject using *t*-tests. Voxels that significantly differed were mapped onto an MRI template. White areas reflect an average increase at a threshold of p<0.001, red areas at a threshold of p<0.01 and orange areas at a threshold of p<0.05. The 12 μg/kg dose resulted in more diffuse increases than the lower dose (Schmidt *et al.*, 1999).

Effect of SSRI treatment on [^{11}C] DASB binding

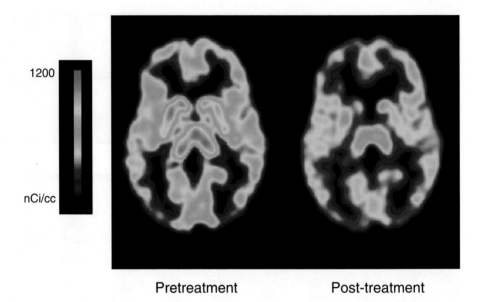

1200

nCi/cc

Pretreatment   Post-treatment

Plate 6.2 A patient has received two PET scans with [^{11}C]DASB (3-amino-4-[(2-dimethylaminomethyl) phenylsulfanyl] benzonitrile), a tracer selective for the serotonin transporter. The first was obtained prior to treatment and the second after treatment with citalopram, 20 mg/day for 4 weeks. Tracer uptake has been reduced in the striatum by approximately 80%, suggesting that 80% of the serotonin transporters are occupied by citalopram with that level of exposure (Meyer *et al.*, 2001)

such signals coupled with filtering the signal for noise and correction for false or lost counts permits an accurate mapping of the signal into image data space. Images are then created that represent the distribution of the tracer. Correcting this for the extent to which the tissue being studied absorbs or attenuates the photon signal ('attenuation correction'), calculating the exposure of the tissue to the tracer estimated from blood samples (the 'input function') and modeling of the relative steady-state concentrations of the tracer in the different tissue compartments can provide a quantitative estimate of the signal in the compartment of interest.

The longer half-life of single-photon-emission computed tomography (SPECT) isotopes and reduced technical requirements for imaging with SPECT make these tracers attractive for use at a very wide range of centers. Anger cameras for imaging with SPECT tracers are used at medical centers throughout the world, making this the more accessible radioisotope technology. At the same time, the greater ability to quantitate the signal through attenuation correction, use of coincidence detection, modeling and the greater versatility of PET isotopes for labeling (without significantly altering the physiological or pharmacological properties of the carrier) have led to PET imaging being more widely used as a research tool in drug development.

Regardless of the tracer and camera used, the images of tracer distribution are often subjected to additional processing. Two common strategies are the co-registration of 'functional' images with structural images of the brain – either magnetic resonance imaging (MRI) or computerized axial tomography (CAT) – to improve the measurement and localization of a signal, and warping of individual data into a common coordinate system (such as the brain atlas by Talairach and Tournoux, 1988) to permit signal averaging across subjects. Reviews of the technology and physiology supporting these methods and discussion of some of the performance characteristics of these isotopes and imaging systems offer more detailed background (Phelps *et al.*, 1986; Burns *et al.*, 1993; Carson *et al.*, 1998).

6.2.2 *FUNCTIONAL IMAGING WITH MAGNETIC RESONANCE*

In addition to radioisotope-labeled compounds, functional imaging can be done using nuclear magnetic resonance (NMR) and MRI. The technical foundations for the signal used in magnetic resonance methods involves quantum physics. What follows is a highly simplified overview of the elements of magnetic resonance using illustrations from classical physics. The interested reader can find a more complete discussion of the technical foundations in a recent text devoted to this subject (Buxton, 2002).

Magnetic resonance imaging ultimately depends on the observation that nuclear particles, including protons, neutrons and electrons, have an intrinsic rotation or spin, creating an electromagnetic field. The magnetic fields associated with protons and neutrons can cancel each other within the atom but in the case of atoms with an odd-numbered atomic weight (such as ^1H, ^{19}F, or ^{31}P) the imbalance in the number of protons versus neutrons leads to a net nuclear spin or magnetic moment. As a consequence, when such an atom is in the presence of an externally generated magnetic field, the magnetic moment of the particle will behave as a dipole (like a small compass needle) and align itself in the direction of the external magnetic field. If these spinning dipoles are perturbed, such as by introducing a change in the direction of the magnetic field or adding energy to the system with another electromagnetic signal, they will tend to rotate or 'precess' at an angle around an axis in the direction of the external magnetic field. This phenomenon can be likened to a gyroscope or a top, precessing at an angle around an axis of gravity as it spins. The frequency of this precession (the 'Larmor frequency') is specific to each atom at a given magnetic field strength. As the atom precesses, it generates its own disturbances in the magnetic field that can be detected as a signal at the Larmor frequency of the atom. In techniques involving *in vivo* MRI, a device is used that has supercooled electrical coils distributed around the bore of the scanner that generate a powerful magnetic field (most commonly 1.5 Tesla for clinical imaging, with 3.0 Tesla machines now being widely introduced), the subject lies within the bore of the machine in the center of the magnetic field and a radiofrequency (RF) coil is placed in some proximity to the tissue of interest. This coil provides the perturbation to initiate signal detection in the form of an RF pulse, as well as detecting the RF signal coming back from the tissue. The initial RF pulse used to perturb the system may be given over a broad frequency range but particles such as protons will absorb the RF energy band that occurs at the same frequency as their Larmor frequency, rather like a tuning fork sounding if a signal is transmitted at the same frequency for which the tuning fork is tuned. It is essentially that 'sound' and its amplitude, from the precessing atoms, that the RF coil receives as an indicator of the presence and amount of particles present. For clinical imaging the magnetic field is not uniform, but is generated as a gradient. The dipoles associated with the atoms generate a signal specific to their location along the gradient, as the Larmor frequency depends on the strength of the field. This permits the source of the signal to be located in space. The RF signal detected has a complex oscillating form that represents populations of nuclear dipoles from locations throughout the detection volume. This complex form is Fourier transformed from changes in signal over time to frequency values in order to map the location of these various populations.

Following perturbation of the system, the dipoles will return to being aligned along the axis of the external magnetic field, referred to as relaxation. The Larmor frequency of an atom can be slightly different depending on the environment of the atom, so that a ^1H atom or proton can have a slightly different frequency depending on whether it is associated with a methyl group,

Table 6.2 Relative relaxation parameters in human brain

Tissue	T_1 (ms)	T_2 (ms)
Cerebrospinal fluid	2500	250
Gray matter	950	95
White matter	700	80

hydroxy group, etc. and it is this difference or chemical shift that permits NMR imaging or magnetic resonance spectroscopy (MRS). In addition, the relaxation time of protons differs depending on the environment, so that different tissues can generate different signals depending on how the experiment is conducted. The relaxation signal can be separated into T_1 (the longitudinal relaxation or that associated with relaxation of the signal that occurs along the direction of the external magnetic field) and T_2 and T_2^* components (the relaxation occurring perpendicular or transverse to the direction of the magnetic field). The T_1 and T_2 times vary significantly between tissues; a selection of those for protons in brain tissues is provided in Table 6.2 to illustrate these differences.

These tissue-specific differences in signal behavior permit the imaging of contrasts and is the basis for clinical imaging and quantitation of brain volumes in different disease states and over time. Because of the slow change in brain structure, 'structural' or 'volumetric' MRI has limited application to pharmacological studies, although changes in structure are being considered as a surrogate measure of drug/treatment effect in multiple sclerosis (Hohol et al., 1997) and Alzheimer's disease (Fox and Freeborough, 1997; Wang et al., 2002).

Subtle differences in the tissue magnetic signal are also the basis for brain blood flow or cerebral blood volume measurement using MRI. Two types of methods are used: those that use an exogenous contrast agent such as gadolinium chelates; and those that rely on an endogenously generated signal such as blood-oxygen-level-dependent (BOLD)-MRI and arterial spin-labeling. Gadolinium (Gd) has a number of unpaired electrons and in tissue causes a decrease in local relaxation time of protons associated with water. This metal can be chelated with DTPA and this agent can be injected as an intravascular contrast agent with a circulation half-life of approximately 1.5 h. Imaging is done by giving this contrast agent intravenously and then estimating the cerebral blood volume (CBV) by measuring the regional decreases in the brain MRI signal compared with the pre-injection scan. In pharmacological, perceptual stimulation or behavioral activation studies the CBV is measured during control and experimental conditions (see Belliveau et al., 1991; Kaufman et al., 1998). The test-retest variability of this method appears to be good (Henry et al., 2001) and has been applied to functional imaging of the effects of psychopharmaceuticals.

The BOLD-MRI approach follows changes in regional brain blood flow by deoxyhemoglobin serving as an endogenous paramagnetic contrast agent. Local hyperemia and increases in venous blood oxygenation accompany increases in neuronal activity. Deoxyhemoglobin has paramagnetic properties whereas oxyhemoglobin does not, and the reduction in deoxyhemoglobin concentration attendant to neuronal excitation is hypothesized to underlie the change in water proton signal observed to occur during visual stimulation experiments (Ogawa *et al.*, 1992). After acquiring rapid serial MRI images during stimulus on and off conditions, one can subtract the paired or averaged images and map the region(s) in the brain where the BOLD signal has changed. This observation is being extended to investigations of cognition, perception, emotion and pain using different stimulus paradigms. Because the signal depends on subtraction of an activated state versus control, it is not as suited for evaluating the effects of drugs during a resting condition and studies of the effects of drug to date have been limited to drugs with very short half-lives or in combination with another activation protocol (see below).

Arterial spin-labeling is another method and involves inducing a magnetization 'label' on arterial blood before entering the brain (Detre *et al.*, 1998). This approach permits quantitation of the signal by knowing the 'input' (the amount of magnetization induced) as well as the 'output' (the measured signal in brain arterial blood) and thus could be used to evaluate 'resting' as well as chronic changes in brain blood flow, although this technique has not been used to date for pharmacological studies.

6.3 TYPES OF FUNCTIONAL IMAGING STUDIES

Functional neuroimaging studies used to characterize psychopharmaceuticals are generally of three classes: those that assess some aspect of brain activity or metabolism; those that assess a specific site in the brain, such as a receptor or enzyme; and those that evaluate distribution of a drug in the brain. The experimental design and imaging method chosen depends on the type of information on drug behavior being sought. Brain metabolism and blood-flow-based methods tend to be adopted by investigators using a neuroanatomic model of drug action. Such an approach is useful for exploring the effect of the drug on behavior as mediated by specific brain regions, although such studies may also provide information on general behavioral states such as sedation or arousal by measuring more diffuse effects. Receptor or site-specific methods generally provide less dynamic information, are most commonly applied to confirm the site and mechanism of action of a drug and typically assume a relationship between site occupancy and pharmacological effect.

To illustrate these differences, a brain activity study of patients with schizophrenia typically involves testing whether a particular brain region, perhaps in the frontal cortex, may be affected by disease process or shows a change in activity during a task different from a control subject. In contrast, a study of patients using a dopamine system tracer would likely focus on the basal ganglia because this brain region provides the best signal-to-noise ratio for many dopamine system tracers. Such a study may acknowledge that basal ganglia function may be germane to the pathophysiology of schizophrenia (Keshavan et al., 1998) but it does not depend on this assumption. Instead, dopamine activity in the basal ganglia serves as a surrogate for dopamine activity throughout the brain. This differs from brain-region-specific mapping of some behavior or cognitive function, because monoamine neurons project diffusely throughout the brain and most likely play a more general role in modulating behavioral states such as attention.

6.3.1 MEASUREMENT OF REGIONAL BRAIN METABOLISM

Assessment of brain activity *in vivo* began with the pioneering work led by Seymour Kety by applying Fick's Principle, a method of estimating the amount of blood flow through a tissue by comparing the arterial and venous concentrations of a gas that enters into the bloodstream at a known rate. Although originally developed to estimate cardiac output, Kety and Schmidt adapted this to estimate whole brain blood flow using inert gases as a diffusion tracer (Kety and Schmidt, 1948). A student of his, Louis Sokoloff, established that the glucose derivative 2-deoxyglucose radiolabeled with ^{14}C could be transported readily across the blood–brain barrier and be taken up by brain cells, and thus could be used to estimate regional brain glucose metabolism. By replacing the hydroxy group with hydrogen on the second carbon, $[^{14}C]2$-deoxyglucose is a substrate for hexokinase to form $[^{14}C]2$-deoxyglucose-6-phosphate but cannot serve as a substrate for isomerase, the next enzyme in the glucose metabolism pathway. Phosphorylation renders the molecule more polar so that it is less likely to move out of the intracellular space. Moreover, dephosphorylation of glucose-6-phosphate or $[^{18}F]$-2-deoxyglucose (*FDG) occurs very slowly *in vivo*. As a consequence, $[^{14}C]2$-deoxyglucose-6-phosphate is effectively trapped and accumulation of this product can be estimated by using the radioactive decay signal generated by the radioisotope. By measuring the arterial input of $[^{14}C]2$-deoxyglucose, the transfer constants of glucose from blood to tissue and the 'isotope effect', the glucose metabolic rate in any tissue can be modeled (Sokoloff et al., 1977). Assessment of tracer uptake follows the injection of isotope-labeled 2-deoxyglucose by about 45 min with ^{14}C-labeled compound and after at least 20 min with ^{18}F-labeled compound to permit assessment at steady state. The estimate therefore integrates metabolism occurring over as many minutes. The ^{14}C technique was developed for evaluation of brain metabolism in rats with quantitation *ex vivo*. The radiolabeled 2-deoxyglucose method was subsequently developed for use *in*

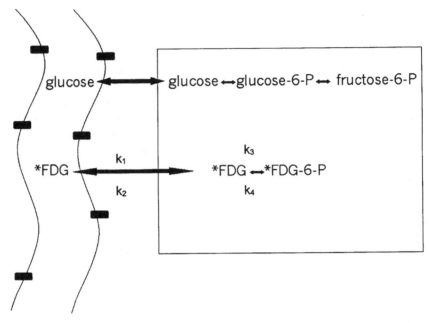

Figure 6.2 Glucose and [^{18}F]-2-deoxyglucose (*FDG) are depicted circulating through the cerebral vasculature. Either compound is readily transported across the blood–brain barrier by an active transport mechanism (■) and into cells including neurons and glia. There, glucose and *FDG enter into the glucose metabolic pathway, with *FDG effectively being trapped after the initial phosphorylation step. As indicated, each process is reversible, although dephosphorylation occurs slowly relative to the time course of an FDG study. Rate constants k_{1-4} are for entry or egress of *FDG across the blood–brain barrier and for phosphorylation and dephosphorylation of *FDG, respectively, used in modeling the brain glucose metabolic rate; P = phosphate

vivo in humans by substituting the positron-emitting ^{18}F isotope for one of the hydrogen atoms on the 2-deoxyglucose molecule (FDG-PET) (Reivich *et al.*, 1979). The basic model for FDG-PET is depicted in Fig. 6.2.

Several distinct features of brain physiology permit application of this technique to the study of psychopharmaceuticals. The brain is highly dependent on glucose oxidative metabolism as a source of energy, utilization of which is directly related to the functional activity of the nervous system. Neuronal activity has been estimated to account for 75% of oxygen consumption in the brain. Most of this energy (80% or more) is required for restoration and maintenance of the ionic gradients as they fluctuate with neuronal firing (Mata *et al.*, 1980; Sokoloff, 1986). The brain has negligible stores of glucose and relies on circulating glucose for its energy needs and an active transport system to move glucose across the blood–brain barrier. The

FDG is readily taken up by this transport system, although the extent of uptake can be influenced by the concentration of plasma glucose, which competes with FDG for uptake. The efficiency of transport across the blood–brain barrier is such that blood flow is generally not limiting for tracer delivery but the potential for a drug to have a direct vascular effect that influences tracer delivery should be considered.

In a prototype experiment evaluating a psychoactive compound, brain metabolism would be measured during a control condition and following acute or chronic administration of a drug. To the extent that a drug interacts with sites that influence the excitability or inhibitory status of neurons, this can be detected as changes in regional brain metabolism. Examples of the results of such an experiment are depicted in Plate 6.1.

This simple experiment can be complicated by a number of issues. First is the relationship between the time course of the imaging method and that of the drug effect, recalling that the estimate of glucose metabolism with FDG-PET reflects an integration of tracer uptake over a period of 20 min or more. This time period provides ample opportunity for polysynaptic and intraneuronal events following interaction between the drug and the primary target. Thus, if the extent and direction of the metabolic effect of the drug are time dependent, this information may be lost in the integrated measure. Some psychoactive drugs have primary targets that include receptors that subtly modulate the excitability of neurons and may be expressed at low densities diffusely throughout the cortex (e.g. some noradrenergic receptors). Signal detection in this situation can be difficult, given the normal levels of intrinsic cortical activity in conscious and alert human subjects. In addition, the 'resting' behavioral state of a conscious human has a significant range and measurements of brain activity can be influenced profoundly by factors such as age, gender and level of arousal (Duara et al., 1987; Yoshii et al., 1988; Camargo et al., 1992; Schmidt et al., 1996). Changes in stimulation or behavior can result in much larger effects on regional brain metabolism than the metabolic effects of tolerable doses of many psychoactive compounds. Thus, unless reasonable efforts are made to control for subject factors and experimental conditions, the between-subject and within-subject variability in regional brain activity will preclude reliable detection of the subtle regional metabolic effects of a drug.

Many compounds have been evaluated for their effects on brain metabolism (London, 1993). A surprisingly limited number of common regional metabolic effects have been seen within drug classes. Antipsychotics, especially the older 'typical' antipsychotics, tend to be associated with changes in striatal metabolism consistent with the high density of D2 dopamine receptors in those brain structures (Cohen et al., 1999). On the other hand, quite different patterns of metabolic effects have been seen following acute doses with paroxetine and fluoxetine, both of which are selective serotonin reuptake inhibitors (Cook *et al.*, 1994; Kennedy *et al.*, 2001), and between α2-adrenoceptor antagonists, with only very minor structural and pharmacological differences (Schmidt *et al.*, 1997, 1999). Cocaine, methylphenidate and amphetamine each block dopamine reuptake as a principal mechanism of action yet result in different regional metabolic effects after acute dosing (London *et al.*, 1990; Matochik *et al.*, 1993; Ernst *et al.*, 1997). These divergent results suggest that even subtle differences in pharmacology and pharmacokinetics may result in markedly different metabolic effects in brain. Subject variables such as age, gender and behavioral state can profoundly influence brain metabolism and can interact with the metabolic effects of drugs (Schmidt *et al.*, 1997; Cohen *et al.*, 1999). One cannot readily extrapolate from any observed metabolic effect of a drug to a behavioral or therapeutic outcome. Nonetheless, metabolic studies of drugs can be very useful for identifying whether a given dose of a drug is likely to have a central effect, has highly regional versus diffuse effects on brain activity and discriminates from other doses or drugs in its effect on neuronal activity.

6.3.2 MEASUREMENT OF CEREBRAL BLOOD FLOW AND VOLUME

Although FDG-PET is the most commonly employed functional imaging method for evaluating functional effects of psychopharmaceuticals, a number of other aspects of brain activity can be assessed and have been tested as indicators of drug effect. Many follow brain blood flow, because regional blood flow is highly coupled to neuronal activity. Radioisotope-labeled blood flow markers that have been used in psychopharmaceutical studies include [^{15}O]H_2O and [^{15}O]butanol. For example, [^{15}O]H_2O PET blood flow has been used in studies of benzodiazepines evaluating global versus regional, acute versus chronic and dose response of the signal (Roy-Byrne *et al.*, 1993a; Matthew *et al.*, 1995).

Contrast-enhanced MRI with Gd-DTPA has been applied to the evaluation of several compounds in man, some focusing on the hemodynamic effects of the drugs on cerebral blood volumes. Kolbtisch and others compared the anesthetic agents nitrous oxide and sevoflurane, noting them to produce compound-specific patterns of diffuse increases in cerebral blood volume (Kolbitsch *et al.*, 2001). Intravenous cocaine, on the other hand, was observed to produce dose-dependent vasoconstriction of cerebral blood vessels (Kaufman *et al.*, 1998).

More recently BOLD-MRI has been employed in studies attempting to test the effect of a drug on regional blood flow at 'rest', and during cognitive tasks or some behavioral paradigm. Breiter and others also tested the effect of acute intravenous cocaine on the BOLD signal and observed regional increases and decreases in signal, some of which were correlated temporally with subjective effects such as euphoria (Breiter *et al.*, 1997). At the same time, the vasoconstrictive effects observed by Kaufman and others using contrast-enhanced MRI suggests that the BOLD signal attributed to brain activity changes could have been confounded by direct vascular effects of the drug. The mixed serotonin agonist/antagonist meta-chlorophenylpiperazine (mCPP) given intravenously was reported by Anderson and others to result in regional increases in the BOLD signal in several subcortical structures compared with pre-injection 'rest', and to result in enhancement and attenuation of the signal generated by a 'go/no-go' task (Anderson *et al.*, 2002). Another notable application of BOLD-MRI to the assessment of psychoactive compounds was that by Stein and others, who measured the effect of rising doses of nicotine on the BOLD signal in human brain. Three doses of nicotine (0.75, 1.50 and 2.25 mg per 70 kg weight) were given intravenously over 1 min to human volunteers who smoked cigarettes. Serial MRI scans were acquired over 20 min, beginning 4 min before the infusion. Voxels were identified that met each of several change-from-baseline criteria. Dose-related increases in the BOLD signal occurred in the nucleus accumbens, amygdala and frontal cortex. This was conducted in the absence of any behavioral challenge during the MRI scans and used contrasts between doses as well as with the baseline to identify a pharmacological signal. Such a study was enabled by the very short half-life of nicotine, permitting repeated exposures within subjects as well as adaptation of the signal detection algorithm to the predicted pharmacokinetics of nicotine (Stein *et al.*, 1998; Bloom *et al.*, 1999).

Although the number and range of studies continues to increase, blood flow methods have not been as extensively used or validated for pharmacological studies and differ from glucose metabolic imaging and from each other in fundamental ways. The temporal resolution of PET and MRI blood flow imaging can be of the order of seconds to minutes, owing to the limited duration of the blood flow signal. To exploit this as well as enhance signal detection, study designs using blood flow measures often employ multiple serial assessments or 'box-car' designs to permit signal averaging. As noted above, blood flow signals from changes in brain activity can be confounded by the direct vascular effects of a drug. For example, ethanol produces different effects on regional cerebral blood flow and brain glucose metabolism, probably in part due to direct effects of ethanol on vascular tone (Volkow *et al.*, 1988; Wang *et al.*, 2000). As noted above, BOLD-MRI signal readouts are semi-quantitative and as such do not measure absolute change. Moreover, MRI blood flow has been suggested to be linked to synaptic activity in contrast to the maintenance of postsynaptic ionic gradients. As such, the MRI signal may be sensitive to neuronal excitation but relatively insensitive to neuronal inhibition (Arthurs and Boniface, 2002). The type of signal detected with these approaches may therefore be fundamentally different. Contrast-enhanced MRI and arterial spin-labeling both permit absolute quantitation of signal and theoretically could be better suited to chronic drug studies requiring measurements separated by days to weeks, and there are fundamental differences in the type of signal used: Gd-DTPA measures cerebral blood volume changes whereas arterial spin-labeling measures blood flow. Different drugs, experimental protocols (e.g. acute versus chronic administration) and disease states can influence these two parameters in distinct ways, which will require thorough understanding of the methods to design the experiments and interpret the data.

Furthermore, the interactions that occur between behavioral activation and pharmacological effect are quite complex and the interpretation of data from such studies is difficult. Positron emission tomography studies have revealed a much greater signal generated by behavioral activations relative to the signal generated by psychoactive compounds at doses that do not cloud consciousness. For example, stimulation of the visual cortex can result in a 50% increase in glucose metabolism or blood flow whereas pharmacological stimulation of the same area with a potent α2-adrenoceptor antagonist may result in a 10–12% increase in regional metabolism (Fox *et al.*, 1987; Schmidt *et al.*, 1999). Drug effects can be distributed throughout the central nervous system, in contrast to the more anatomically delimited activations associated with many of the behavioral tasks and perceptual stimuli employed. Moreover, pharmacological effects follow a much different time course than behavioral activation, so partitioning of the signal contributed by the two interventions will be challenging. Nonetheless, brain blood flow experiments that skilfully combine pharmacological and behavioral activation could be very informative in determining how psychoactive compounds modulate brain activity during tasks or perception, and thus influence behavior.

In addition to general measures of brain metabolism and activity, several methods are available for specifically evaluating the activity of the dopaminergic system. These include radiolabeled tracers evaluating presynaptic, synaptic and postsynaptic activity. Presynaptic dopaminergic function can be assessed with ^{18}F-labeled dihydroxyphenylacetic acid ([^{18}F]DOPA), the amino acid derivative that serves as a substrate for dopa decarboxylase. [^{18}F]DOPA is taken up readily by the brain and in dopaminergic neurons is decarboxylated to form [^{18}F]dopamine which is stored along with endogenously formed dopamine in intraneuronal vesicles. Owing to the slow turnover of newly synthesized dopamine relative to the time interval of the PET study, the labeled DOPA is 'trapped' as labeled dopamine in dopaminergic neurons. Thus, the rate of brain uptake and accumulation of tracer in dopamine neuron-rich areas can be regarded as a valid estimate of the capacity or activity of dopa decarboxylase (Garnett *et al.*, 1978). Primates previously given MPTP to produce an animal model of Parkinson's disease and patients with Parkinson's disease show a significantly lower uptake of labeled dopa in striatum and ventral tegmentum compared with controls (Leenders *et al.*, 1986; Doudet *et al.*, 1989). Presynaptic function can also be assessed with radiolabeled tracers that bind to the dopamine transporter, such as [11]C- or ^{123}I-labeled CIT (*N*-(3-fluoropropyl)-2-carbomethoxy-3-(4-iodophenyl)nortropane). The most common application of these methods is evaluation of the dopaminergic system in patient samples for evaluating disease severity and progression, although they have also been considered for assessing the chronic effects of treatment with dopamine agonists on dopaminergic neuron integrity (Brooks, 2000; Doudet, 2001). Synaptic and postsynaptic function following acute or chronic drug treatment can be assessed by dopamine-receptor-specific tracers, and some of the applications of these have been reviewed elsewhere (Schmidt, 2001). Understanding these methods requires an introduction to receptor occupancy theory and the assumptions that underlie the use of receptor-specific tracers.

6.3.3 RECEPTOR OCCUPANCY THEORY

In addition to the measurement of brain activity, ligands have been developed labeled with positron- or single-photon-emitting isotopes targeted to sites in the brain such as neurotransmitter systems or receptor populations. Using these methods, receptor tracer studies have been used to measure receptor distributions and binding potentials as possible markers of pathophysiology of disease, to optimize drug treatment and to understand the clinical pharmacology of antipsychotic drugs.

The concept of substrate-specific receptors in the brain evolved in part from theories about the mechanism of action of drugs. The foundation of this concept was laid as early as 1685 by Robert Boyle, who postulated that certain medicaments were more 'fit' to be detained by a particular organ based on the drug size, shape and motion. Specific 'substances' or receptors were proposed by Langley in 1878 to account for the opposing effects of the muscarinic agonist pilocarpine and antagonist atropine (Parascandola, 1986). Receptor theory as an explanation of drug action continued to evolve as theories of brain organization moved from a holistic concept, assuming direct connectivity between neurons, to a model of the brain championed by Ramon y Cajal that recognized neurons to be independent. Sir Charles Sherrington gave this additional support when he demonstrated that neurons were able to communicate at synapses by chemical rather than electrical means (Finger, 1994).

A. J. Clark formulated receptor occupancy theory as a quantitative model in 1933 in his doctoral dissertation. This model describes the binding of a ligand (either a drug or endogenous substrate) to a receptor and then links this occupancy to responses. According to mass action, the binding of a ligand to a receptor is a function of the product of their respective concentrations at equilibrium. The theory assumes that the binding is reversible, proceeds at a rate dictated by the affinity of the receptor for the ligand and that there are a finite number of receptors rendering the process saturable. This model is summarized by Equations (6.1) and (6.2):

$$[L] + [R] \overset{k_1}{\underset{k_2}{\Longleftrightarrow}} [LR] \tag{6.1}$$

$$\frac{[LR]}{[L] + [R]} = K_A \tag{6.2}$$

where [L], [R] and [LR] are the concentrations of ligand, receptor and bound receptor, respectively, and k_1 and k_2 are the association and dissociation constants, respectively, and K_A is the equilibrium association constant.

The conservation equation for receptors defines the total number of receptors as the sum of bound and free receptors (Equation (6.3)). Although the receptor population is in fact made up of subpopulations of receptors in high- and low-affinity states, this is most relevant for modeling agonist interactions. Because most tracers are radiolabeled antagonists, this simplified model is sufficient for most tracer studies. The conservation and mass action equations (Equations (6.3) and (6.4)) can be rearranged to calculate the number of bound receptors:

$$[R_T] = [R] + [LR] \tag{6.3}$$

$$[LR] = \frac{[L][R_T]}{K_A + [L]} \tag{6.4}$$

where $[R_T]$ is the total receptor concentration.

Using this model, K_A and the maximum quantity of bound receptors (B_{max}) can be calculated using a Scatchard plot. This is done *in vitro* by using a range of concentrations of ligand applied to a constant number of receptors in a single compartment, either tissue slices or homogenates. When using a radioisotope-labeled ligand as an *in vivo* tracer, the concentration of tracer is very low relative to other receptor substrates so that the effect of the tracer on the physiological conditions is negligible. Nonetheless, the activity of the tracer is held to be an accurate marker for the process of interest, whether it is the relative density of the receptor or the occupancy of the receptor pool by the drug or endogenous substrate (Fekarny, 1998).

Assaying brain receptors with a radioisotope-labeled ligand *in vivo* was developed from *in vitro* methods of measuring brain receptors using autoradiography, although *in vivo* measurements are significantly more complex. Rather than the single compartment used for *in vitro* measurements, most full compartmental models used to describe *in vivo* conditions use two or more compartments in which to measure tracer concentrations. The distribution of tracer is first divided into intravascular (blood or plasma) and extravascular compartments. The extravascular compartment is further divided into the amount of tracer bound to the receptor of interest ('specific binding'), the free tracer and the tracer bound to other sites ('non-specific binding'). The latter two segments can be collapsed into a single 'non-displaceable' component (Huang and Phelps, 1986). This is described in Equation (6.5):

$$
\begin{array}{ccccc}
& \| \; \| & & & \\
& k_1 & & k_3 & \\
[L_P{}^*] & \longleftrightarrow & [L_{ND}{}^*] & \longleftrightarrow & [L_S{}^*] \\
& k_2 & & k_4 & \\
& \| \; \| & & & \\
& \text{BBB} & & &
\end{array}
\tag{6.5}
$$

where BBB is the blood–brain barrier, $[L_P{}^*]$, $[L_{ND}{}^*]$ and $[L_S{}^*]$ are the concentrations of tracer in plasma and in non-displaceable and specifically bound domains, respectively, k_1 and k_2 are the transport rate constants in and out across the blood–brain barrier, respectively, and k_3 and k_4 are the on and off rate constants, respectively.

In imaging brain receptors, the movement of tracer from the intravascular to the extravascular compartment is a function of the blood–brain barrier penetrability of the carrier. Even for lipophilic compounds that enter the brain readily via passive diffusion, this occurs at rates much slower than the binding of the tracer to the receptor. This requires the measurement and correction of image data for the intravascular or 'blood flow' signal. Moreover, tracers are simply labeled drugs or analogs of endogenous substrates, rendering them subject to the vicissitudes of distribution and metabolism. This can require the measurement of lipophilic metabolites that may retain the isotope label in order to correct the image data.

In vitro methods determine receptor kinetics by comparing binding across a range of ligand concentrations. The limits for radiation exposure from the radioisotope and the logistics required for performing these imaging studies generally do not permit the use of a range of tracer or cold-challenge drug concentrations within subjects for human *in vivo* studies. In theory, K_A and B_{max} could be calculated by estimating the high specific-activity tracer concentrations in the extravascular compartment at several time points or using low specific-activity tracer infusions over an extended period of time. However, these methods are not sufficiently accurate or practicable to use in a single PET experiment, so B_{max} and K_A cannot be determined properly. As a compromise, the ratio B_{max}/K_A is frequently calculated. This ratio corresponds to the ratio of k_3/k_4 and is referred to as the binding potential (Mintun *et al.*, 1984). The binding potential of a tracer can be obtained using a full or reduced compartmental model and fitting the rates of distribution of the tracer in the different compartments (from the time–activity curves) and calculating k_3 and k_4. For selected tracers it can be approximated using a reference tissue method.

Following this method, the tracer activity in a region with high concentrations of a receptor (e.g. basal ganglia for D2 receptors) is essentially corrected for non-specific binding by using the time–activity curve measured in a region with low or negligible concentrations of the receptor (such as cerebellum for D2 receptors) (Lammertsma and Hume, 1996). A commonly used 'correction' involves simply calculating the ratio of integrated activity in the region of interest relative to the reference region.

Receptor-specific tracers have been used to estimate the dose/occupancy relationships for a number of psychopharmaceuticals, including dopamine D2 receptor antagonists (Nyberg *et al.*, 1996), serotonin 5-HT2a and 5-HT1a receptor antagonists (Gefvert *et al.*, 1998; Rabiner *et al.*, 2000), benzo-diazepines (Shinotoh *et al.*, 1989), neurokinin NK1 receptor antagonists (Bergstrom *et al.*, 2000), drugs acting at muscarinic cholinergic receptors (Raedler *et al.*, 1999), inhibitors of dopamine and serotonin transporters (Meyer *et al.*, 2001; Volkow *et al.*, 2002) and opiate receptor agonists (Sadzot *et al.*, 1990). These studies are conducted after single-dose challenges in dose-ranging studies or after chronic treatment. An example of such a study is depicted in Plate 6.2. Chronic treatment with the selective serotonin reuptake inhibitor (SSRI) citalopram, at a dose predicted to be in the therapeutic range, results in the occupancy and presumed blockade of approximately 80% of the available serotonin transporters in brain.

In addition to estimating occupancy at steady state, by conducting serial studies after treatment is stopped one can estimate the duration of occupancy (Grunder *et al.*, 1997). One may thus calculate the central clearance of active drug in the brain, which often will be much slower than peripheral clearance due to the lipophilic nature of many psychopharmaceuticals. These types of studies can be extraordinarily informative for understanding the relationship between drug dose and efficacy and safety. At the same time, the inventory of tracers available for such studies is quite limited. Whereas a number of tracers are available for the dopaminergic system, no tracer is currently available for imaging many of the other systems in brain. As drug development begins to explore the potential of new targets such as the excitatory amino acids and peptide receptors, there will be a critical need for the parallel development of tracers directed at these targets.

6.3.4 DRUG DISPOSITION

Disposition of a drug in the brain can be assessed by estimating the distribution of the drug labeled with a radioisotope (Farde *et al.*, 1996) or, in selected cases, with MRS. Distribution using radiolabeling is the most commonly used approach and generally involves substitution of ^{11}C for a ^{12}C atom in the molecule, the site being determined by the ease in the radiolabeling (such as a methyl group) and the likelihood of generating significant amounts of brain-penetrant metabolites bearing the label during the time course of the PET study. The principle is the same as drug distribution studies in peripheral compartments using ^{14}C-labeled drug except that the measurement is in the brain with all the technical requirements and constraints of PET. A very small amount of the radiolabeled drug is given intravenously and PET images of the brain are acquired almost immediately after. The data are corrected for the amount of tracer circulating in the bloodstream, which also contributes to the brain signal, and then the amount and distribution of the tracer in brain tissue can be estimated. The objective of these studies is often to characterize how easily and rapidly a drug enters the brain – a critical issue in developing new psychopharmaceuticals – and this does not depend on whether the binding of the drug is specific or not. Indeed, most psychoactive drugs that are developed for clinical use are very lipophilic and distribute principally into brain lipid such as white matter. Although the concentration of tracer is nanomolar with this technique, the plasma to brain ratio can be used to predict the relative concentrations of 'cold' drug given at pharmacological doses. The short half-life of ^{11}C allows estimation of brain penetration for a little over an hour and would not predict poorly but still penetrant compounds.

6.3.5 ASSESSING DRUG DISPOSITION WITH MRS

As noted above, NMR or MRS can be used to detect any atom with an 'odd' atomic weight and therefore can be used to measure several other atoms in brain tissue besides protons. Clinical imaging with MRI relies on protons for the signal because of their great abundance (especially associated with water) and diffuse distribution. Other atoms of interest in psychopharmaceutical studies have included ^{19}F and ^{7}Li, provided that they are 'mobile' (visible to MRS) and present at micromolar concentrations. Such concentrations are achieved during chronic treatment with lithium salts and many fluorinated psychotropic compounds such as fluoxetine and fluphenazine. The advantage of this technique is that the signal does not require the introduction of a radioisotope, it estimates concentrations under chronic (steady state) conditions and serial scans can be conducted to look at the clearance of these compounds between doses or after dosing has stopped (Henry et al., 2000; Moore et al., 2002). Moreover, because MRS can detect the clinical form of the drug, uses clinical doses and conducts the study at steady state, one can estimate the absolute concentration of the drug in the brain. The caveat to this statement is that lipophilic metabolites that are brain penetrant and retain the fluorine atom will also be measured by MRS. Drug disposition studies using MRS are limited to drugs with these atoms, and the concentrations in the brain of even highly lipophilic compounds are such that the resolution is limited. However, MRS can provide pharmacokinetic information in the brain, where these compounds have their therapeutic effect. Similar to studies with radiotracers, MRS studies have shown that the clearance from the brain is generally much slower than the clearance from the bloodstream. This knowledge is critical for determining the appropriate dose and dosing interval for these compounds.

6.4 FUTURE DEVELOPMENTS

The full potential of any of the methods described has not been realized and much remains to understand and validate more fully the information yielded by these techniques. As an accepted measure of hexokinase activity, FDG-PET provides a model for the development of other approaches to evaluating brain physiology. Other enzyme systems that have been explored include the labeling of monoamine oxidase (MAO) A and B with 'suicide' inhibitors (clorgyline and deprenyl, respectively), revealing important information on the time course of the effect of MAO inhibitors and the unexpected finding of significant downregulation of MAOs in cigarette smokers (Fowler et al., 1996, 1998). ^{11}C-labeled rolipram is currently being investigated as a potential measure of change in phosphodiesterase enzyme type 4, an important link in the second-messenger cascade initiated by many antidepressants (Lourenco et al., 2001). Other enzyme systems also might be explored with suitable radiolabeled substrates. Most studies of brain activity have been conducted after single doses, yielding valuable information about acute pharmacology, but chronic effects are generally more relevant to the therapeutic and safety characteristics of drugs. Magnetic resonance spectroscopy has only begun to be explored as a means of evaluating drug effects in the brain. Beyond the studies of ^{7}Li and ^{19}F, MRS can be used to explore the effect of drugs on endogenous molecules carrying ^{31}P, such as the various forms of phosphorylated adenosine used as energy in the cell, and proton-rich biomolecules (other than water) that are involved in cellular metabolism and neuronal signaling. For example, ^{1}H-MRS was successfully applied to estimating the exposure response relationship between vigabatrin and brain GABA concentrations (Petroff et al., 1996).

A rich library of tracers exists for the dopamine system and perhaps also the serotonin system; however, little or nothing currently exists for the assessment of many other neurotransmitter systems in the brain, some of whose receptors have been identified only recently. Pharmaceutical and biotechnology industries are major sources not only of new compounds that target these sites as candidate therapeutics but also of compounds that may serve as radiotracers to evaluate these sites and the effects of disease and treatment. The incentive and raw materials for continued development of functional imaging of the human brain will depend on the establishment of sustained collaborations between academic and government research centers and the pharmaceutical industry.

7

Psychotropic Drugs and Cognitive Function

7.1 INTRODUCTION

Human behavior traditionally has been conceptualized in terms of three functional areas: *cognition*, designating the information-handling aspect of behavior; *emotionality*, comprising feelings and emotions; and *executive functions*, which are related to the way behavior is expressed. As formulated by Deutsch Lezak (1995, p. 20), components of each of these three sets of functions are as integral to every bit of behavior as are the length and breadth and height to the shape of an object, i.e. none of them takes priority over the others. Referring to the computer operations of input, storage, processing and output, Deutsch Lezak (1995, p. 22) distinguishes the following cognitive functions:

- *Receptive functions*: the ability to select, acquire, classify and integrate information.
- *Memory and learning*: information storage and retrieval.
- *Thinking*: the mental organization and reorganization of information.
- *Expressive functions*: the means through which information is communicated or acted upon.

This chapter deals with the question of how psychotropic drugs act upon cognitive functions in man. Some of the pertinent information, i.e. how single doses of these pharmaceuticals affect cognitive performance in healthy volunteers under experimental conditions, has been reviewed and discussed in Chapter 3. However, when dealing with drug effects in patients suffering from schizophrenia, depression, anxiety disorders, etc. one must expect a much

Psychopharmacology, Fourth Edition. By R. Spiegel
© 2003 John Wiley & Sons, Ltd: ISBN 0 471 56039 1: 0 470 84691 7 (PB)

more complex picture to emerge: owing to their beneficial action upon mental disorders and a variety of symptoms, psychotropic drugs are likely to have direct or indirect beneficial effects on some disturbed cognitive functions; on the other hand, it appears likely that certain aspects of cognitive performance can be impaired due to the sedative or anticholinergic effects of many of these drugs.

The structure of this chapter follows the classification of psychotropic drugs into antipsychotics, antidepressants and mood stabilizers, anxiolytics, psycho-stimulants and antidementia drugs. In view of the variety of conditions treated with these compounds, the different clinical significance of cognitive symptoms within the diseases treated, the differences in drug use (prophylactic, short-term symptomatic, long-term symptomatic, maintenance) and other factors, one may anticipate a rather heterogeneous picture to emerge as far as the effects on cognitive performance are concerned.

7.2 ANTIPSYCHOTIC DRUGS

7.2.1 COGNITIVE CHANGES IN SCHIZOPHRENIA

Schizophrenia designates a group of mental disorders rather than a uniform disease. Eugen Bleuler (1911), who coined the term schizophrenia, disputed the then current Kraepelinian concept of 'dementia praecox' because he had recognized that the disorders in question could have very different courses and outcomes. Specifically, not all patients with schizophrenic psychoses ended up in dementia praecox, i.e. with a premature loss of their mind. Carpenter and Buchanan (1994) suggested that the clinical manifestations of schizophrenia could be grouped into three relatively separate core domains of psychopathology (the 'three-compartment model' of schizophrenia):

(1) Psychotic symptoms: hallucinations, delusions.
(2) Cognitive impairment: positive formal thought disorder such as: tangentiality, loss of goals, incoherence, looseness of associations, neologisms.
(3) Negative symptoms: restricted affect, diminished emotional range, poverty of speech, curbing of interests, diminished sense of purpose, diminished social drive.

According to this model, a discussion of potential therapeutic drug effects on cognitive function in schizophrenia should focus upon the correction of abnormalities in thought and speech. Other authors, e.g. Schultz and Andreasen (1999), appear to subsume a much wider range of schizophrenic symptoms under the umbrella of cognitive abnormalities: "Several cognitive and emotional functions are impaired, such as perception (hallucinations), inferential thinking (delusions), motivation (avolition) and thought and speech (alogia)... Many negative symptoms are cognitive, such as alogia, avolition, and attentional impairment...". This broader interpretation of cognitive disturbances implies that all patients with schizophrenia suffer from some kind of cognitive impairment and that a discussion of positive drug effects on cognitive functions would comprise most of the symptomatic spectrum of the disorder.

Depending on the criteria applied and the specific neuropsychological tests used there is great variation in the reported frequency of cognitive impairment in schizophrenic patients. Deutsch Lezak (1995, p. 324) cautioned that 'the majority of persons diagnosed as schizophrenics have neither the neurological stigmata nor significant neuropsychological deficits'. Meltzer and Fatemi (1998) estimated that about 40% of patients with schizophrenia have major deficits in measures of attention, executive function, verbal learning and memory, spatial and verbal working memory, semantic memory and psychomotor performance. Palmer et al. (1997) reported that only about a quarter of schizophrenic patients in their study sample could be considered 'neuropsychologically normal'. Bilder et al. (2000) provided mean values, standard deviations, etc. of psychomotor performance scores but no estimation of the percentage of schizophrenic patients showing significant cognitive deficit.

Much of the current knowledge about cognitive impairment in schizophrenia was summarized by O'Carroll (2000) as follows:

(1) Significant cognitive deficit affects up to 75% of patients with schizophrenia (this estimation may be very much on the high side; see Rund and Borg, 1999).
(2) A wide range of cognitive functions are affected, particularly memory, attention, motor skills, executive function and intelligence. In contrast, implicit learning appears to be unaffected (Danion et al., 2001).
(3) The cognitive impairment often predates the illness onset. It is an intrinsic part of the illness and is also observed in young, drug-naïve patients. According to a number of cross-sectional and longitudinal studies (e.g. Heaton et al., 2001; Norman et al., 2001), cognitive deficits do not show significant progression in the majority of schizophrenic patients.
(4) Efforts to explain core clinical features of schizophrenia as a consequence of specific neuropsychological abnormalities have been disappointing.
(5) Cognitive impairment is related to social and functional outcome.

Egan et al. (2001) reported that mentally healthy siblings of schizophrenic patients had weaker performance than unrelated healthy controls on a number of tests on which the schizophrenic patients showed significant deficit (Wisconsin Card Sorting, Trail Making B and some verbal tests). Impairment on one test only weakly predicted impairment on other tests, suggesting that there are specific familial and possibly heritable cognitive deficiencies that may act as individual risk factors. According to Egan *et al.* these 'cognitive phenotypes' may identify distinct, familial traits associated with schizophrenia. If applied to therapeutic trials, this concept could provide more individualized analyses of therapeutic outcomes: in addition to group means, standard deviations, etc. one would then consider individual performance deficits at baseline as well as their changes following treatment, and provide separate analyses with subgroups of patients characterized by similar deficits at baseline.

7.2.2 EFFECTS OF ANTIPSYCHOTIC DRUGS

According to an early overview by Davis and Casper (1978), the cognitive performance of schizophrenic patients usually improves during the course of treatment with antipsychotic drugs. Textbook authors such as Baldessarini (1985) Hinterhuber and Haring (1992) and Janicak *et al.* (1993) did not specifically address the effects of antipsychotic drugs on cognitive functions in schizophrenic patients. Delirious states were mentioned as an occasional side effect of antipsychotic drugs with pronounced anticholinergic action such as thioridazine and chlorpromazine; the incidence of such events is highest in elderly patients. Cassens *et al.* (1990) noted that the available literature contained no conclusive evidence of an adverse effect of antipsychotics on the learning and memory functions of patients. Rund and Borg (1999) stated that "there is not yet sufficient empirical evidence for dramatic effects of conventional neuroleptics with regard to either improvement or impairment [of cognitive function]".

Major interest in the beneficial effects of antipsychotic drugs on cognitive function in schizophrenic patients emerged after 1990, and most of the recent reports therefore focus on the newer, atypical drugs rather than on traditional antipsychotics. A critical review of studies published up to 2001 (Weiss *et al.*, 2002) lists 17 papers dealing with clozapine (8 studies), risperidone (7 studies), olanzapine (3 studies) or quetiapine (4 studies). Some of the papers contained data from exploratory open trials whereas others dealt with findings from comparative studies with more than one antipsychotic drug. The results reported by Weiss *et al.* are summarized in Table 7.1; however the authors made it clear that the underlying studies were heterogeneous with regard to size, design, duration and other relevant factors. As a consequence, they "provide conflicting results and have a variety of methodological limitations. It appears that the findings from many exploratory studies can now be distilled into more focused, hypothesis-driven study design". Harvey and Keefe (2001) shared the critical attitude of Weiss *et al.* and noted that "the methodology for assessing the treatment of cognitive deficits [in schizophrenia] is still being developed".

Table 7.1 Improved cognitive performance after atypical antipsychotics[a]

	Clozapine	Risperidone	Olanzapine	Quetiapine
Reaction time	Yes	No	n.a.	n.a.
Visuomotor tracking	n.a.	Yes	Yes	Yes
Verbal fluency	Yes	n.a.	Yes	Yes
Attention	Yes	Yes	Yes	Yes
Executive function	(Yes)	Yes	Yes	Yes
Verbal learning and memory	Mixed results	Yes	Yes	Yes
Immediate recall	n.a.	Yes	n.a.	Yes
Visual learning and memory	No/n.a.	Mixed results	Yes	n.a.

[a]Summary of findings reported by Weiss *et al.* (2002); see text concerning the quality of the underlying studies; n.a. = no data available.

More recently, two methodologically advanced studies have been published: a comparison between four antipsychotic drugs in a trial of 14 weeks duration (Bilder *et al.*, 2002, see Box 7.1); and a study of 2 years duration comparing an atypical with an older 'typical' antipsychotic drug (Green *et al.*, 2002). Perhaps the most striking finding in the study by Bilder *et al.* is the superior performance of risperidone on learning and memory and the somewhat disappointing effect of clozapine on cognitive functioning in these chronic, therapy-resistant patients. Both observations are in contrast to clinical observations made in the same study and reported by Volavka *et al.* (2002): risperidone was found to be less clinically effective than clozapine and olanzapine, and clozapine proved superior to the other treatments with regard to negative symptoms. These discrepant observations would support statements made by, for example, O'Carroll (2000) and Potkin *et al.* (2001), that clinical symptoms and cognitive performance of schizophrenic patients may show almost independent courses. On the other hand, one should also keep in mind that the findings originate from a relatively short-term study and that it is perhaps unrealistic to expect clear-cut and reliable cognitive improvement in patients who had been ill for many years before being included in this study.

The study by Green *et al.* (2002) included 62 patients, almost exclusively males, mean age 43 years, mean age of onset of the disease about 25 years, with a diagnosis of schizophrenia or schizoaffective disorder. In contrast to the patients studied by Bilder *et al.* (2002), these individuals were not treatment-resistant and they were stabilized on antipsychotic drugs for at least 2 months before entering the trial. The doses of medication used in this maintenance trial were much lower than those reported by Bilder *et al.*: the mean daily dose of haloperidol was 5 mg or slightly less and the mean daily dose of risperidone was about 6 mg. The planned study duration was 2 years, with about half of the patients completing the trial; a neurocognitive battery providing 13 key variables was administered at baseline and then at weeks 4, 24, 48, 72 and 104.

Box 7.1 A Controlled Comparison between Four Antipsychotic Drugs

In a cooperative study of four US state psychiatric hospitals, Bilder *et al.* (2002) compared three atypical antipsychotic drugs (clozapine, olanzapine, risperidone) with haloperidol in a double-blind, parallel-group trial. Patients (n = 101) had a diagnosis of treatment-resistant schizophrenia or schizoaffective disorder according to DSM-IV; treatment resistance was defined as "persistent positive symptoms (hallucinations, delusions, or marked thought disorder) after at least 6 contiguous weeks of treatment, presently or documented in the past, with one or more typical antipsychotics at doses $\geqslant 600$ mg/day chlorpromazine", plus "a poor level of functioning over the past 2 years, defined by the lack of competitive employment or enrollment in an academic or vocational program . . ." Patients also had to have a baseline total score of at least 60 on the PANSS (Positive and Negative Syndrome Scale; Kay *et al.*, 1987). Mean age in the four groups was comparable (about 40 years), as was mean duration of illness (about 20 years) and the mean number of previous hospitalizations; more than 80% of the patients were male, more than 50% were black and less than 30% were white.

The four drugs were administered by psychiatrists blinded to treatment group assignment of patients. The 14-week study consisted of an 8-week dose escalation and fixed dose and a 6-week variable-dose period. The mean dose levels (mg/day) of the four compounds after the first 8 weeks were 452 for clozapine, 20.2 for olanzapine, 8.3 for risperidone and 19.6 for haloperidol. Patients on haloperidol received prophylactic anticholinergic medication to prevent extrapyramidal symptoms, and a few other drugs were permitted to treat agitation and insomnia.

The neurocognitive test battery consisted of 10 tests that provided 16 individual measures. By using principal component factor analysis of baseline values, a global score and four domain scores were calculated; these were termed 'declarative verbal learning and memory', 'processing speed and attention', 'simple motor functioning' and 'general executive and perceptual organization'.

The main findings with regard to drug effects on cognitive performance were as follows:

- Patients treated with olanzapine improved in global score, in general executive and perceptual organization and in processing speed and attention.

- Patients treated with risperidone improved in global score.
- Patients treated with clozapine improved in simple motor functioning.

With regard to the global score, and taking into account the number of patients with 'clinically significant' neurocognitive improvement, patients on olanzapine and risperidone fared better than those on haloperidol; patients on clozapine were between those on risperidone and haloperidol. The average effect sizes were judged as being in the small to medium range. There were several significant correlations between the clinical (PANSS) variables, notably the negative symptom subscale scores, and the neurocognitive changes. On the other hand, when partialed out, the PANSS scores had little influence on the main neurocognitive effects, indicating that treatment-related changes of cognitive function and psychiatric symptoms proceeded with considerable independence.

In contrast to earlier studies clozapine had significant beneficial impact on motor performance but not on memory function. According to the authors, this could be due to the anticholinergic effect of clozapine. Risperidone, a drug without anticholinergic properties, showed the strongest effect on declarative verbal learning and memory, whereas olanzapine, which also has strong anticholinergic effects, was not better than clozapine and haloperidol with regard to its effect on memory.

The neurocognitive findings were summarized in a general composite score and separately in three cluster scores, one standing for perceptual discrimination, one for memory and fluency, and the third one for executive functioning. Improvement from baseline after 2 years was observed in both treatment groups for the general composite score and for the memory and fluency cluster, but there were no significant differences between the patients treated with risperidone and haloperidol. The time course of cognitive improvement was different in the two groups: patients on risperidone showed a gradual and continuous increase in performance; patients on haloperidol displayed initial improvement and subsequent stabilization at the higher level. Interestingly, patients on haloperidol had more tremor and akathisia, but these adverse events did not appear to have a relevant impact upon cognitive performance. The authors speculated "that conventional [antipsychotic] medications may have neurocognitive benefits at lower doses that are neutralized or reversed at higher doses".

7.2.3 COMMENTS

A preliminary conclusion that one can draw from the studies quoted in this section is that antipsychotic drugs often have modest positive effects on the cognitive functions of schizophrenic patients. As Green (2002) has pointed out, the second-generation (atypical) antipsychotics may convey advantages over the conventional ones if used at standard doses, but even with these more recent drugs neurocognitive performance is often not brought up to that of normal controls. Many questions are still unanswered, however (see Harvey and Keefe, 2001): the extent, specificity and practical significance of cognitive deficits in different subtypes of schizophrenia (Brazo *et al.*, 2002), their temporal relation-ship to the clinical symptomatology and its changes on drug treatment and, at least in the case of acutely psychotic patients, the reliability and validity of psychometric measurements performed on individuals suffering from delusions, hallucinations, thought disorder and associated affective symptoms.

7.3 ANTIDEPRESSANT DRUGS

7.3.1 COGNITIVE CHANGES IN DEPRESSION

Mood disorders are frequently associated with cognitive impairment. In younger depressives attention and concentration are primarily affected, and responses in speed-related tasks may be abnormally slowed. Complaints about serious cognitive dysfunction, which are particularly frequent in older patients with depression, cannot always be fully substantiated by means of objective tests (O'Hara *et al.*, 1986). Nevertheless, significant deficits in the following areas have been found:

- Episodic memory and learning, involving both explicit verbal and visual memory performance; in contrast, recognition and implicit memory tasks appear to be spared.
- Executive tasks, e.g. tests of verbal fluency and attentional set-shifting (such as card sorting tasks), are significantly impaired in patients with more severe depression and in elderly depressed patients.

The severity of the disorder appears to contribute to the neuropsychological deficits; this relationship is most clearly recognized in the so-called melancholic subtype of depression. Another relevant factor is age: cognitive deficits are generally more severe and more widespread in old than in younger depressed patients (Butters *et al.*, 2000).

There have been different approaches to explain the cognitive deficits in depression. Weingartner and Silbermann (1982), noting that depressed patients had more difficulty with 'effortful' than with 'automatic' memory tasks (e.g. verbal recall vs. recognition), hypothesized that an 'altered motivation state' characteristic of depression was responsible for the cognitive deficiencies observed. Austin *et al.* (2001) consider this view ("if patients feel unwell they will not try so hard") somewhat dated; in their view the fact that there may be persistent cognitive impairment even upon recovery in mood disorders, particularly in older subjects, provides "important evidence that enduring brain abnormalities are implicated in the etiology of depressive disorder". Studies using neuroimaging techniques suggest that structural, mainly subcortical abnormalities in aged depressed patients frequently underlie the observed cognitive deficits. However, in a discussion of the possible neural localization of cognitive dysfunction in aged depressive patients, Austin *et al.* (2001) caution against premature allocation of abnormal neuropsychological test results to specific neuroanatomical defects: most neuropsychological tasks relate to more than one cognitive domain, making diagnoses based on test performance and aiming at specific structural deficits rather doubtful.

7.3.2 EFFECTS OF ANTIDEPRESSANT DRUGS

Antidepressants differ from one another in at least two areas of pharmacological activity that are relevant to cognitive function: their degree of sedative action (which may be due to different mechanisms) and their central anticholinergic effects. Sedative drug action might be evident as impairment of cognitive performance in general, whereas central anticholinergic effects might manifest themselves more specifically as impairments of learning and memory (see Section 7.5). Experimental study results gathered in healthy volunteers and summarized in Table 3.6 (Chapter 3) support the first assumption but not necessarily the second one: impairment on a variety of cognitive performance parameters is seen after sedative antidepressants, yet there is no strong evidence of a specific action of anticholinergic agents, such as amitriptyline and imipramine, on measures of learning and memory. Previous reviewers (Deptula and Pomara, 1990; Thompson, 1991; Curran, 1992a) drew similar conclusions and stressed the close association between general sedative drug effects and impairment of cognitive performance seen in healthy subjects. It should be noted, however, that two studies in non-depressed volunteers, published by the same group of investigators (Curran *et al.*, 1988; Sakulsripong *et al.*, 1991) did suggest a memory-impairing action of the antidepressant amitriptyline going beyond what could be expected on the basis of its sedative effects alone.

Although states of confusion and delirium are well known side effects of some older antidepressants, textbooks of psychopharmacology before 1990 hardly mentioned any specific actions of these drugs upon cognitive function in patients. Hollister (1978) reported an incidence of confusional states in 10–15% of all patients treated with tricyclic antidepressants, rising to 35% and more in patients aged over 40 years. Schatzberg *et al.* (1978) described a phenomenon occasionally noted in individuals over 40 years old and receiving antidepressants, to which they gave the term *speech blockage*: patients had difficulty in finding the next logically following thought in a discussion or in expressing an idea in words. The appropriate words would usually occur to them after a pause of a few seconds, but the unexpected interruptions in thought and speech processes often caused anxiety and worry. An experimental study (Branconnier *et al.*, 1987) comparing the sedative antidepressant maprotiline with the sedative and anticholinergic drug amitriptyline in patients with major depressive disorders confirmed the occurrence of speech blockage after amitriptyline in patients over 55–60 years but not in younger age groups.

Because antidepressants help to resolve depressive episodes and also may have sedative and anticholinergic actions, the question of practical importance arises as to whether the use of specific antidepressant compounds is associated with improvement in depressive cognitive dysfunction or with additional deterioration. An early, often quoted study by Sternberg and Jarvik (1976, see Box 7.2) suggested that amitriptyline and imipramine led to clinical improvement in the majority of depressive patients that, despite the strong anticholinergic effects of both compounds used, was accompanied 4 weeks later by an improvement in memory function. This somewhat reassuring finding has been supplemented and partially confirmed by results obtained in studies with other antidepressant drugs (see review by Thompson, 1991). Furthermore, a longitudinal investigation in a population-based sample of 1488 adults (Podewils and Lyketsos, 2002) failed to support the concept that the use of tricyclic antidepressants is related to measurable long-term (median 11.5 years) cognitive deficits; it should be mentioned, however, that the assessment scale used in this observational study, the MMSE (Mini-Mental State Examination; Folstein *et al.*, 1975), provides only a crude estimate of cognitive function, and that the amount and duration of antidepressant drug use in the population studied were not specified.

Although deleterious effects of antidepressants with anticholinergic action upon cognitive functions have not really been proven in controlled clinical trials, there are other medical reasons to restrict the use of these drugs in elderly and old patients (Chapter 1). Consequently, strong educational efforts are made in some countries to replace, at least in older depressed patients, drugs such as amitriptyline, clomipramine, doxepin and imipramine with compounds having similar efficacy but less or no anticholinergic action (van Eijk *et al.*, 2001). Preferred antidepressants with minor or no anticholinergic effects according to these authors comprise a number of tricyclic compounds (e.g. desipramine, nortriptyline, trimipramine), the selective serotonin reuptake inhibitors (SSRIs), the monoamine oxidase inhibitors (MAOIs) and several other compounds such as trazodone, venlafaxine and mirtazapine.

Proven or alleged lack of negative effects upon cognitive function, especially memory performance, is occasionally used as an argument to support the use

Box 7.2 Anticholinergic antidepressants: Improvement or Deterioration of Memory?

Sternberg and Jarvik (1976) studied 26 patients with endogenous depression and 26 healthy subjects matched for age, gender and education. The patients were newly hospitalized and had not yet received any antidepressants at the time of the first examination. Three tests of learning and memory were performed by the patients and subjects: learning of 15 weakly associated pairs of words; recognition of 15 previously shown drawings of familiar objects among 30 drawings; and association of three portraits with three fictitious descriptions of people.

The depressed patients were found to be inferior to the healthy subjects in pair-associate learning and in linking portraits with descriptions of people. Picture recognition did not differ significantly because both groups had near-maximum performance. When the tests were repeated 3 h later, both groups of subjects performed worse than before and the differences between the patients and healthy controls were significantly reduced. This was interpreted by the authors as an indication that immediate memory but not the ability to retain learned material was affected in the depressed patients. The patients then were treated with either imipramine or amitriptyline at doses of 150–300 mg/day. Four weeks later, the therapeutic results were evaluated and patients were divided into four groups:

- Group A: fully remitted ($n = 4$).
- Group B: considerable improvement ($n = 8$).
- Group C: moderate improvement ($n = 8$).
- Group D: no noticeable improvement ($n = 6$).

At this time the tests of learning and memory were repeated with groups A, B and C, i.e. with 20 patients showing at least moderate clinical improvement, as well as with some of the healthy volunteers to estimate the effect of training. Compared with their performance at baseline, the 20 patients showed highly significant improvement in the two recall tasks immediately after presentation but not 3 h later (i.e. the time point when their performance had not differed much from that of the reference group at baseline). The authors also noted a correlation between the improvement in clinical state and the improvement in memory, because performance was improved most markedly in groups A and B.

> This study, notwithstanding its imperfect design, is often quoted
> as evidence to show that improvement of depression and normal-
> ization of cognitive performance are likely to go together, and that
> antidepressants with strong anticholinergic action are not really
> harmful for the cognitive function of depressed patients.

of newer antidepressants, not just in older patients but in depressed individuals
generally. It is of interest, therefore, to consider briefly the published evidence
relevant to this issue:

- A critical review by Olver *et al.* (2001) on so-called "third-generation
  antidepressants" (venlafaxine, reboxetine, nefazodone, mirtazapine) covered 30 controlled therapeutic trials and a number of relapse prevention
  studies. Questions addressed were overall efficacy, speed of onset and safety
  but, according to this review, none of the third-generation antidepressants
  was specifically tested with respect to its potential effects on cognitive
  function in depressed patients.
- A meta-analysis of 32 controlled studies comparing venlafaxine with several
  SSRIs and other antidepressants (Smith *et al.*, 2002) demonstrated some
  modest efficacy advantage for venlafaxine. Tolerability was considered
  comparable to that of the reference compounds but no information is
  provided on the effects of venlafaxine on cognitive function in depressed
  patients.
- A number of SSRIs and SNRIs were tested for their effects on cognitive
  function in repeated-dose studies in healthy, non-depressed volunteers.
  Studies with SSRIs before 1999 have been reviewed by Lane and O'Hanlon
  (1999) and some more recent reports deal with nefazodone, paroxetine and
  sertraline (Furlan *et al.*, 2001; Schmitt *et al.*, 2001; van Laar *et al.*, 2002).
  However, considering the populations studied in these trials (non-depressed
  subjects), the duration of drug administration (1–2 weeks) and the mostly
  low drug doses used, the relevance of these studies for a clinical situation
  may be questioned.

With regard to its effects on cognitive performance in the target population, the
SSRI sertraline appears to be the most thoroughly studied newer antidepressant. Lane and O'Hanlon (1999) listed three controlled clinical studies with
fluoxetine and three with sertraline; however, all three trials with fluoxetine and
one of the trials with sertraline were not sufficiently powered to demonstrate
reliable differences between treatments. One of the two adequately powered
studies, a comparison between nortriptyline and sertraline in elderly depressed
patients (Bondareff *et al.*, 2000; see Box 7.3), supports the notion that
antidepressants with anticholinergic action (such as nortriptyline) are similarly

effective as SSRIs against depressions of old age but may impair cognitive function, particularly memory performance. The other study was a comparison lasting 12 weeks between two SSRIs, sertraline and fluoxetine, in 236 outpatients 60 years of age or older who met the DSM-III-R criteria (APA, 1987) for major depressive disorder (Newhouse *et al.*, 2000). In this trial the two compounds produced similar improvement on the Hamilton Rating Scale for Depression scores, resulting in almost identical responder rates; patients treated with sertraline were found to be transiently superior to those on fluoxetine on a memory test (shopping list) and significantly better in the digit symbol substitution task (DSST) after 6 and 12 weeks of treatment. Together with similar observations made in several smaller comparative studies (e.g. Levkovitz *et al.*, 2002), these results suggest that antidepressants without anticholinergic effects, such as SSRIs and SNRIs, do not negatively affect cognitive performance and ought to be given preference in the treatment of elderly depressed patients.

Box 7.3 Effects of Two Antidepressants on Cognitive Function in Older Depressed Patients

In a double-blind, parallel-group study, Bondareff *et al.* (2000) compared the SSRI sertraline and the tricyclic compound nortriptyline with regard to their efficacy and safety in a group of 210 outpatients 60 years and older. The patients met the DSM-III-R criteria for major depressive episode and had a minimum score of 18 on the Hamilton Rating Scale for Depression. Their mean age was about 68 years, most patients were white and about 60% were female; the severity of depression was rated as 'moderate' in more than 70% and as 'severe' in more than 20% of the cases. The daily doses of sertraline were between 50 and 150 mg, and those of nortriptyline were 25–100 mg; the treatment lasted 12 weeks. In addition to clinical rating scales and self-assessment instruments, patients took the following tests of cognitive performance:

- The DSST from the Wechsler Intelligence Scale.
- A shopping list task, presented as a selective reminding procedure.
- The MMSE (Folstein *et al.*, 1975).

About 70% of the patients in both treatment groups completed the trial, with similar therapeutic efficacy (Hamilton Rating Scale for Depression) shown for both compounds. The pattern of adverse events was different, with more patients reporting diarrhea, nausea and insomnia on sertraline, and more patients on nortriptyline reporting dry mouth and constipation. Significant differences in favor of sertraline were found in all three cognitive measures used:

- The MMSE showed some improvement on sertraline and some minor decline on nortriptyline; the difference between treatments was statistically significant ($P < 0.01$).
- Performance on the DSST was improved on both drugs, but more so on sertraline ($P = 0.002$).
- The number of items recalled on the shopping list task increased on sertraline and decreased on nortriptyline ($P < 0.001$).

These differential findings would support the concept that nortriptyline (which has modest anticholinergic action) may have negative effects on cognitive functioning, especially memory performance, in elderly depressed patients, whereas sertraline (which is devoid of anticholinergic effects) has no or perhaps slightly favorable effects on cognitive function in these patients. According to the authors, the observations "may reflect the selective vulnerability of older adults to the central anticholinergic activity of nortriptyline".

7.3.3 EFFECTS OF LITHIUM AND OTHER MOOD STABILIZERS

According to Lenox and Manji (1998) the "cognitive effects of lithium appear to be some of the most problematic for patients, yet they remain the least studied". A number of early observational studies were concerned with the question of whether lithium, which is normally administered for months or years, leads to detectable cognitive disturbance, particularly memory impairment. A starting point for these studies was the observation that many patients treated with lithium complained of being mentally slower, less attentive and also more forgetful than they used to be before they were put on lithium.

In healthy subjects lithium leads to slight psychomotor slowing, which is usually accompanied by a subjective feeling of impaired performance and learning capacity (Judd *et al.*, 1987) and can last for several weeks. Greil and Van Calker (1983) reviewed the then available clinical literature and concluded that the actions of lithium on the cognitive functions, including memory, of patients on continuous treatment are slight. This view was supported by subsequent studies by Engelsmann *et al.* (1988) and Joffe *et al.* (1988). However, most of the available evidence stems from observational studies that do not allow definitive conclusions: baseline measurements of cognitive performance obtained before starting lithium treatment were presented in only a few studies; in addition, practically all of these investigations lack a control group not treated with lithium, with the consequence that a definitive evaluation of the observed effects is not possible.

Observations of patients treated with lithium for 10 years or more have provided the somewhat comforting finding that, even after long-term treatment, these individuals did not show memory disorders going beyond the expected age-related changes (Engelsmann et al., 1988).

Most antiepileptic drugs with approved or out-of-label use in affective disorders have been more or less systematically tested with regard to their effects on cognitive performance. The results listed below are from studies in epileptic patients. Because the doses used in bipolar disorder are generally similar to those used in epileptic patients, the findings can probably be extrapolated to bipolar patients. In mania, however, the doses needed are often higher, meaning that the results do not necessarily apply. Reports are available on the following:

- Carbamazepine: small risk of cognitive impairment on chronic doses; some reports on cognitive improvement (Loiseau, 2002).
- Gabapentin: no negative effects reported (Ramsay and Pryor, 2002).
- Lamotrigine: no negative effects reported (Stephen and Brodie, 2002).
- Tiagabine: some improvement in therapy responders (Schachter, 2002; Sommerville, 2002).
- Topiramate: cognitive slowing, impairment of verbal memory, word-finding difficulties, reduced psychomotor speed (Sachdeo and Karia, 2002).
- Valproic acid: generally minimal effect on cognitive function; individual cases with clinically relevant impairment (Genton and Gelisse, 2002).

In conclusion and, although specific studies in patients with affective disorders are lacking, the majority of these compounds do not appear to cause significant problems with regard to their impact upon cognitive function.

7.4 ANTIANXIETY DRUGS

7.4.1 COGNITIVE CHANGES IN ANXIETY DISORDERS

Stage fright and its consequences on cognitive performance, e.g. sudden forgetting of previously well-remembered material in a test situation, illustrate that states of intensive emotional arousal, including situational anxiety, can lead to transient partial amnesia, i.e. the inability to retrieve information from memory. Despite these common experiences there appears to be a lack of systematic study of cognitive deficiencies in patients suffering from generalized anxiety disorder, panic disorder or social anxiety disorder. According to Hindmarch (1998) "it is possible to argue that cognitive dysfunction of one sort

or another is a characteristic feature of anxiety in all its manifestations";
however, there does not seem to be much clinical or experimental evidence to
support and specify this statement. Similarly, although there is a vast literature
on the pathophysiology and biology of anxiety disorders (e.g. Stein and Uhde,
1998), the relationship between the hypothetical biological pathways underlying panic disorder, social phobia, post-traumatic stress disorder (PTSD), etc.
and the mechanisms of cognitive failure have not been elucidated.

A recent review (Belanoff *et al.*, 2001) lists some 50 studies dealing with
short- and long-term relationships between circulating corticosteroids and
cognitive function in patients with affective disorder, Alzheimer disease or
Cushing's syndrome as well as in young and old healthy volunteers – but not a
single investigation on one of the anxiety syndromes. Needless to say that
studies in patients with anxiety disorder would be of great interest because
glucocorticoids such as cortisol are released by the adrenal cortex in response
to a wide range of stressors, including acute and chronic anxiety, and there is
evidence that excessive circulating levels of corticosteroids can be associated
with cognitive impairment in healthy subjects and in patients with mental
disorder. In the absence of published findings from patients with anxiety
disorder it is noteworthy that studies in young and old healthy subjects pointed
toward a negative relationship between (pharmacologically manipulated or
physiologically changing) cortisol levels and cognitive performance (table 1 in
Belanoff *et al.*, 2001). Based on these experimental findings and on clinical
observation, it appears safe to assume that at least some patients with anxiety
syndromes experience shorter or longer episodes of cognitive impairment.

7.4.2 EFFECTS OF BENZODIAZEPINES

Benzodiazepine anxiolytics and hypnotics such as diazepam, oxazepam,
lorazepam, nitrazepam and flurazepam have dose-dependent sedative, myorelaxant and memory-impairing activities, and the question arose early on as to
whether the effect of the drugs on learning and memory is part of their general
sedative action (Chapter 3) or should be considered a specific effect. If the
amnestic effect of benzodiazepines were specific, it would arise even with low
and possibly subtherapeutic doses; if non-specific, amnesia could in principle
be avoided by careful individual dosage adjustment. Another question
concerns the duration of the memory-impairing activity of benzodiazepines
during therapeutic use: is there attenuation of these effects after a few days in
the same way as with general sedation, or are learning and memory
impairments to be expected even after weeks or months of chronic
administration?

The fact that single-dose administration of benzodiazepines could have
marked amnestic effects was first recognized in anesthesiology where these
drugs are used to relax and sedate patients prior to surgery. It was found that,

after surgery and on waking from anesthesia, patients had mostly forgotten events occurring between the benzodiazepine premedication and the operation (Box 7.4).

Box 7.4 Amnestic Effects of Benzodiazepines: a Clinical Experiment in Anesthesiology

In a controlled clinical experiment George and Dundee (1977) used various benzodiazepines in groups of between 10 and 20 female patients immediately before minor surgery in order to achieve preoperative sedation. The drugs used were diazepam (10 and 20 mg), flunitrazepam (1 and 2 mg) and lorazepam (4 mg). After intravenous injection of the benzodiapezine, each patient was shown ten pictures at fixed intervals, the content of which they had to name while the nurse showing the pictures simultaneously noted the degree of sleepiness. Six hours after the operation, when the patients had recovered, they were asked which pictures they remembered (free recall) and were subsequently shown 20 pictures from which they could select those previously shown (recognition). The experiment yielded the following results:

(1) Some amnesia occurred after all three benzodiazepines, although there were pronounced differences between the three drugs with regard to the time of onset of action, peak effect and duration of action. For example: the amnestic effect of diazepam occurred as soon as 1 min after injection but had abated completely 60 min later.

(2) There was a close relationship between the extent of the memory impairment for a specific picture and the degree of sleepiness recorded by the nurse at the time when this picture had been presented.

(3) No patient suffered total amnesia for the entire period of the investigation and recognition performance was always superior to free recall.

Clinical experiments such as that conducted by George and Dundee (1977) allow the following interpretation: intravenous (and, similarly, high oral) doses of benzodiazepines cause sleepiness and eventually induce sleep. Despite being sleepy immediately after the injection, the patients were able to perceive and correctly name pictures shown to them before full anesthesia, but they had only a limited ability to remember the pictures later, once the effect of the substance had ceased. Thus, when given before or during the acquisition phase, benzodiazepines impair the acquisition and consolidation of new material, the transition from a short-term to a long-term store. The impairment concerns not only visually presented content but also verbally presented words and other materials (Lister, 1985). The action of benzodiazepines in the acquisition phase was shown to be dose dependent (Ghoneim *et al.*, 1984a,b) and, as seen in the experiment of George and Dundee (1977), has a different duration with different compounds, i.e. is related to the biological half-life of the drug in question.

Put in more clinical terms, benzodiazepines can induce *anterograde amnesia*, i.e., they will negatively affect the registration phase in the information processing scheme reported on p. 68. The question then arises as to whether, if administered after the registration phase, benzodiazepines can also affect encoding processes, i.e. the phase of further processing of new information and its linking with existing memory content. This phenomenon, called *retrograde amnesia*, does not seem to occur with benzodiazepines (Curran, 1991): information acquired before drug administration remains accessible even at a later date. It should be noted, however, that the temporal relationships in the recording and processing stages of new information and their precise relationship to the administration and action of drugs are complex, and that observations made in single-dose experiments performed under circumscribed, laboratory-like conditions may not be representative of the more typical chronic use of anxiolytic drugs.

Questions of specificity of the amnestic action of benzodiazepines were discussed by Curran (1991). Based on her own work and studies by other authors she concluded that the amnestic effects of benzodiazepines cannot be explained fully by their general sedative effects. Furthermore, different types of learning and memory performances are not altered in the same way by benzodiazepines: episodic memory is affected more than semantic memory, and voluntary cognitive processes more than automatic processes. In contrast, the learning of skills and procedures is hardly affected by benzodiazepines at all. With regard to another important issue, that of the persistence of the amnestic effects, Taylor and Tinklenberg (1987) stated that this undesirable activity of benzodiazepines undergoes rapid habituation on repeated administration. However, in the case of the benzodiazepine anxiolytics, this statement was based almost exclusively on clinical impressions and studies in healthy subjects. Thus, in one of the few controlled clinical trials with anxiolytics, Lucki *et al.* (1986) found that, even after years of administration of benzodiazepines in medium to large doses, each additional individual dose could lead to mild anterograde amnesia. This observation suggests that, although tolerance to the sedative effects of benzodiazepines may develop in some areas of performance, there is less tolerance with regard to memory performance.

Golombok *et al.* (1988) reported on a retrospective study in long-term (more than 1 year) users of benzodiazepines. They found a negative correlation between the cumulative dose of medicine over 1 year and the performance in some attention and learning tests. The higher the cumulative anxiolytic dose, the poorer the performance. On the other hand Curran (1992b), in a study of long-term benzodiazepine consumers (7 months to 28 years!), established that an individually adjusted normal daily dose had little influence on most aspects of performance, including learning and memory tests. The only exception was a two-stage word-pair association test that indicated some decrement after benzodiazepine anxiolytics. In a review of various studies, Curran concluded "that the repeated use of benzodiazepines over weeks does not lead to tolerance of episodic memory impairments" (1991, p. 6). In another review article, King (1992, p. 84) commented that, with regard to habituation, the amnestic action of benzodiazepines lay between the general sedative action (which showed rapid habituation) and the anxiolytic action (which did not show habituation).

There has been discussion as to whether some benzodiazepines may, perhaps as a consequence of particularly high affinity for specific benzodiazepine subreceptors, be able to induce greater or less important disturbance of cognitive functions than others. According to Hindmarch (1998), the benzodiazepine clobazam has anticonvulsant and anxiolytic but no sedative and amnestic properties at the usual doses and should be given preference, particularly in the treatment of elderly patients with anxiety disorder. Unresolved issues around benzodiazepines include the observation that some of these compounds with short plasma half-lives have prolonged effects on cognitive function including memory, whereas other derivatives with long-lived and pharmacologically active metabolites do not show these effects (Ghoneim and Mewaldt, 1990). Ghoneim (1992) also reported that the sedative–hypnotic actions of benzodiazepines could be abolished with benzodiazepine antagonists, whereas the amnestic effects of these drugs were at least partially resistant to antagonists. Another controversial issue that will be dealt with in Chapter 8 are the possible consequences of benzodiazepine action on learning and memory when a patient is receiving concomitant psychotherapy, i.e., is expected to acquire new behaviors and cognitive patterns.

In conclusion, although there has been extensive research into the cognitive effects of benzodiazepines for more than 30 years, knowledge in this area of psychopharmacology remains patchy. There is a consensus, however, that old patients in particular are at risk for cognitive disturbances when being prescribed benzodiazepines (Foy *et al.*, 1995; Ranstam *et al.*, 1997; Hanlon *et al.*, 1998), and that alternative anxiolytic drugs should be given preference if possible.

7.4.3 OTHER ANXIOLYTIC DRUGS

As indicated in Chapter 1 some antidepressant drugs, particularly SSRIs and SNRIs, are being used increasingly for the pharmacotherapy of anxiety

disorders. Although these drugs are not devoid of adverse effects, they appear
to have little effect on cognitive functions (Section 7.3.2). Their use for the
long-term treatment of obsessive–compulsive disorder (OCD) and panic
disorder, notably in elderly patients, is therefore encouraged.

Another alternative is buspirone, a non-benzodiazepine anxiolytic that
seems to be free of untoward effects on cognitive performance (Ninan *et al.*,
1998). As indicated in Chapter 1, the anxiolytic effect of this compound may
take a few weeks to occur (and is often rather weak), meaning that buspirone is
better suited for long-term treatment of anxiety syndromes than for immediate
anxiolysis.

7.5 PSYCHOSTIMULANTS

7.5.1 COGNITIVE ABNORMALITIES IN ATTENTION DEFICIT HYPERACTIVITY DISORDER

The most frequent psychiatric use of psychostimulant drugs is in children and
adolescents with attention deficit hyperactivity disorder (ADHD). Given this
preferential use, and in view of the controversies around the chronic
administration of potentially addictive drugs in a juvenile population, the
following section will focus on the effects of psychostimulants on cognitive
function in children and adolescents with ADHD. When addressing this topic
it is important to recall that the three cardinal symptoms required for a
diagnosis of ADHD – developmentally inappropriate hyperactivity, impulsivity and inattention – do not explicitly comprise cognitive dysfunction. It is,
however, easy to imagine that all three behavioral characteristics are likely to
translate into deficient performance in a variety of tasks, including tests of
cognitive function.

The DSM-IV (APA, 1994), which distinguishes three subtypes of ADHD – a
predominantly inattentive type, a predominantly hyperactive–impulsive type
and a combined type – lists nine behavioral criteria of which six must be
fulfilled for the diagnostic label of 'inattention':

- Failure to give close attention to detail
- Difficulty with sustained attention
- Does not seem to listen
- Does not follow through on instructions
- Has difficulty organizing tasks and activities
- Avoids tasks that require sustained mental effort
- Loses things he/she needs for tasks or activities
- Is easily distracted by extraneous stimuli
- Is often forgetful

In the context of tests of cognitive function, most or all of these behavioral characteristics are likely to interfere with optimal performance. However, poor performance on tests of cognitive function are neither necessary nor sufficient for a diagnosis of ADHD: the DSM-IV stipulates that clinically significant impairment in social, academic or occupational functioning (due to the above symptoms) must be notable in two or more settings for a diagnosis of ADHD to be made.

Neuropsychological testing of children with ADHD suggests deficits in executive functioning and working memory (Stubbe, 2000). Poorer performance than in age-matched healthy children is recorded on a wide variety of tasks such as perceptual discrimination, reaction time, vigilance, continuous performance, rote learning, paired associate learning, etc. According to one current school of thinking (see Crosbie and Schachar, 2001), "deficient inhibition" constitutes a core disturbance in ADHD: deficient inhibitory control is assumed to be responsible for a number of impairments in behavior, working memory, impulse regulation and internalization of speech. These deficits underlie the abnormalities of conduct exhibited by ADHD individuals in everyday life, as well as the impulsive, inattentive and inconsistent behavior exhibited on a variety of tasks. Deficient inhibitory control can be operationalized and measured by means of the stop-signal paradigm (Schachar et al., 2000), a laboratory task that requires a rapid ongoing motor response and the sudden cessation of that response following a specified signal. However, not all children with ADHD perform poorly on the stop-signal task, and by far not all ADHD children and adolescents show consistently deficient performance on cognitive tasks and in school.

7.5.2 EFFECTS OF PSYCHOSTIMULANTS

There is a large number of double-blind, randomized, placebo-controlled studies demonstrating the efficacy of psychostimulant drugs in improving behavioral symptoms and cognitive dysfunction in ADHD patients (for review see Wilens and Biederman, 1992; Greenhill et al., 1999). Methylphenidate is the drug most frequently studied, but amphetamine and pemoline show similar efficacy. The vast majority of clinical trials included children between 5 and 12 years of age, and it is generally recognized that studies in children will produce more consistently positive results than trials in adolescents or adults. Responder rates in children are as high as 75%; children with comorbid anxiety and those who have less severe symptoms generally do not respond as well (Gray and Kagan, 2000). Most published studies lasted up to 12 weeks, with improvement seen in the following areas of cognitive functioning:

- Attentiveness and on-task behavior. More specifically, stimulant drugs improve the ability of children with ADHD to sustain both attention and effort under challenging circumstances, i.e. on very demanding cognitive tasks (Berman *et al.*, 1999) and with the experience of failure, e.g. when confronted with an unsolvable word-puzzle task (Pelham *et al.*, 1997).

- Significant improvement in performance is seen on many laboratory measures of attention, learning, information processing, short-term memory and vigilance (Elia *et al.*, 1999).
- Response variability and impulsive responding on cognitive tasks decrease and the accuracy of performance increases. According to Klorman *et al.* (1994), methylphenidate and chronological age had generally similar effects in a Sternberg (continuous short-term memory) task: greater accuracy and speed (as well as more 'mature' event-related potential patterns) were seen after methylphenidate both in ADHD and in non-ADHD children.

It is also recognized that scholastic achievement of children with ADHD improves significantly on psychostimulant treatment, although not as dramatically as behavior: according to Greenhill *et al.* (1999) effect sizes on cognitive measures are typically between 0.6 and 0.8, whereas those on behavioral measures, based on teachers' reports, are slightly higher (0.8–1.0). On the other hand it generally takes lower doses of stimulant drugs to improve cognitive and scholastic performance than to obtain better behavioral manageability (Cantwell, 1996; Elia *et al.*, 1999). Regarding the optimal dosing and scheduling of psychostimulant drugs, several issues have been discussed repeatedly:

(1) Dose–response relationship on cognitive tasks: although some early studies suggested a plateau or even a reversed effect at higher drug doses, most controlled trials with methylphenidate support a linear dose–response relationship up to 0.9 mg/kg. Higher doses of methylphenidate (0.9 mg/kg) were found to be particularly effective on tasks with high cognitive processing load (Berman *et al.*, 1999).

(2) Paradoxical effects: cognitive impairment and perseverative behavior are occasionally seen in children treated with psychostimulants. According to Greenhill *et al.* (1999) such phenomena are indicative of a drug overdose and will improve at dose reduction. Constriction of attention or 'overfocusing' as a consequence of treatment with psychostimulants has been another critical issue (Breggin, 1999). Based on an extensive review of the literature and their own experience, Wilens and Biederman (1992) assert that there is no evidence of such phenomena at doses up to 1.0 mg/kg of methylphenidate.

(3) Rebound effects: methylphenidate and amphetamine are short-acting drugs and, consequently, one often observes reappearance of symptoms in the afternoon if the drug is taken early in the morning. Controlled studies with staggered administration of active drug and placebo have shown that a return of symptoms during the day is due to waning of the drug action after a few hours and not to a rebound effect. Currently available

---

Box 7.5 A Swedish Long-term Study with Amphetamine in ADHD

A trial published by Gillberg *et al.* (1997) comprised 62 children (52 males, 10 females), aged 6–11 years and meeting DSM-III-R criteria for ADHD. The children suffered from severe attention deficits and 42% had comorbid diagnoses including mild mental retardation, autistic features, oppositional defiant disorder and tic disorder. They were included in a parallel-group, randomized, double-blind, placebo-controlled study of amphetamine treatment.

All patients had a 3-month single-blind baseline amphetamine titration period and all 62 patients improved significantly during this time. They were then randomized to amphetamine or placebo. During the 12-month double-blind phase, 71% of the children in the placebo group and 29% in the amphetamine group stopped treatment or were switched to open treatment. Most of these dropouts occurred in the first 3 months of the double-blind trial. Thirty-two children (8 on placebo and 24 on amphetamine) completed the study as planned. Early dropouts were considered in a separate statistical analysis.

Behavioral symptoms were assessed by means of a parent rating scale (Conners, 1990). There were highly significant differences between the children taking amphetamine and those taking placebo on the total behavior score as well as on all subscores. Teacher classroom scores (Conners, 1990) followed the same pattern, clearly favoring amphetamine. Improvements were 43–47% on the parent scores and 27–40% in the classroom. Clinical results were similar in the pure ADHD and in the comorbid group. Changes in cognitive performance were measured by means of the Wechsler Intelligence Scale for Children, 3rd edition revised (WISC-R; Wechsler, 1992). Data available from eight children taking placebo for 6 months or longer were compared with those having taken amphetamine for 9 months or more ($n = 35$) and indicated a slight advantage for the children on amphetamine (change of 4.5 points from baseline to month 15, compared with a change of 0.7 on placebo during the same time interval; $P < 0.05$, one-tailed). Verbal and performance scores on the WISC-R showed similar results.

The small but statistically significant effect seen in the amphetamine group on the WISC-R was probably a real finding, i.e. not an artifact of retesting. Overall, this study shows that the positive clinical effects of amphetamine on behavioral symptoms and cognitive performance are maintained after 15 months of treatment.

slow-release formulations of methylphenidate and amphetamine facilitate drug administration once daily without the reappearance of symptoms later in the day.

(4) One issue that attracted much interest some 30 years ago is *state-dependent learning (SDL)* and memory (p. 68), which deals with the question of whether any material or behavior acquired under specific conditions (e.g. under the influence of a drug) will be accessible under different, e.g. drug-free, conditions (Weingartner, 1978). Several controlled studies on SDL, with conflicting results, were also performed in ADHD children (Spiegel 1996, p. 203); despite its potential importance, it appears that the topic has not been revisited in the last few years.

Probably the two most contentious issues in the treatment of ADHD with psychostimulants are the long-term efficacy of these drugs and the long-term outcome of patients. Beneficial effects of methylphenidate and similar drugs on symptoms of ADHD were typically demonstrated in controlled trials of a few weeks duration; however, ADHD is a chronic condition and its symptoms usually reappear upon discontinuation of pharmacological treatment. Two questions thus arise: are stimulant drugs effective long-term, i.e. after years of use; and what is the long-term prognosis of children with ADHD? Scientifically sound answers to both questions would necessitate long-term, placebo-controlled studies, yet it is ethically problematic and practically not feasible to keep ADHD patients with clinically relevant symptoms without active treatment for years. As far as the efficacy of psychostimulants beyond a few months is concerned there are now several published controlled studies, all lasting 12 months or longer, indicating that the efficacy of stimulant drugs is maintained. Two of these studies, one with amphetamine and one with methylphenidate, are summarized in Boxes 7.5 and 7.6.

Box 7.6 The MTA Study (Multimodal Treatment Study of Children with ADHD)

Probably the largest and most thoroughly prepared, performed and analyzed treatment study in ADHD was sponsored by the US National Institute of Mental Health (NIMH) and the US Department of Education in response to public concern regarding the use of stimulant medication use in children and adolescents (MTA Cooperative Group, 1999). A total of 579 children (80% boys; screened from more than 4500 candidates) were recruited in six centers having extensive experience with ADHD; the children were between 7 and 9.9 years of age and had a diagnosis of ADHD, combined type. After extensive baseline investigations they were assigned randomly to 14 months of four different management strategies:

(1) Medication only: individual titration of methylphenidate, followed by monthly visits.

(2) Behavioral treatment: intensive parent training, school-based intervention and child-focused treatment, with therapist involvement gradually reduced over time.

(3) Combined medication and behavioral treatment.

(4) Community care: treatment by community mental health providers (about two-thirds of these children received stimulant medication through their doctors).

Clinical outcomes before, during and after treatments were assessed in six multiple domains represented by 19 separate measures. The domains were: ADHD symptoms; aggression-oppositional defiant disorder; internalizing symptoms; social skills; parent–child relations; and cognitive performance (measured with three subscales of the Wechsler Individual Achievement test: reading, mathematics, spelling).

All four treatment groups showed sizable reductions in symptoms over time, with significant differences between the groups in degrees of change. For most ADHD symptoms, children in the combined treatment and medication management groups showed significantly greater improvement than those given behavioral treatment or community care. Combined and medication management treatments did not differ significantly on any direct comparisons, but in several instances the combined treatment proved superior to behavioral treatment and/or community care while the medication management did not.

With few exceptions the Wechsler scores showed small positive average changes within all four groups. The combined treatment group had the largest and the community care group had the smallest baseline-adjusted change scores on all three cognitive measures. Statistically significant differences were found between the combined and the behavioral treatment groups and between the combined treatment and the community care groups, both on the reading achievement score. In addition to the main findings regarding the best average treatment effects, this study shows that the cognitive performance of ADHD children was slightly enhanced as part of a more general clinical improvement on several of the treatments, and that clinical improvement as well as slight cognitive enhancement is observed after months of treatment with a stimulant drug used alone or in combination with an intensive behavioral treatment program.

The Swedish study (Gillberg *et al.*, 1997) as well as the MTA study (MTA Cooperative Group, 1999) from the USA showed that the stimulant drugs used maintained their efficacy on behavioral as well as cognitive measures in ADHD for at least 1 year. This supports observations made in naturalistic long-term studies that tolerance to the effects of amphetamine and methylphenidate does not develop in children and adolescents suffering from ADHD. The picture is less clear with regard to the outcome of ADHD in adulthood: several long-term, controlled follow-up studies suggest that the syndrome may persist in 10–60% of young adults diagnosed as having ADHD in childhood (Wilens *et al.*, 1998). The actual contribution of drug therapy to these long-term outcomes is difficult to estimate because medication used for some time in childhood may have been discontinued and resumed again for some time, and many non-drug-related factors are likely to have intervened between childhood, adolescence and early adulthood.

7.6 ANTIDEMENTIA DRUGS

7.6.1 COGNITIVE CHANGES OF AGING AND DEMENTIA

Some change in cognitive functioning with advancing age is considered normal. Older people are thought of as being forgetful: they may not remember events and conversations, keep asking the same question, sometimes have problems finding words, go out shopping and forget what they wanted to buy. These lapses are part of a complex of changes that occur in the sensory, motor and cognitive faculties of people as they grow older: accuracy and speed of sensory perception and voluntary motor activity diminish, and attentiveness, interests and motivation change during the course of life (Craik and Salthouse, 1992). Interindividual variation increases with age in practically all areas examined, and the normal range of physiological as well as psychological functioning is wider in older than in young persons. Cognitive performance in older age also depends on education and previous professional activities; it is additionally affected by the general state of health of the individual.

However, aging is not related to a general decline in intellectual abilities. Losses occur mainly in areas of performance that are directly dependent on intact sensory and motor abilities. Older persons also tend to encounter difficulties when called upon to perform cognitive and other tasks under pressure of time. The subjective significance of a task and a person's familiarity with the conditions under which performance is evaluated are further factors that assume greater importance in older people than in the young.

When an elderly, physically healthy person shows a generalized decline in cognitive functioning that "causes significant impairment in social or occupational functioning and represents a significant decline from a previous

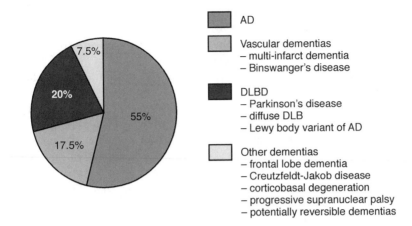

AD

Vascular dementias
– multi-infarct dementia
– Binswanger's disease

DLBD
– Parkinson's disease
– diffuse DLB
– Lewy body variant of AD

Other dementias
– frontal lobe dementia
– Creutzfeldt-Jakob disease
– corticobasal degeneration
– progressive supranuclear palsy
– potentially reversible dementias

Figure 7.1 Differential diagnosis of dementia (AD = Alzheimer's disease; DLBD = dementia with Lewy body disorder; DLB = dementia with Lewy bodies)

level of functioning" (APA, 1994), there is the possibility of *dementia*. Dementia ('loss of mind') designates a syndrome characterized by "global deterioration in all aspects of mental functioning, including memory, general intellect, emotional attributes and distinctive features of personality" (Roth, 1980). A diagnosis of dementia presumes deterioration in several areas of mental functioning and not just of memory (although memory impairment is a necessary condition for a diagnosis of dementia). Dementias are common in the very old: about 5% of all persons over 65 years and about 20% of all those aged 80 years are to be classed as demented (Henderson, 1986). According to present-day views, the number of individuals over 65 years affected by dementia doubles for every 5 years or so of life.

A dementia syndrome may be caused by a number of underlying diseases that can be detected or excluded by medical, neurological and psychiatric examinations (Small *et al.*, 1997). The most common cause, accounting for 55% of all chronic cases of dementia, is Alzheimer's disease (AD). Other brain disorders that may underlie dementia are cerebrovascular disease, Lewy body disorder (McKeith and Burn, 2000), frontotemporal degeneration (Snowden and Neary, 1999) and others (Fig. 7.1). Reversible causes of dementia syndromes include depression (Geerlings *et al.*, 2000), some endocrine disorders, dietary deficiencies and drug overdosage (Starr and Whalley, 1994).

7.6.2 ALZHEIMER'S DISEASE

The clinical hallmark of AD is gradual and irreversible cognitive decline. This manifests initially with symptoms of memory failure and 'mild cognitive impairment' (MCI) that is insufficient to significantly affect daily functioning. The MCI is often, but not always, followed by more severe mental decline: it is estimated that 10–15% of individuals with MCI will convert to dementia within 1 year (Petersen *et al.*, 2001a). For this reason, a recent practice guideline (Petersen *et al.*, 2001b) recommends the evaluation and clinical monitoring of persons with MCI.

Dementia due to AD steadily worsens, typically over the course of about 10 years, but survival in some patients may be as short as 3–4 years. In late stages AD leads to what is sometimes called a vegetative state, i.e. the patient is bedfast and totally dependent on others for all basic living activities. Patients with AD typically die from bronchitis or pneumonia. Risk factors of AD are age, female gender and presence of the apolipoprotein ε4 (APO ε4) allele. Higher levels of education, moderate levels of daily wine consumption and higher levels of fish in the diet have been associated with a lower risk for AD (Cummings and Cole, 2002).

Alzheimer's disease is a chronic, progressive and degenerative brain disease. It is macroscopically characterized by atrophy of the cerebral cortex, which, at least in advanced stages, can be detected by computer-assisted tomography (CAT) or magnetic resonance imaging (MRI). So-called neuritic plaques (extracellular deposits of beta-amyloid in the brain), neurofibrillary modifications (tangles), neuron loss and other abnormalities are characteristic microscopic features (Katzman, 1986). Because there is as yet no specific clinical, biochemical or neurological test for a diagnosis of AD in the living patient, unequivocal diagnosis can strictly be made only by postmortem examination of the brain. Using a set of diagnostic rules (McKhann *et al.*, 1984) one can reach about 80–90% agreement between the clinical and postmortem diagnosis.

The symptoms of AD are not restricted to the cognitive domain but include the following:

- Apathy is apparent early in the clinical course, with diminished interest and reduced concern.
- Agitation and aimless activity become increasingly common as the illness advances and are a frequent precipitant of nursing home placement.
- Depressive symptoms are present in about 50% of patients, and approximately 25% exhibit delusions at some stage of the disorder.

Assessment methods that determine mental functioning (attention, orientation, memory, speech, understanding of speech, psychomotor functions) in a simple, practical way are recommended for a rough estimation of the severity of dementia. The best-known instrument is the Mini-Mental State Examination (MMSE, Folstein *et al.*, 1975), which allows the grading of dementia on a 30-point scale on the basis of a simple 5–10-min examination. Other, rather more involved procedures include the Dementia Rating Scale (DRS) of Mattis (1976) and the Alzheimer Disease Assessment Scale (ADAS) of Rosen *et al.* (1984). The

Consortium for the Establishment of a Registry of Alzheimer's Disease (CERAD; Heyman *et al.*, 1997) has worked out a minimum standard battery to describe the cognitive dysfunction of patients with AD. Specific neuropsychological techniques can be applied for a more detailed description of the mental functions that are still retained and those that are impaired (see Deutsch Lezak, 1995).

7.6.3 CHOLINERGIC AGENTS

In addition to containing markedly increased numbers of amyloid plaques and neurofibrillary tangles, brains of patients with AD also show significant disturbance of chemical neurotransmission. The noradrenergic, serotoninergic and several other neurotransmitter systems are affected, but the most pronounced dysfunction is found in the cholinergic brain systems. As discussed in Chapter 2 (pp. 53 f.), the *cholinergic hypothesis of AD* integrated numerous clinical, neurochemical and pharmacological findings and was a basis for rational drug development to treat the disease. Most currently approved antidementia drugs are cholinesterase inhibitors (ChE-Is), i.e. compounds that inhibit the enzymatic breakdown of acetylcholine and thus raise the availability of the neurotransmitter. The three most frequently used ChE-Is are donepezil (Aricept®), rivastigmine (Exelon®) and galanthamine (Reminyl®) (Table 7.2).

When treated with one of the ChE-Is the majority of patients with AD will show stabilization or slight improvement of their remaining cognitive abilities and everyday functioning for at least 6 months (Wolfson *et al.*, 2002) or even longer (Giacobini, 2000; Gauthier, 2002). About one in five patients is likely to manifest clinically relevant improvement of cognitive performance and ADL (activities of daily life) when treated with a ChE-I. However, mental and functional decline will continue unchanged in about 25% of patients despite pharmacological treatment. The effect size of treatment with ChE-Is depends on the severity of the disorder when therapy is initiated: in controlled clinical studies, patients with more severe dementia showed a much greater therapeutic effect, i.e. a greater difference between active drug and placebo, than patients with mild AD (Burns *et al.*, 2002; Potkin *et al.*, 2002). This is probably due to the fact that the brain cholinergic deficit is more pronounced in severe AD (Davis *et al.*, 1999), leading to faster and more profound loss of cognitive and functional abilities in these patients if left untreated. On the other hand, there is also evidence that treatment with ChE-Is should be initiated as early as possible because the cognitive and functional losses incurred early in the disease cannot be recovered fully when pharmacological intervention is delayed (Doraiswamy *et al.*, 2002).

Many AD patients, especially those in advanced stages of the disorder, suffer from serious behavioral and psychiatric symptoms of dementia (acronym: BPSD), making their own life and that of their family or professional caregivers difficult. Studies in institutionalized AD patients with BPSD indicate

Table 7.2 Commonly used cholinesterase inhibitors (for details see Jann *et al.*, 2002)

	Donepezil	Rivastigmine	Galanthamine
Chemical class	Piperidine	Carbamate	Phenanthrene alkaloid
Origin	Synthetic compound	Synthetic compound	Natural product (from the flower snowdrop)
Enzymes inhibited	Acetylcholinesterase (AChE)	AChE, butyryl-cholinesterase (BuChE)	AChE
Inhibition type	Rapidly reversible	Slowly reversible	Rapidly reversible
Brain selectivity	Yes	Yes	No
Administration	Once daily	Twice daily	Twice daily
Dosage	Start with 5 mg/day; increase to 10 mg/day after about 1 month; maximum 10 mg/day	Start with 3 mg/day; increase to 6 mg/day after about 1 month; maximum 12 mg/day	Start with 8 mg/day; increase to 16 mg/day after about 1 month; maximum 24 mg/day
Metabolism route	Cytochrome P-450 isoenzymes	Target enzymes: AChE and BuChE	Cytochrome P-450 isoenzymes

that ChE-Is can be effective against symptoms such as hallucinations, delusions, aggressiveness and aimless wandering. In some cases ChE-Is may even replace the psychiatric drugs, e.g. antipsychotics, that are used routinely to deal with BPSD but are likely to produce serious side effects in old patients. A placebo-controlled study with rivastigmine in patients suffering from dementia with Lewy bodies (a form of degenerative dementia accompanied by serious psychiatric and neurological symptoms) demonstrated significant clinical benefit (McKeith *et al.*, 2000) and thus supports the use of ChE-Is in patients with BPSD.

7.6.4 NON-CHOLINERGIC APPROACHES TO AD

Cholinesterase inhibitors are the only class of drugs currently approved by most Health Authorities and recommended by professional associations (e.g. Doody *et al.*, 2001) for the symptomatic treatment of AD. However, ChE-Is intervene at a late stage of the pathophysiological cascade leading to AD (Fig. 7.2); furthermore, their efficacy is limited and they may cause a number of side effects, most frequently nausea, vomiting, diarrhea, anorexia and dizziness. For these reasons, major efforts are being made to alter the biological processes

Genetic base   Missense mutations in APP and presenilin genes

⇓

Core pathological   ***Increased Aβ42 production and accumulation*****
process   ⇓

Aβ42 oligomerization and deposition as **diffuse plaques**

⇓

Subtle effects of Aβ oligomers on synapses

⇓

Inflammatory process   ***Microglial and astrocytic activation:***
complement factors, cytokines, etc.**

⇓

Progressive synaptic and neuritic injury

⇓

Altered neuronal ionic homeostasis; oxidative injury

⇓

Altered kinase/phosphatase activities → **tangles**

⇓

Widespread neuronal/neuritic dysfunction and cell death with transmitter deficits

Figure 7.2 Amyloid cascade hypothesis (modified after Hardy and Selkoe, 2002. Reprinted with permission. American Association for the Advancement of Science) *Cholesterol is thought to be involved in the formation of β-amyloid (Aβ) in the brain. Inhibitors of cholesterol formation could then prevent the formation of (neurotoxic) β-amyloid.
**The inflammatory step in the pathophysiological process of AD is thought to be blocked by NSAIDs.

leading to AD at an earlier stage, and eventually to prevent the outbreak of the disorder. From the many approaches that are currently discussed (Jacobsen, 2002), two relatively advanced ones will be mentioned briefly in the following paragraphs: the use of anti-inflammatory drugs and cholesterol inhibitors.

Anti-inflammatory drugs

Regular consumption of non-steroidal anti-inflammatory drugs (NSAIDs) such as diclofenac, ibuprofen or naproxen may reduce the risk of developing AD. Retrospective case–control investigations show that individuals who used these drugs for some time against rheumatic or arthritic conditions were significantly less frequently diagnosed with AD. These observations support the concept that inflammatory processes and mediators are involved in the complicated sequence of pathogenetic events (Figure 7.2; Hoozemans *et al.*, 2002) that ultimately lead to AD. Specific issues that remained open until a few years ago were the doses of NSAIDs needed, the minimum duration of NSAID use required and the optimal timing (beginning and end) of NSAID consumption to attain maximum protection against AD. A recently published investigation from Holland appears to answer some of these questions: In't

Veld *et al.* (2001) followed a sample of almost 7000 subjects aged 55 years and older and not suffering from dementia at baseline, i.e. in 1991. Within an average follow-up period of 6.8 years, 394 of the study participants developed dementia (293 AD, 56 vascular dementia, 45 other types of dementia). The observed risk of developing AD then was related to the use of NSAIDs as documented in pharmacy records, resulting in the following relative risks of developing AD:

- Patients with short-term (up to 1 month) use of NSAIDs during the observation period had a relative risk of 0.95 (95% confidence interval 0.70–1.29).
- Patients with intermediate-term (more than 1 month, up to 2 years) use of NSAIDs had a slightly reduced relative risk of 0.83 (95% confidence interval = 0.62–1.11).
- Patients with long-term (at least 2 years) use of NSAIDs had a substantially reduced relative risk of 0.20 (95% confidence interval = 0.05–0.83).

Age and apolipoprotein E status did not alter these relationships, and the risk of developing vascular dementia was not affected by NSAID consumption. According to In't Veld *et al.* the protective effects of NSAIDs did not depend on the dose used, and the calculated benefit was greater when the drugs were taken at least 2 years before the (model-based) onset of AD. As pointed out by Breitner and Zandi (2001), these observations suggest that there is a critical period for intervention in the disease process leading to AD, i.e. preventive treatment with NSAIDs should be initiated at an early prodromal stage of the disorder, e.g. in MCI. It is hoped that ongoing trials with NSAIDs will provide evidence for or against these assumptions.

Cholesterol Inhibitors

Possibly still further up the pathogenetic cascade (see Fig. 7.2), evidence has accumulated that a specific class of cholesterol-lowering drugs may inhibit the formation of beta-amyloid and thus prevent the development of AD. As mentioned earlier, brains of AD patients show an accumulation of plaques that are composed mainly of β-amyloid, a peptide consisting of 40–42 amino acids derived from the (non-pathological) amyloid precursor protein (APP). It is widely accepted today that excessive formation and accumulation of β-amyloid in the brain is critical for the initiation and progression of AD (Hardy and Selkoe, 2002). Increased cholesterol levels in blood and/or brain are thought to facilitate the pathological enzymatic step from APP to β-amyloid, implying that patients with abnormally high levels of cholesterol in blood (hyperlipidemia) run a greater risk of developing AD. Epidemiological studies have in fact revealed an association of hyperlipidemia and AD, and it has been shown also that hyperlipidemic patients treated with lipid-lowering agents (HMG-CoA reductase inhibitors, so-called statins) have a significantly smaller incidence of AD than untreated or non-statin-treated hyperlipidemic patients (Wolozin, 2002). Although the mechanisms underlying the preventive effect of statins in AD still need to be elucidated (Crisby *et al.*, 2002), these generally well-tolerated drugs deserve to be tested systematically in persons with a higher risk of AD, e.g. individuals with MCI. As is the case for anti-inflammatory compounds, Phase II studies with several statins are currently underway and are expected to provide the necessary clinical information within a few years.

7.7 CONCLUDING REMARKS

Cognitive impairment is seen in many psychiatric and neurological disorders. For disorders such as AD, cognitive decline constitutes a key diagnostic and psychopathologic feature; in other cases, e.g. in depression and anxiety disorders, cognitive impairment may be an epiphenomenon rather than a core pathognomonic element. These differences also imply different expectancies with regard to the drugs used to treat mental and neurological diseases: AD patients' cognitive performance should definitely profit from treatment with antidementia drugs; patients with depression and anxiety disorder should primarily not deteriorate when being treated with antidepressants and anxiolytics. As shown in the preceding paragraphs, the distinction between direct, beneficial drug effects, e.g. on symptoms of schizophrenia and depression, and direct or indirect (positive and negative) effects of these drugs on cognitive function is not always straightforward. Although this may be an attractive area for many more sophisticated studies, in clinical practice deleterious effects of drugs on performance must be monitored carefully and balanced against the therapeutic benefit noted in the individual patient.

8

Psychopharmaceuticals and the Treatment of Mental Disorders

Revision by
HOSSEIN FATEMI

8.1 INTRODUCTION

In Chapter 1 of this book, psychopharmaceuticals were introduced as effective medicines that primarily have a symptomatic action but are problematic in several respects. Antipsychotics can cause serious side effects and antidepressants often exert their therapeutic effects only after a delay of weeks and in many cases have unpleasant side effects. With anxiolytics, hypnotics and, in particular, psychostimulants, there are problems with habituation and the potential of dependency. It is therefore not surprising that psychopharmaceuticals do not enjoy a very high reputation among many doctors and the general public (see Box 8.1) and have been given names such as 'chemical strait-jackets' for the older neuroleptics (Szasz, 1957) or 'chemical blinkers for the mind' for tranquillizers. Elomaa (1993) even posed the question of whether the long-term use of conventional antipsychotics should be considered a crime against humanity.

A visit to a psychiatric hospital is also rarely suited to dispelling reservations about psychopharmaceuticals. Some patients wander around like robots, their movements lack natural animation, their expressions are rigid and they appear pale and apathetic, cut off from their surroundings. An encounter with a relative or friend suffering from a mental illness and being treated with psychopharmaceuticals can be shocking and confusing, and the layperson is usually not in a position to evaluate whether the signs that they see and hear are expressions of the illness being treated or the effects of the medicines administered.

Psychopharmacology, Fourth Edition. By R. Spiegel
© 2003 John Wiley & Sons, Ltd: ISBN 0 471 56039 1: 0 470 84691 7 (PB)

Box 8.1 The Negative Image of Psychopharmaceuticals: a Summary

(1) In hospitals, psychopharmaceuticals, especially antipsychotics, are sometimes used as a disciplinary measure: patients are forcibly subdued by means of medication. Medication may be used as a form of punishment for rebelliousness.

(2) Psychopharmaceuticals are employed for brainwashing: under the influence of psychopharmaceuticals the patients become indifferent, lose their own will and adapt themselves to circumstances in an environment that is itself mentally sick.

(3) Psychopharmaceuticals encourage 'revolving door' psychiatry: patients are often sent home as being 'cured' too soon and swiftly return to the clinic. As time goes by, they cease to believe in a cure and in themselves.

(4) Many doctors prescribe psychopharmaceuticals in order to get rid of difficult patients and so that they do not have to become more involved in the problems of their patients.

(5) For doctors and patients, psychopharmaceuticals are often the simplest way out of a difficult situation: drugs suppress a few acute symptoms but do not lead to a permanent solution for the basic underlying problems.

On the other hand, nurses and doctors who lived through the period before 1953/54 and then saw the introduction of modern psychopharmaceuticals could hardly believe the unprecedented therapeutic advances that these medicines provided: how much suffering, anxiety and waste of human life could be eliminated inside and outside of psychiatric hospitals. Relief and sometimes elation, together with new therapeutic optimism, can be sensed in the early publications on the discovery of antipsychotics and antidepressants (see Chapter 2).

In the following paragraphs we will attempt to determine more precisely the value and position of psychopharmaceuticals in the treatment of mental disorders. This will be done on the basis of a literature survey referring, with few exceptions, to comparative studies between two or more forms of therapy. Historically, the following tendencies can be detected in this area of comparative therapeutic research:

- In the 1960s and early 1970s, the studies often related to the question of whether and in which particular therapeutic indications psychopharmaceuticals show superiority over placebo.

- At about the same time, studies were performed to determine whether psychopharmaceuticals or specific psychotherapeutic procedures produced better results in the treatment of mental disorders, especially schizophrenia and depression.
- In the last two decades, interest has been directed primarily to the question of how psychopharmaceuticals and non-drug procedures relate to one another and how they can best be combined.

Problems of optimal dosage and duration of drug treatment for mental disorders have also been addressed in numerous controlled studies and are presented separately below for antipsychotics, antidepressants, mood stabilizers, anxiolytics and psychostimulants. This division again makes sense because the disorders treated and the therapeutic approaches used differ in significant aspects and the empirical studies carried out in the individual indications show major qualitative and quantitative differences.

8.2 ANTIPSYCHOTICS AND THE TREATMENT OF SCHIZOPHRENIA

8.2.1 PROOF OF EFFICACY

The efficacy of antipsychotics for the symptomatic treatment of schizophrenic psychoses is not disputed: a tranquillizing, emotion-subduing and antihallucinatory effect can be seen clearly in the majority of patients and has been confirmed in a large number of comparative studies versus placebo. According to a compilation by Davis and Casper (1978), even before 1969 there had been 66 placebo-controlled studies performed in the USA with chlorpromazine, 18 with trifluoperazine, 15 with fluphenazine, 10 with triflupromazine, 9 with haloperidol and 7 with thioridazine: a vast majority of these studies demonstrated the superiority of the active product over placebo. The therapeutic effect of the antipsychotics arose in 60–75% of patients during the first 6 weeks of treatment, although later improvements were also observed. The symptoms most perceptibly improved by the use of antipsychotics were:

- psychotic thought disorder, paranoid ideation
- hallucinations
- mannerisms
- autism
- general slowness or motor hyperactivity
- withdrawal, hostility
- affective blunting and indifference

According to a formulation of Heinrich (1976, p. 27), "psychotic syndromes which are characterized by a lively emotional mobility, wealth of symptoms, active confrontation with one's own disease and with one's surroundings, react from experience appreciably better to neuroleptic drug therapy than do those syndromes which are, as it were, burnt out, torpid, lacking in symptoms, and emotionally frozen". The prospects for patients with schizophrenia simplex and with schizophrenic defect or residual syndromes are less favorable than for patients having catatonic and paranoid–hallucinatory schizophrenias (Crow, 1982).

In connection with the introduction of newer, 'atypical' antipsychotics, the question arose as to whether and to what degree these drugs have a beneficial effect not only on the positive (or productive) symptoms of schizophrenia but also on the negative part of the schizophrenic syndrome (apathy, social withdrawal, emotional blunting, impoverishment of thought and speech). Möller (1995) emphasized that *negative symptoms* are observed at various stages of schizophrenic psychosis and are therefore to be evaluated differentially also. Depending on the type and stage of psychosis, they occur in association with positive symptoms or are separate, and they also respond in a differential way to antipsychotics. One can speak of a particularly marked or even a specific effect of an antipsychotic on negative symptoms only when a preparation acts on apathy, social withdrawal, etc. after the acute positive symptoms have faded, but especially in patients with schizophrenic defect or chronic deficit state. This type of effect has been obtained convincingly with the atypical antipsychotic clozapine, which also is used successfully in cases of so-called treatment resistance (Farmer and Blewett, 1993). Additionally, Dugan *et al.* (2001) compared several studies of olanzapine against typical antipsychotics and found advantages for olanzapine in terms of positive and negative symptoms, depression and extrapyramidal side effects (EPS). In contrast, a recent meta-analysis (Geddes *et al.*, 2000) did not produce clear evidence that atypical agents are more effective or better tolerated than conventional antipsychotics. Geddes *et al.* concluded that "conventional antipsychotics should usually be used in the initial treatment of an episode of schizophrenia unless the patient has previously not responded to these drugs or has unacceptable extrapyramidal side effects". Nevertheless, the overall clinical wisdom based on recent evidence is that, because of the propensity for atypical antipsychotics to cause fewer EPS, the potential benefit in amelioration of both negative and positive symptoms and the superiority in treating treatment-unresponsive patients, atypical agents should be tried initially in any patient with psychosis (Bradford *et al.*, 2002).

8.2.2 QUESTIONS OF DOSAGE AND DURATION OF TREATMENT

There may be considerable differences between the lowest and the highest recommended doses for antipsychotics (see Table 1.2 in Chapter 1). The major factors responsible for the wide dosage range are the weight and age of the patients, their general physical health and the type and severity of the mental disorders. Baldessarini emphasized (1985, p. 48) that "there have been very few systematic investigations of dose–effect relationships, or comparisons of specific types of agents, in large numbers of psychotic patients diagnosed by reliable methods". The published doses for antipsychotics therefore should be seen only as rough guidelines and the dosage must be tailor-made individually on the basis of the symptoms to be treated and tolerability.

Two dose–effect studies with haloperidol allow a statement to be made regarding adequate doses, at least for this antipsychotic: a double-blind comparison between daily doses of 10, 30 and 80 mg of haloperidol in 87 recently hospitalized patients with schizophrenia revealed no advantage of the two higher doses over the dose of 10 mg per day (Rifkin *et al.*, 1991), and a study by McEvoy *et al.* (1991) in 106 patients with schizophrenia and schizoaffective psychoses showed that an increase in dose above an individually optimal level (mostly less than 10 mg per day in this study) produced no additional therapeutic effect but rather an increase in side effects, especially EPS.

Despite the clear trend towards lower doses seen in recent years, one should also warn against experimenting with inadequate doses *at the beginning of a treatment*: especially in younger, physically healthy patients it is important to achieve a rapid antipsychotic action that is also clearly perceptible to the patient. (For specific questions of so-called 'high-dose' antipsychotic medication see Thomson, 1994.)

Dosage during Long-term Treatments

Baldessarini and Davis (1980) attempted to clarify whether there is a significant relationship between the antipsychotic maintenance dosages administered and the risk of relapse in the case of chronic schizophrenics. Correlations calculated for 23 controlled studies showed no relationship between the administered doses of antipsychotics and the risk of relapse within a wide range. Based on this result, the authors ruled that the maintenance dosage for each individual patient should be kept as low as possible in order to prevent antipsychotics from causing undesirable delayed effects.

Kane and Lieberman (1987) critically discussed the possibility of dose reduction during long-term treatments. From several controlled studies it clearly emerged that the reduction of an originally administered antipsychotic dose and the risk of relapse are closely correlated. On the other hand, patients on lower antipsychotic doses were described as less emotionally withdrawn, livelier, more relaxed and less sluggish. Because these patients also showed fewer signs of incipient tardive dyskinesia, Kane and Lieberman drew the following conclusion: "Dosage reduction can lead to a diminution in adverse effects and improvement in some subjective and objective measures of well-being; however, the risk of psychotic exacerbation increases, and patients must be observed carefully with a readiness to increase medication when necessary and usually on a temporary basis" (Kane and Lieberman, 1987, p. 1107).

In a double-blind, multicenter, prospective study, Csernansky *et al.* (2002) showed that among patients with clinically stable chronic schizophrenia or schizoaffective disorder the risk of relapse was significantly lower with risperidone than with haloperidol (34% vs. 60%, $P < 0.001$). The means of daily doses of risperidone ($\sim$4.9 mg) and haloperidol (11.7 mg) were similar to those used in clinical practice (Csernansky *et al.*, 2002). The reduced risk of relapse found with risperidone could be due to its superior efficacy, better tolerability or both (Csernansky *et al.*, 2002).

Duration of Treatment and Compliance

In discussions of the necessary and sensible duration of treatment of schizophrenic patients with antipsychotics, two tendencies compete: the desire to keep each patient in hospital for as short a time as possible and to keep exposure to potentially harmful antipsychotics as short as possible; and the endeavour to avoid relapses and symptomatic deteriorations as far as possible.

According to Heinrich (1976), the hospital treatment of productive schizophrenic psychoses usually lasts about 6 weeks, sometimes less in the case of catatonic syndromes and 2–4 months with schizophrenia simplex. Discharge from the hospital is striven for as early as possible so that the patient is less likely to become used to the protective atmosphere in hospital and so that the family and other social contacts are not unnecessarily hindered. On the other hand, patients may be discharged only when their state has stabilized to the extent that they are capable of coping with the stresses that will unavoidably occur on return into their usual environment. Each patient must be prepared thoroughly for discharge: he must be made to understand clearly that he has to take his medication in the prescribed manner and must learn to recognize signs of deterioration in his state as being possible premonitions of a psychotic episode. Inner unrest, increased anxiety, sleep disturbances, a dejected or irritable mood lasting over some period of time, prolonged tiredness and disturbed concentration are warning signs that should quickly bring the patient to the doctor's surgery (Herz and Melville, 1980; Jorgensen, 1998), although psychotic episodes may also occur without identifiable prodromal symptoms (Malla and Norman, 1994).

A large percentage of patients take the antipsychotics prescribed for them either irregularly or not at all. Precise figures are unknown but doubtless very high and many relapses and readmissions to hospital for schizophrenics are attributed to 'non-compliance', i.e. to the failure to observe therapeutic instructions. Revolving door psychiatry would thus seem to be partly due to the patient's rejection of treatment. One possible remedy is to prescribe notoriously unreliable patients *depot antipsychotics*, i.e. injectable galenic formulations of antipsychotics that are released over a period of weeks from the muscle tissue and then exert their therapeutic action. The most frequent cause of the failure to take medication as instructed – the often unsatisfactory tolerability of conventional antipsychotics arising particularly with high doses – is, however, not eliminated by this procedure. Antipsychotics frequently lead to motor and vegetative disturbances (Chapter 1): tremor, stiffness, palpitations, outbreaks of sweating, impotence, dizziness and the typical feeling of neuroleptic constraint are all phenomena that remind the discharged patient that he is actually still sick and may cause him to discontinue the orally administered medication on his own initiative.

The intramuscular administration of antipsychotics acting for weeks prevents this independent action and improves compliance; on the other hand, only highly potent antipsychotics such as fluphenazine, flupenthixol and haloperidol are suitable for depot administration and it is precisely these medicines that lead more frequently to EPS and dysphoric mood (van Putten *et al.*, 1984).

8.2.3 DISCONTINUATION TRIALS WITH ANTIPSYCHOTICS

The question of the optimal duration of antipsychotic treatment of schizophrenic patients has been investigated in so-called discontinuation trials: depending on the study, the medicine that had been administered for months or years was abruptly or gradually withdrawn and, in the better-controlled studies, replaced by placebo. According to Gardos and Cole (1978) and Woggon (1979), who discussed the literature relating to older neuroleptics, the mean relapse rate in schizophrenic patients 6 weeks after drug discontinuation is as high as 50%. Observations for 2 years show that chronic schizophrenic patients who had been switched to placebo experienced a relevant deterioration of their state 2.5–3 times more frequently than those patients who continued to take their original neuroleptic. Studies in which depot antipsychotics were discontinued confirm these figures (Odejide and Aderounmu, 1982; Wistedt *et al.*, 1982; Gilbert *et al.*, 1995).

The risk of relapse in discontinuation trials depends on many non-pharmacological, often poorly controllable factors, notably the expectations of the patients, doctors and nurses, other environmental factors, the duration of hospitalization and prior treatment, and the time interval since the last acute psychotic episode. On the basis of an analysis of 14 discontinuation trials, Kane and Lieberman (1987) found that the relapse rate varied greatly from study to study: depending on the trial, relapse rates of 30–86% with clustering around 60–70% have been reported in the first 12 months after placebo substitution. According to Kane and Lieberman, this scatter is a result of the different inclusion criteria applied and the different definitions of 'relapse'.

They therefore proposed that a quantifiable increase in symptoms be used as the dependent variable instead of the relapse rate in future studies of this type.

In a 2-year maintenance study by Schooler *et al.* (1997) 313 patients with schizophrenia who had been stabilized on depot fluphenazine were randomized to one of three medication strategies using fluphenazine decanoate under double-blind conditions: continuous moderate dose (12.5–50 mg every 2 weeks); continuous low dose (2.5–10 mg every 2 weeks); or targeted, early intervention (fluphenazine only when symptomatic). Subjects were also randomized to one of two family treatment strategies, supportive or applied. Both continuous low-dose and targeted treatment increased the use of rescue medication and relapse in comparison with a continuous moderate dose, with targeted treatment increasing the rehospitalization rate significantly; there were no significant differences between family treatments (Schooler *et al.*, 1997). Overall, this study clearly confirms the value of maintenance antipsychotic medication in the prevention of relapse and rehospitalization.

More important in practice than percentages would be an answer to the question of whether the relapse or exacerbation tendencies of individual patients can be estimated on the basis of specific features even *before* the planned withdrawal of antipsychotics. Unfortunately, the answer is largely negative. According to present knowledge there are no reliable clinical features that speak for or against the maintenance of antipsychotic therapy in individual cases (Möller, 1992).

Consequently, in most cases the recommendation remains that the anti-psychotic treatment of schizophrenic patients should be continued for at least 12 months after the termination of the acute episode and then, if this concerns the first psychotic episode and productive symptoms are no longer detectable, to reduce gradually and eventually discontinue the antipsychotic drug (Kissling, 1991). Monthly check-ups by psychiatrists are necessary after this withdrawal of medication in order to recognize an impending relapse and to prevent it with initially low doses of antipsychotics. In patients with frequent relapses, continuous treatment with antipsychotics is preferred and efforts should be directed at finding the minimum dose that is still effective (Schooler, 1991). Other factors that are also decisive in individual cases include the patient's relationship with the treating doctor, the attitude of the patient and relatives to the side effects of antipsychotics and to the possibility of renewed hospitalization, and the ease of access to outpatient and inpatient psychiatric services.

Prodromal signs of schizophrenia, such as sleep disturbance, agitation, preoccupation with odd ideas and disorganized thinking, may be recognized in at-risk populations and if treated could potentially lower the risk of developing full-blown schizophrenia (Wyatt and Henter, 2001). Although it is still difficult to identify accurately all at-risk preschizophrenic patients, the consensus appears to be that early intervention with low-dose antipsychotics (preferably atypical agents), stress reduction and psychosocial intervention may reduce both the risk and the severity of developing psychosis (Wyatt and Henter, 2001; Zipursky and Schulz, 2002).

8.2.4 DRUG THERAPY AND PSYCHOTHERAPY OF SCHIZOPHRENIA

The introduction of antipsychotic drugs represented such a decisive advance in the treatment of schizophrenia that the endeavors made in the 1940s and 1950s concerning individual psychotherapy of schizophrenic patients were largely pushed into the background. Whereas older textbooks of psychiatry refer respectfully to the psychoanalytically orientated attempts at therapy for schizophrenics undertaken by Rosen and Benedetti, they generally qualify their remarks by adding that the results of these often heroic efforts were quantitatively modest and that the wider application of such methods is out of the question on practical grounds. Over a period of 10 years a qualified therapist could treat only 40–60 schizophrenic patients (Müller, 1972).

Early Comparative Studies: Psychotherapy vs. Drug Treatment

According to an often-cited review of studies provided by May (1968), antipsychotics represent considerably more effective treatment for acute forms of schizophrenia than do various types of psychotherapy:

- *Antipsychotics versus psychotherapy* (two comparative studies). Both studies covered large, statistically equivalent groups of patients with productive symptoms: one study compared group psychotherapy and antipsychotics; the other compared analytically orientated individual therapy and antipsychotics. The results were similar inasmuch as both trials showed the drug therapy to be markedly superior in almost all clinically relevant characteristics and symptoms.
- *Antipsychotics versus combined antipsychotic therapy and psychotherapy* (five studies). Here, too, the results were clearly in favor of drug therapy because there were virtually no relevant differences between patients receiving antipsychotics alone and those treated with antipsychotics plus psychotherapy. Three of the five studies involved group therapy and the other two individual psychotherapy: neither of these forms of psychosocial treatment augmented the effect of the simultaneously administered antipsychotics to any demonstrable extent.
- *Psychotherapy versus combined psychotherapy and drug therapy* (two studies). In both studies the patients received analytically orientated individual therapies with the result that the effect of the combined therapies was appreciably superior to that of psychotherapy alone. It was found in both studies that the administration of drugs had no unfavorable effect on

the course of, or the results of, the psychotherapy that had been going on for up to 2 years.

The conclusion that May reached on the basis of this analysis was quite clear: " ... if one were faced with the hypothetical choice of using one and only one form of treatment in addition to the usual hospital care, the objective evidence would indicate that, for the average *hospitalized* schizophrenic patient, drug therapy would at present, generally speaking and on the average, be the treatment of choice over other physical and non-physical forms of treatment" (May, 1968, pp. 1170–1171). Interestingly, this statement also holds true for so-called environmental therapies, i.e. for occupational therapy, group activities, preparation for a profession, therapeutic community models, patient self-government and other hospital-run programs. In the opinion of May, eight additional controlled trials clearly showed the superiority of antipsychotic therapy compared with such measures that, although somewhat increasing its prospects of success, come nowhere near to taking the place of drug therapy.

Two Long-term Studies from the 1970s

May's survey related almost exclusively to studies with hospitalized patients who, as experience shows, have quite variable outcomes: some of these patients will stay in the protected environment of a clinic for a long time or even permanently, whereas the majority of schizophrenics can be discharged and perhaps will never return to the hospital again.

One aspect of great importance in the long term, namely a reduction in the relapse risk *after the remission of an acute schizophrenic episode*, forms the subject of two comprehensive studies involving schizophrenic patients who had been discharged from hospital (Hogarty and Goldberg, 1973; May *et al.*, 1976); see Boxes 8.2 and 8.3.

More Recent Studies

In more recent studies, the therapeutic efforts have probably emphasized more than before the individual requirements of the patients and their social relationships. As an example of a project directed to individual requirements and thus 'uncontrolled' in various respects, a therapeutic study published by Alanen *et al.* (1986) in 100 schizophrenic patients in Turku, Finland, can be cited. Three-quarters of these cases were hospitalized initially and almost all received antipsychotics, at least at the start of treatment, mostly in rather low doses. They were subsequently incorporated into various psychotherapeutic and sociotherapeutic programs that were greatly individualized and adapted to the resources available in the participating institutions: intensive individual

Box 8.2 Pharmacotherapy and/or Psychotherapy in Remitted Schizophrenic Patients

In a study conducted by Hogarty and Goldberg (1973), a sample of 374 schizophrenic patients, who had been discharged after showing marked improvement and had adjusted to ambulatory treatment with an antipsychotic for 2 months, was divided into four different treatment groups: chlorpromazine plus psychotherapy; placebo plus psychotherapy; chlorpromazine alone; placebo alone.

The psychotherapy consisted of regular individual sessions dealing with the patient's family as well as social and professional problems. With the number of relapses during the following 12 months used as the criterion of therapeutic success, the results were as follows:

- chlorpromazine plus psychotherapy: 26% relapse
- chlorpromazine without psychotherapy: 33% relapse
- placebo plus psychotherapy: 63% relapse
- placebo without psychotherapy: 73% relapse

These results unequivocally confirm the efficacy of antipsychotic therapy in preventing new schizophrenic episodes, whereas the protective benefit of psychotherapeutic efforts was demonstrable but quantitatively less impressive. A second evaluation after a further 12 months, i.e. after a total follow-up of 2 years, confirmed the first year's findings: at this point in time considerably fewer of the patients being treated with antipsychotics had suffered a relapse in comparison with those treated with placebo and there was further, albeit numerically less important, confirmation of the efficacy of psychotherapy. In a subsequent publication (Hogarty *et al.*, 1976) the authors considered whether the effect of the psychotherapeutic measures in the group receiving combined therapy was at best due to the fact that the respective patients took their medication more regularly than did the remaining patients, with the result that the presumed effect of the psychotherapy was in reality a consequence of the more reliable intake of the medication. It emerged that there was no difference between the average daily doses prescribed for the groups and that the compliance reported by patients and relatives was more or less the same for both groups. The protective effect of the psychotherapy was consequently deemed a real one and not merely the result of a more regular intake of the medication.

Box 8.3 Long-term Follow-up of Schizophrenic Patients

May *et al.* (1976) published follow-up examinations over several
years from a sample of 228 patients who had participated in a
comparative treatment study in the 1960s. During their stay in
hospital the patients (schizophrenics of both sexes hospitalized for
the first time) had received one of the following therapies according
to a randomized experimental design:

- analytically orientated individual psychotherapy
- an antipsychotic (trifluoperazine)
- psychotherapy plus antipsychotics
- electroshocks
- environmental therapy, i.e. none of the four therapies named

After 3, 4 and 5 years the long-term effects of these treatments were
examined. The criterion of success was taken to be the number of
days spent by the patients in psychiatric hospitals since the first
hospitalization and since their discharge from first hospitalization.

After 3 years, 203 patients could be followed up: the total
number of days spent in hospital in the case of the groups treated
with psychotherapy and with environmental therapy alone was
significantly greater than in the other three groups. The results
were similar for the number of hospital days since discharge:
patients on analytical psychotherapy had, on average, to be
rehospitalized more frequently and/or for longer periods than the
other patients.

After 4 years, when 113 patients could be examined, the result
was about the same and a similar tendency was observed in 61
patients 5 years after commencement of the study: in all cases the
catamnestic findings were least favorable for those patients treated
with psychotherapy or environmental therapy.

In this study, psychotherapy was clearly inferior to both drug
therapy and to electroshock treatment; the patients treated with
psychotherapy and environmental therapy were, on average,
hospitalized for 50% longer than the other groups and, as noted
by the authors, this clearly contradicts a popular prejudice against
antipsychotics: "it was simply *not* true that patients who had been
initially treated with drugs relapsed more rapidly and spent more
time in hospital in the end than non-drug-treated patients. On the
contrary, the initial advantages of drug treatment seemed to persist

for at least three years and, to a lesser extent, up to five years"
(May *et al.*, 1976, p. 86).

A critical remark that should be made in this context is that the
authors merely took as independent variables the treatments
applied at the time of first hospitalization, neglecting other factors
that had arisen in subsequent years. If the patients really were
schizophrenics, it is almost certain that the majority of them would
have received further treatment that – contrary to the original
experimental plan – could no longer be introduced in the sense of a
controlled trial. The results after 4 and 5 years must be regarded
rather cautiously for this reason.

psychotherapy, occasional psychotherapy of an essentially supportive nature,
care in day clinics, family and husband/wife therapy, support in occupational
rehabilitation. Five years after the start of this program, more than half of all
patients and about one-third of the typical schizophrenics were asymptomatic,
and clear psychotic features could be detected only in a minority. In many
cases the antipsychotics had been discontinued without a relapse occurring, a
result that was particularly clear in those patients who had received occasional
or intensive individual psychotherapy. In all, the monograph by Alanen *et al.*
provides a rather optimistic picture of the therapeutic outcome for
schizophrenic patients.

Schooler and Hogarty (1987) summarized a large proportion of the works
published since 1978 in which drug treatment and psychotherapy or
sociotherapy were combined, and drew the following conclusions with regard
to the treatment of schizophrenia:

- *Individual psychotherapy.* One controlled comparative study with four
  treatment groups (depot antipsychotics vs. orally administered antipsychotics, intensive vs. less intensive psychotherapy directed to interpersonal
  problems) had been published. Marked differences could not be detected
  between the four treatments during the course of 2 years, although the
  group given depot antipsychotics plus intensive psychotherapeutic care
  tended to do best: none of the patients in this group suffered further relapses
  after the first 8 months of study.
- *Social and life skills training.* The four available studies were of short
  duration (5 days, 7 weeks, nine weeks, 12 weeks) and showed an
  improvement in the parameters of interest (eye contact, self-assertion).
  There was no detailed information on the antipsychotics administered and,
  according to the authors, it is also unclear how long the stated behavioral
  changes lasted.

- *Group psychotherapy.* In this area there was a well-documented study by Malm (1982) in 80 recently hospitalized schizophrenics. All patients were receiving depot antipsychotics and underwent a 3-month course to improve their social skills; half of the patients also participated in communication-orientated group therapy for 1 year; in this group there was an additional improvement in features relating to ability for emotional contact, general well-being, leisure activities and social contacts.
- Particularly interesting are treatment trials directed to the *relatives of schizophrenic patients,* with the objective of modifying family dynamics. Four of the six studies cited by Schooler and Hogarty were based on the concept of expressed emotions (EE), i.e. they started from the observation that schizophrenic patients who return from the hospital to families with markedly expressed feelings of criticism, hostility or even excessive care suffer relapses more frequently than others. In a study by Leff *et al.* (1982) it emerged that the relapse rate was reduced from 50% to 9% within 9 months by eliminating or attenuating this behavior of the relatives and the simultaneous administration of antipsychotic drugs to patients.

Müller and Schöneich (1992) also reported on favorable experience with intensive outpatient psychotherapy combined with antipsychotic drug treatment. On the basis of a before-and-after comparison over 2×5 years in a university outpatient clinic, they were able to show that the duration of rehospitalizations required by 89 patients could be reduced from a mean of 10 weeks to 2 weeks per year when a special schizophrenia outpatient service offering individualized psychotherapy and psychosocial treatment was available to the patients instead of the routine psychiatric outpatient service. A beneficial effect of psychotherapy was demonstrated both in those patients taking antipsychotics continuously for long-term prophylaxis and in those taking the drugs intermittently when prodromal symptoms appeared in order to prevent relapse.

The view of combined drug therapy and psychotherapy in schizophrenia has thus changed fundamentally since May's review (1968) classified psychotherapy as being of very little value. Whether given orally or in depot form, whether used for long-term maintenance or intermittently, antipsychotic drugs form the backbone of schizophrenia therapy but at the same time it is now recognized that individualized psychotherapy and psychosocial therapy of hospitalized patients and especially of outpatients is essential because these measures decisively improve the quality of life of patients and their families and help to prevent rehospitalizations and thus improve the long-term prognosis of schizophrenic psychoses (see Sellwood *et al.*, 1994; Mojtabai *et al.*, 1998; Bustillo *et al.*, 2001 for more references and a critical discussion of various psychosocial treatment models).

8.3 ANTIDEPRESSANTS AND THE TREATMENT OF DEPRESSION

8.3.1 TREATMENT OF DEPRESSIVE EPISODES

The drug therapy of depression differs in a number of critical points from that given to schizophrenics. Depressions are phasically occurring deviations from the norm that, in the majority of cases, show spontaneous remission, although this often may be only after a period of some months. The majority of depressives can be treated as outpatients – a fact that explains why the illness generally does not make as severe an encroachment into the family and social surroundings of the patient as does schizophrenia. Outsiders are able to imagine what a depression must be like, or at least believe that they can: everyone is occasionally sad, disappointed or devoid of hope. In the eyes of his fellow men and women a depressive consequently tends to be a person to be pitied but not one who is necessarily mad.

The efficacy of antidepressants has been demonstrated statistically (Table 1.5 in Chapter 1) and confirmed also in a meta-analysis of about 300 published clinical studies (Davis *et al.*, 1993): a positive therapeutic result is to be expected in almost two-thirds of cases with imipramine, amitriptyline, amoxapine and newer antidepressant drugs (Anderson, 2001), whereas a good one-third of all patients show a clinically relevant improvement with placebo. According to Davis *et al.* (1993), these figures prove the therapeutic utility of antidepressants "beyond the shadow of a doubt" and also show that there are hardly any quantitative differences in efficacy between the various substances licensed as antidepressants. But what is to be done with the 35% or so of patients who do not obtain a beneficial effect within 6 weeks of medication and who are thus 'refractory to therapy'? Poor compliance must be assumed in some of these patients, perhaps as a result of side effects of antidepressants, and in others the prescribed dose may be inadequate; both of these factors could be monitored by measuring drug levels in the plasma. In the other cases with 'true refractoriness to treatment', leading authors first advise a change of antidepressant, then combined drug therapy (Fatemi *et al.*, 1999) and finally a change to other forms of treatment. Suitable staged plans or strategies are reported by Janicak *et al.* (2001, chapter 7) and, more recently, by a Task Force of the World Federation of Societies for Biological Psychiatry (Bauer *et al.*, 2002).

None of today's antidepressants are devoid of side effects, which, for their own part, can intensify the feeling of illness and concern felt by the patient. Doctors consequently will not prescribe antidepressants unnecessarily, especially in older patients who react particularly sensitively to the central and peripheral effects of these substances. Many doctors even seem to tend to insufficient prescriptions: according to a survey reported by Keller *et al.* (1982), in the USA more than half of patients suffering from a depressive illness for at least 1 month were either receiving no antidepressants or antidepressants in insufficient doses. Two-thirds of these patients were receiving psychotherapy and more than half were taking anxiolytics, but only about one-third had been treated with antidepressants for at least 4 weeks. Whether this situation was the consequence of insufficient familiarity with the diagnosis and therapy of depression (as the authors of the study assume) or whether it reflected wise restraint (Uhlenhuth, 1982) remained open. A more recent survey in the USA (Druss *et al.*, 2000) supported earlier findings by Keller *et al.*: in a national sample of 7589 young adults, 312 (4.1%) fullfilled DSM-III criteria for current major depression, but only 7.4% of these were being treated with an antidepressant. Underreporting of depressive symptoms to health providers, mainly general practicioners, and limited access to general medical care appeared to be the main reasons for this situation. An earlier study from Sweden (Isacsson *et al.*, 1992) showed the potentially tragic consequences of inadequate antidepressant prescription. Of 80 representative suicide victims selected in the period 1970–1984, at least 40 had consulted a doctor in the 3 months before their death. Of these, 27 received a prescription for psychopharmaceuticals, mostly anxiolytics or sleeping pills (i.e. the patients must have complained of mental symptoms), but an antidepressant was prescribed in only eight cases. The authors of this study therefore saw a clear relationship between inadequate psychopharmaceutical prescription and successful suicide, and they demanded an improvement in the training of general practitioners with regard to psychiatric diagnosis and drug therapy.

Treatment of Depression with Newer Generation Antidepressants

Although the efficacy of tricyclic antidepressants in the treatment of unipolar depression is beyond reproach, the side-effect profile of these agents makes them less desirable as first-line therapeutic agents. Introduction of selective serotonin reuptake inhibitors (SSRIs) such as fluoxetine, paroxetine, sertraline, citalopram and fluvoxamine in the past decade has revolutionized the treatment of depression universally. The side-effect profile of SSRIs, such as nausea, diarrhea and sexual dysfunction, is considerably more benign than that of tricyclic drugs. Multiple controlled trials have proven the efficacy of SSRIs vs. placebo (Nemeroff, 1994). Recently, a number of SNRIs (serotonin and noradrenaline reuptake inhibitors) and so-called atypical antidepressants have been marketed that may have additional advantages over SSRIs, such as more rapid onset of action (venlafaxine, mirtazapine) and low sexual side-effect potential (bupropion, nefazodone). Additionally, it appears that venlafaxine may be more efficacious in cases of treatment-refractory depression (Clerc *et al.*, 1994; Fatemi *et al.*, 1999). Finally, in a recent report (Thase *et al.*, 2001), venlafaxine was shown to be superior to SSRIs and placebo in attaining remission in depressed patients (Nemeroff and Schatzberg, 2002).

8.3.2 PROBLEMS OF MAINTENANCE THERAPY

According to modern treatment guidelines, episodes of endogenous depression are treated with antidepressants for 6–12 months, both in hospital and at home. In cases of doubt the medication is given for a longer period because the restored subjective feeling of well-being does not necessarily reflect the abatement of a depressive episode and is often only the expression of transient symptom suppression. Short-term prospects are good for the acutely depressive because remission occurs within 1 year in 85% of patients. In the medium and long term the prognosis is less favorable: up to 65% of all patients receiving no further treatment suffer a relapse of greater or lesser severity within one year. About half of all depressives experience more than one severe depressive episode in the course of their lives and are thus at risk for years (Klerman and Weissman, 1992), and about 15% of all depressed patients commit suicide. In view of the fact that depression is a recurring illness or even a chronic illness in a proportion of patients, the question of maintenance therapy arises in many cases.

Continuation Therapy of Depressive Episodes

Controlled discontinuation trials show that about half of all depressive patients suffer a serious relapse within 6 months if their antidepressant medication is withdrawn shortly after the disappearance of acute symptoms; with continuation therapy, only about one-fifth of patients experience a relapse in the same period. The difficulty for the treating doctor is to estimate reliably how long he should continue to prescribe antidepressants for patients who have overcome depression. Consensus groups suggest that this period should be *between four and six months* after the symptoms of depression have resolved (Montgomery, 1997); even mild continuing symptoms may indicate that a depressive episode has not ceased completely and that the treatment should be continued further (Lader, 2001).

Because the continued symptoms of a treated episode cannot always be separated from the prodromal symptoms of a subsequent episode (Fava and Kellner, 1991), the continuation or rapid resumption of drug therapy is advisable in all such cases. A prerequisite is close cooperation between doctors, patients and relatives so that symptoms are recognized early and reported, and the necessary measures can be taken (CINP Task Force, 1993).

PreventiveTherapy (Secondary Prevention)

Unipolar depressions occur more frequently than manic–depressive or bipolar disorder (see next section) and are etiologically heterogeneous. The question of maintenance therapy is consequently a complex one in such cases and some aspects are as yet unsolved. Lithium provides a certain amount of protection against further episodes of unipolar endogenous depression but it is still unclear whether depressive episodes can really be prevented or merely attenuated sufficiently to prevent the need for hospitalization. Many clinicians regard the protective effect of lithium in cases of unipolar depression to be too weak to merit its routine use. Instead, the long-term administration of antidepressants is frequently recommended. Several studies have shown that these drugs not only suppress or curtail acute depressive phases but also can prevent the reappearance of previously resolved episodes or, when administration is continued for years, the appearance of new episodes (Kupfer *et al.*, 1992). *Chronic treatment* with antidepressants is generally considered to be justified when episodes of depression have occurred at least twice in 5 years within the context of unipolar depression (CINP Task Force, 1993; Kennedy *et al.*, 2002).

8.3.3 TREATMENT OF BIPOLAR DISORDER WITH MOOD STABILIZERS

Some 10–15% of all affective illnesses are manic–depressive or bipolar psychoses (ICD no. F31). Treatment of bipolar disorder may vary depending on the symptoms of patients and whether they are acutely manic, depressed or mixed. The compilation and review of clinical reports is quite revealing regarding the efficacy of a number of medications in use in the USA, Europe and elsewhere.

Treatments during Acute Mania

The superiority of lithium over placebo has been shown in five controlled studies (see Keck and McElroy, 2002), which indicate that 70% of treated patients experiencing acute manic symptoms can obtain partial response. Lithium non-response as well as intolerance of lithium's side effects provided the impetus to try a number of agents that may have efficacy in the acute treatment of mania. One such agent is valproic acid, which has been shown to exhibit a broad spectrum of efficacy in acute mania. Eight controlled trials confirm that valproic acid is effective in acute treatment of manic and mixed episodes and is comparable in efficacy to lithium and haloperidol in overall antimanic activity (Keck and McElroy, 2002). Another anticonvulsant agent that possesses antimanic efficacy, is carbamazepine; numerous controlled studies have found this medication to be efficacious in the acute treatment of manic symptoms (Keck *et al.*, 1992; Keck and McElroy 2002). Several antipsychotic agents also may exhibit antimanic activity, e.g. olanzapine, chlorpromazine, risperidone and ziprasidone. Among these drugs, olanzapine has been shown to exhibit robust antimanic activity based on double-blind, randomized controlled trials (Berk *et al.*, 1999; Tohen *et al.*, 2001). This led to recent FDA (US Food and Drug Administration) approval of olanzapine as an antimanic agent. Controlled studies indicate that lamotrigine, an anticonvulsant with GABAergic and Na channel stabilizing effects, may have antimanic activity (Frye *et al.*, 2000; Ichim *et al.*, 2000). Finally, two controlled studies indicate that nimodipine, a calcium channel blocker, may be effective in ultrarapidly cycling manic patients (Pazzaglia *et al.*, 1993, 1998; Keck and McElroy 2002).

Treatments during Acute Bipolar Depression

Results of crossover studies indicate that lithium is efficacious in treating acute depression in bipolar subjects unequivocally (36%, 29/80) and partially (43%, 34/80), respectively (Zomberg and Pope, 1993; Keck and McElroy, 2002). Various antidepressants have shown variable rates of efficacy in the treatment of acute bipolar depression, i.e. desipramine (50%), maprotiline (67%), imipramine (40–60%), tranylcypromine (87%), moclobemide (53%) and fluoxetine (60%) (Keck and McElroy, 2002). Among the anticonvulsants, valproic acid and lamotrigine appear to have some potential efficacy in the treatment of acute bipolar depression (Calabrese *et al.*, 1992, 1999; Fatemi *et al.*, 1997).

MaintenanceTreatments for Bipolar Disorder

Several controlled trials have shown that lithium is efficacious in the maintenance treatment of bipolar disorder, with higher serum levels (0.8–1 mol/l) being more indicative of successful prophylaxis (Keck and McElroy, 2002). Valproic acid also appears to have efficacy in maintenance therapy, specifically in bipolar patients with mixed mania and rapid cycling (Bowden *et al.*, 1995). The results concerning carbamazepine's efficacy as a maintenance medication are controversial (Stuppaeck *et al.*, 1994). Other potential agents with some evidence of good maintenance value include clozapine and olanzapine. A combination of lithium and carbamazepine or other anticonvulsants is recommended under certain conditions if an adequate preventive effect cannot be obtained with the substances individually (Bauer *et al.*, 2002).

8.3.4 DRUG THERAPY AND PSYCHOTHERAPY OF DEPRESSIONS

Numerous investigations have been published concerning the question of the contributions that psychotherapy and drug therapy can make to the treatment of depressions, which psychotherapeutic procedures are particularly suitable for depressions and whether combined drug therapy and psychotherapy is sensible for depressions.

Studies from the Early 1970s

The first such investigation, the so-called Boston–New Haven Study, has been described in several complementary individual reports (Klerman *et al.*, 1974; Weissman *et al.*, 1974; Paykel *et al.*, 1976). This started out with 150 ambulatory female depressed patients and involved a comparison between six forms of treatment:

- For at least 1 h per week, 75 of the patients saw psychotherapeutically trained female social workers with whom they were able to discuss the problems preoccupying them at the time. These therapies were supportive and not primarily analytically orientated (high-contact group). The remaining 75 patients saw a psychiatrist for about 15 min per month, told him how they felt and discussed any changes in the medication (low-contact group).
- One-third of the patients in each of the two groups were then given an antidepressant (amitriptyline) in doses of 100–200 mg per day, one-third were given placebo and the remaining one-third received no tablets at all.

Cells were formed (Table 8.1) on the basis of this 2×3 design receiving different forms of treatment. The patients (mean age 38 years) were suffering from depressions of moderate severity, most of which were classified as neurotic, i.e. not endogenous. The women, usually from low- or middle-class backgrounds, had been selected from an original sample of 278 depressive patients, the selection criterion being a pronounced symptomatic improvement under amitriptyline therapy within 4–6 weeks (Fig. 8.1). After 4 and 8 months the patients were evaluated on the basis of the criteria of 'relapse rate' and 'social adjustment and satisfaction': relapse was defined as the renewed return of a depression rating score to the pretreatment level, and social adjustment was assessed on the basis of an extensive interview. Results were as follows:

(1) At the end of the trial (6 months after randomization) the relapse rate in both amitriptyline groups was $> 50\%$ lower than in the four non-drug groups. In the high-contact groups the relapse rate was some 25% lower than in the low-contact groups (this difference was not statistically significant). Both forms of therapy – drug and psychotherapy –

Table 8.1 Cells showing the 2×3 design receiving different forms of treatment

	Amitriptyline	Placebo	No medication	Total
High contact	25⟶19	25⟶18	25⟶18	75⟶55
Low contact	25⟶20	25⟶15	25⟶16	75⟶51
Total	50⟶39	50⟶33	50⟶34	150⟶106

The cells show the respective numbers of patients at the beginning and end of the trial.

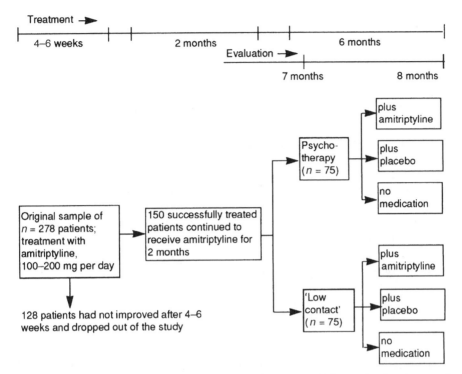

Figure 8.1 Design of the study by Klerman *et al.* Treatment of depression by drugs and psychotherapy **131** 186–191 (1974). 1974 the American Psychiatric Association; http://AJP.psychiatryonline.org. Reprinted by permission

consequently had favorable effects on the relapse rate, the impact of amitriptyline being numerically superior.

(2) After 4 months' treatment (whereof 2 months in the assigned group) there was no difference between the groups in respect of social adjustment and satisfaction. After 8 months, significantly better results were observed in the high-contact groups than in the other patients, there being no difference between those patients receiving medication and those receiving no medication.

In the authors' views drug therapy was clearly superior to psychotherapy with regard to the prevention of relapses, although social adjustment – and hence also long-term prognosis – was improved in those patients receiving psychotherapy. It was striking to note the difference in the effect between the two forms of treatment over time: amitriptyline worked more rapidly and strongly on the actual depressive symptoms, whereas psychotherapy acted more slowly and on different mental aspects. The two therapies were additive, as seen in the amitriptyline–high-contact group. The authors concluded: "Psychotherapy is not an alternative to antidepressant treatment and does not prevent relapse or the recurrence of symptoms. Alternatively, continued amitriptyline has no effect on social adjustment and is no better or worse than a placebo or no pill" (Weissman *et al.*, 1974, p. 778).

Several points need to be noted in the interpretation of this often-cited study. Firstly, the 150 female patients included in the study constituted a selection in that they had responded favorably to amitriptyline given in a trial of several weeks' duration before the actual study, thus implying that drug treatment was favored from the outset. Secondly it was not the immediate, antidepressive action of the two modes of treatment that was compared, but their maintenance effect once symptomatic improvement had already occurred. The higher incidence of relapses in the groups receiving placebo or no medication therefore could have been the result of the premature discontinuation of the medicament to which the patients had responded favorably. It is consequently all the more interesting to note the effect, found as a trend but not statistically significant, of psychotherapy on the relapse rate. On the other hand, the improved social adjustment in the groups receiving psychotherapy is not surprising: these patients had been treated for 6 months with a view to their social adjustment and the resolution of interpersonal conflicts, and they evaluated themselves at the end of the study; their hopes and expectations therefore must have spilled over into the assessments (Spitzer, 1976).

Despite these limitations, the following conclusions can be drawn from the Boston–New Haven Study and two other, similarly extensive studies published at the same time – one with analytically orientated group therapy (Covi *et al.*, 1974) and one with family therapy (Friedman, 1975):

(1) The treatment of depressive patients using either drugs or psychotherapy appears to influence different symptoms or personality areas. The antidepressants acted in particular on symptoms in the somatic, drive/ motivation and mood sectors, with psychotherapy affecting more the relationship between the patients and their families and their wider surroundings.

(2) Combined treatments had mainly additive effects. Patients being treated pharmacologically and psychotherapeutically benefited in two ways. There was no evidence of a negative interaction between drug treatment and psychotherapy.

Both conclusions apply to outpatients with neurotic (i.e. rather lighter and generally non-endogenous) forms of depression. Two of the three investigations dealt with maintenance therapy of patients who had already shown pronounced symptomatic improvement with antidepressant treatment.

In the following studies, psychotherapeutic techniques were applied that had been specifically developed for the treatment of depressions, namely cognitive therapy, interpersonal therapy and a behaviorally orientated technique known as social skills training.

Studies with Cognitive Therapy

Cognitive therapy (CT) is based on a theory developed by Beck (1991) according to which some typical symptoms of depression (despair, sadness, suicidal tendencies) reflect pathological changes in the cognitive organization of an individual. Patients suffering from depression regard themselves, their world and the future in a negative light (= depressive triad). Their distorted thinking is a result of logical and conceptual errors, including arbitrary conclusions, over-extensive and thus false generalizations and simplifications. The purpose of CT is to make the patients aware of their cognitive errors on the basis of typical examples and, by means of specific training and guidance, to enable them to correct their false attitude. Cognitive therapy is sometimes combined with social skills training and is then called, by some authors, cognitive–behavioral therapy (CBT).

A trial carried out in Scotland (Blackburn et al., 1981; see Box 8.4) supported the use of CT in mild to moderately severe depression. In a subsequent study carried out by Beck et al. (1985) in Philadelphia, the efficacy of CT alone was compared with that of CT plus drug treatment. Eighteen of the 33 outpatients (9 men, 24 women) with mild to moderately severe depression received a maximum of 2 h of CT in 12 weeks; 15 patients also received CT with additional amitriptyline individually dosed within a range of 50–200 mg/day. At the end of treatment there were no significant differences between the two groups with regard to the various rating scales, i.e. the antidepressant administered in addition to CT had neither a beneficial nor an adverse effect overall. A follow-up examination 12 months later showed a slight tendency in favor of the combined CT plus antidepressant treatment.

Murphy et al. (1984) could only partially confirm these results in a study involving 87 depressive outpatients. Their mostly middle-class, predominantly female and rather young patients with moderately severe to severe depression were allocated randomly to one of the following treatment groups:

- CT: two sessions of 50 min per week for 8 weeks, then one session per week for 4 weeks
- drug therapy: an individually adjusted dose of the antidepressant nortriptyline up to a previously established therapeutic window
- CT plus drug therapy

Box 8.4 Cognitive Therapy, Drug Treatment and their Combination

Blackburn *et al.* (1981) studied 49 patients with mild to moderately severe depressions in a psychiatric outpatient department and 39 patients from a general practice in Edinburgh, i.e. a total of 88 patients, of whom 64 (14 men, 50 women) completed the study. The patients were selected on the basis of the Research Diagnostic Criteria (Spitzer *et al.*, 1978) as well as various rating and self-rating scales; one-third of the patients each received one of the following, randomly allocated treatments for a maximum of 20 weeks:

- CT: 2 h per week for 3 weeks, then 1 h per week
- drug therapy: generally amitriptyline or clomipramine at 150 mg/ day
- CT plus drug therapy: a combination of both procedures

Patients with a decrease in their symptoms by less than 50% after 12 weeks were considered therapeutic failures. Major results of a rather complex statistical evaluation were as follows:

(1) Patients from both the psychiatric outpatient unit and from general practice showed the best results with combined CT and drug therapy.
(2) The poorest results in both subgroups were obtained with drug therapy alone.
(3) In the general practice patients, CT was significantly better than drug therapy.
(4) Endogenous and non-endogenous depressives showed similar rates of success or failure with the three types of treatment.

In all, this study suggested the *suitability of CT in mild to moderately severe depressions* and tended to speak against the drug treatment of patients whose mental illness is conditioned primarily by their life situation. The study also confirmed that drug therapy and non-drug treatments can be combined in depressions.

- CT plus 'active placebo' (atropine and phenobarbitone in very small doses to imitate the concomitant effects of the antidepressant)

Seventy of 87 patients ended the study as intended, and most of the premature terminations concerned patients given the antidepressant or CT plus antidepressant. Comparisons within the four groups undertaken at the end of treatment and then again 4 weeks later showed a highly significant decrease in symptoms relative to baseline in all four groups, but no difference between the groups. This means that all four treatments were approximately equally effective and that the combination of an antidepressant with CT provided no additional benefit, unlike the observations of Blackburn *et al.* (1981). Also of interest are the results published by Simons *et al.* (1986) concerning a follow-up of these patients 12 months later: most relapses occurred in the group of patients treated with drugs alone, whereas the patients treated with CT (with or without additional antidepressant) showed relevant deterioration less frequently.

In all, and despite the considerable differences between the cited studies, these results suggest that CT is an effective therapeutic procedure for ambulatory patients with mild to moderately severe depressions. It also appears that CT and drug therapy may have similar efficacy in these cases, although the small numbers typical of these trials leave the possibility of type 2 errors open. It remains to be determined whether a combination of CT with an antidepressant provides a significant additional benefit, and it is also unclear what the precise indications are for the two forms of therapy (see Hollon *et al.*, 1991). Two more recent studies also have not provided definitive answers to these questions:

- In a multicenter study with exemplary methodology involving 250 patients, Elkin *et al.* (1989) found that drug therapy with imipramine, together with the usual clinical care, tended to be more effective than 16 weeks of treatment with CBT (one session per week) in patients with 'major depressive disorder', and that CBT in turn had greater efficacy than placebo treatment plus the usual clinical care. Superiority of drug therapy over CBT was particularly seen in severely ill patients. Re-analysis of the findings (Elkin *et al.*, 1995) showed that all treatment modalities were similarly effective in milder cases, and that therapy with imipramine was significantly more effective than CBT and the usual clinical care in more severe cases (patients with Hamilton Rating Scale for Depression scores of $\geqslant 20$). Interpersonal therapy showed a slight advantage over CBT and the usual clinical care in the more severe cases.
- On the other hand, the results of a study by Hollon *et al.* (1992) suggested that 12 weeks of CT is as effective as the same duration of treatment with imipramine. In this comparison between CT, imipramine and a combination of CT plus imipramine in 107 ambulatory depressives, the combination treatment tended to be superior to the two single therapies, but without achieving the threshold of statistical significance. The superiority of drug therapy reported by Elkin *et al.* (1989, 1995) was thus not confirmed in this study. However, the high dropout rate (about 40% of all patients) was a notable feature and affected all three treatment groups to roughly the same degree.

In another study of interest in this connection, Mercier *et al.* (1992) noted that the majority of patients with so-called atypical depression not responding to CT did respond favorably to treatment with a monoamine oxidase (MAO) inhibitor or imipramine following CT. They concluded that both CT and drug therapy can be considered effective treatments for different groups of depressed patients and possibly have differential indications. However, the small number of cases in this study does not allow a conclusion to be reached regarding possible prognostic factors for successful therapy with CT or antidepressants. In a trial published by Scott *et al.* (2000) patients with residual symptoms of major depression ($n=158$) were randomized to receive clinical management alone or clinical management plus 18 sessions of CT, and were followed for 16 months. This study indicated that the addition of CT to pharmacotherapy may produce modest improvements in social and psychological functioning. More importantly, there were also fewer relapses occurring in the patient group receiving CT in addition to clinical management.

Studies with 'Interpersonal Therapy'

The techniques of interpersonal therapy (IPT) developed by Klerman, Weissman and other authors are based on the concept that depressions have their origin in the area of interpersonal relationships and that they also run their course in that area (see Klerman *et al.*, 1984). The purpose of IPT is to restore the patients within a short time to a position in which they can better understand their interpersonal problems and are able to change their unsatisfactory behavior towards others that leads to conflicts and frustrations. An early IPT study is presented in Box 8.5.

Prusoff *et al.* (1980) and Klerman *et al.* (1982) analyzed the outcome of this investigation in still another way by classifying the patients according to types of depression. On the basis of Research Diagnostic Criteria (Spitzer *et al.*, 1978) they formed several subgroups, the most important of which was a group of endogenous depressive patients ($n=20$) and a group of depressives whose illness was labeled situative ($n=31$). Situative depressions were diagnosed when the illness developed after an event or in a situation that probably contributed to the appearance of the depressive episode at that particular time. This led to the following insights:

- Endogenous depressives responded best to a combination of drug and psychotherapy. Drug therapy alone was only marginally better than free appointments. Psychotherapy alone was less effective than free appointments.
- In the case of situative depressives, psychotherapy and combined drug and psychotherapy achieved approximately the same result and both were markedly better than drug therapy alone, which in turn was better than free appointments.

Box 8.5 Interpersonal Therapy, Drug Treatment and their Combination

A first study with separate and combined use of IPT and antidepressants (Weissman *et al.* 1979) comprised 81 outpatients (12 men, 69 women) aged 18–65 years (mean approximately 30 years) suffering from moderately severe unipolar depressions and classified as neurotic depressions. Half of the patients received at least one session of 50 min of IPT per week for 16 weeks; the other patients were given the name and telephone number of a psychiatrist at the clinic and could call him whenever they wanted to make an appointment. They were granted a maximum of one therapy session per month. Half of each of the two psychotherapy groups received amitriptyline in individually adjusted daily doses of between 100 and 200 mg, or placebo.

Clinical assessments were made by specialized raters not involved in the treatment after 1, 4, 8, 12 and 16 weeks. The study was intended to include 96 patients, 15 of whom withdrew at the very beginning when they heard what treatment they were to be given. Most of those withdrawing were in the psychotherapy group. In addition, patients who failed to show any pronounced improvement in their symptoms within 8 weeks or whose condition even deteriorated were withdrawn from the study. In the case of those patients withdrawing from the study, scores recorded at the time of withdrawal were used for purposes of evaluation; this represents a last observation carried forward (LOCF) analysis. Withdrawals from the study occurred rather frequently and showed the following distribution:

	Withdrew	Withdrew during the first week	% Completed
Psychotherapy group	13/25	8	48
Drug therapy group	16/24	4	33
Psychotherapy plus drug therapy group	8/24	1	67
Free appointments group	16/23	2	30
Total	53/96	15	45

According to this criterion, the combined therapy was superior to the other three treatments, and drug therapy alone was little different from the control conditions with free appointments. An additional assessment directed at target symptoms (DiMascio *et al.*, 1979) showed that the drug therapy had a particularly rapid and thorough effect on sleep disorders, whereas anxiety and other affective symptoms only showed a significant improvement at a later stage. The effect of psychotherapy on anxious and depressive mood was of rapid onset, whereas vegetative and somatic symptoms showed little change. No negative interactions were observed between the two forms of therapy, the treatment effects thus being differential and additive. The results indicated that drug therapy was particularly suitable for those patients whose symptoms were mainly vegetative–somatic in nature. Furthermore, the authors concluded from their findings that a patient rejecting one of the two forms of therapy (drug or psychotherapy) can be offered the other form of therapy with good prospects of success.

Viewed as a whole, this investigation supports the view that tricyclic antidepressants are particularly effective in cases of endogenous depression, whereas psychotherapy, possibly in conjunction with drug therapy, constitutes the best solution in cases of situative depression (which would probably be termed reactive depression in the terminology used hitherto). It is interesting to note that the combination of drug therapy with psychotherapy provided additional benefit in patients with endogenous depression. It must, however, be stated that this final conclusion is only based on a fairly small subsample.

In a large multicenter study published by Keller *et al.* (2000), patients with chronic non-psychotic forms of depression (n=681) were randomized to one of three groups: treatment with nefazodone; cognitive–behavioral analysis system of psychotherapy; or combined treatment. Among the 519 patients who completed the study, 55% in the nefazodone group and 52% in the psychotherapy group, as compared with 85% in the combined treatment group ($P < 0.001$), responded favorably (with either a remission or a 50% improvement of their symptom scores) to the treatment modality. The rates of withdrawal were similar in the three groups, supporting the superiority of combined pharmacological and psychotherapeutic treatment.

Social Skills Therapy

This behavior-orientated form of therapy is based on the assumption that depressions are attributable to the inability of patients to provide themselves with positive 'reinforcement' through suitable modes of behavior (Kovacs, 1980). As Bellack *et al.* (1981) stated, depressive persons often have disturbed relationships within their marriage or families, cannot affirm themselves and create widespread unease in their surroundings, inducing hostile feelings and rejection in others. Social skills therapy or training (SST) attempts to overcome the behavioral deficit and thereby to increase affectively satisfactory social contacts with family members, friends, colleagues and others.

Bellack *et al.* (1981) reported on a comparative study involving 72 women with non-psychotic unipolar depression, of whom 60% came from a psychiatric outpatient clinic and 40% answered advertisements for treatment in the press and radio. They were aged 20–60 years with a mean age of 36 years. The patients were divided into the following treatment groups at random:

- Amitriptyline: the dose was increased from an initial 50 mg to 200 mg/day within 2 weeks. The patients saw their psychiatrist for 15–20 min each week, mainly to discuss the medication.
- SST plus placebo: the patients received 1 h of SST each week for 12 weeks with an experienced SST therapist. They also received placebo tablets.
- SST plus amitriptyline: in addition to SST, the patients received amitripty- line in individually adjusted doses.
- Psychotherapy plus placebo tablets: the patients in this group received 1 h of individual, generally psychodynamically orientated psychotherapy by experienced psychotherapists each week for 12 weeks.

The most striking result of this study was the high dropout rate in the two groups treated with amitriptyline: more than 50% of these patients and almost 30% of those receiving SST plus drug interrupted the treatment prematurely, whereas only 15% of the SST plus placebo group and 24% of the psychotherapy plus placebo group dropped out. The patients remaining in the study showed similar degrees of improvement in their symptoms after 12 weeks. In the discussion of their results, the authors considered the possibility that the numerous dropouts in the amitriptyline groups resulted from the recruitment procedure and the disappointed expectations of the patients: presumably many of them had wanted a helper or ally and were disappointed when only medication and an occasional short interview were offered to them.

Concluding Comments on Drug Therapy and Psychotherapy of Depressions

As Weissman *et al.* (1987) emphasized in a review some years ago, the utility of several psychotherapeutic procedures in the treatment of unipolar non-psychotic depressions has been shown convincingly in a number of independent, controlled studies. Clearly structured procedures with time limits, such as CT, IPT and SST, represent valuable alternatives or a supplement to drug therapy with antidepressants, especially in outpatients. This view is supported by the large, carefully controlled study by Keller *et al.* (2000, see above), which resulted in very similar response rates for drug treatment and psychotherapeutic intervention. In a more recent review of literature, Cascalenda *et al.* (2002) identified six multiple-cell, randomized, controlled double-blind trials and determined the rates of full remission in 883 outpatients with mild to moderate non-melancholic, non-psychotic major depression after treatment with antidepressants, psychotherapy (mostly CBT and IPT) or control (i.e. no treatment). Both therapeutic approaches proved similarly effective and superior to control conditions, with percentages of remission for patients assigned to medication, psychotherapy and control conditions being 46.4%, 46.3% and 24.4%, respectively. Moreover, more patients dropped out of control conditions (54.4%) than of either treatment group.

However, Meterissian and Bradwejn (1989) drew a rather different conclusion after critical analysis of a large number of studies comparing drug therapy and psychotherapy of depression. Although they did not generally question the value of non-drug procedures, they maintained that in most comparisons the drug treatment was not applied with the same care and specialist knowledge as used in the case of psychotherapy. Depending on the study, inadequate antidepressant doses were used, plasma levels of the drug were not monitored or hardly any of the known methods for improving the therapeutic success of drugs (change of drug, combination with lithium, etc.) were used. Because it is a matter of finding the specific indication for various treatments, these authors consider it essential to apply all the compared procedures optimally. It is obviously very demanding to compare psychotherapy and drug therapy in a reliably blind and unbiased manner; according to Meterissian and Bradwejn, this requirement was not fullfilled in most of the available studies.

Drug therapy with antidepressants usually cannot be dispensed with in the case of hospitalized patients with severe depression. There have been only sporadic controlled studies performed to determine whether psychotherapeutic measures provide a significant effect in these patients. Tölle (1985) emphasized the need for psychotherapeutic effort specifically in melancholic patients, who frequently consider themselves not to require or not to be worthy of treatment. Although these patients often feel themselves to be lost, rejected and valueless, therapeutic attention can get through to them and give them the feeling that they are not entirely alone, given up by everybody and fully misunderstood. A study by Miller *et al.* (1989) in 45 hospitalized patients with mainly severe depressions seems to support this view: patients who had received CT or social skills therapy in addition to drug therapy responded better to the antidepressant treatment and after 1 year also showed fewer relapses than patients who had received only antidepressants in addition to the usual hospital care.

In conclusion, as summarized by Kupfer and Frank (2001), many randomized controlled trials have "established that pharmacological and psychotherapy intervention provides excellent short-term benefit in terms of both reduced symptoms and suffering and improved functioning... treatment usually is not complicated and can be administered by both psychiatrists and primary care physicians.... Long-term treatment appears to be effective across the adult and geriatric life span. Regardless of the choice of treatment, treatment adherence is very important and clearly makes a difference in outcome." (Kupfer and Frank, 2001, p. 136).

8.4 TREATMENT OF ANXIETY SYNDROMES

Introductory Comments on Nomenclature

Chapter 1 introduced the benzodiazepine anxiolytics as drugs with a very broad but not always clearly delimited range of indications in almost all branches of medicine. In the present connection we are concentrating on the most common uses of these drugs in psychiatry, i.e. on anxiety disorders. According to DSM-IV (APA 1994), these are:

- Panic disorder with and without agoraphobia.
- Specific phobias.
- Social phobia.
- Obsessive–compulsive disorder.
- Post-traumatic stress disorder.
- Acute stress disorder.
- Generalized anxiety disorder.
- Substance-induced anxiety disorder, e.g. due to alcohol, opiate or sedative abuse.
- Anxiety disorder due to general medical conditions, e.g. due to metabolic, infectious, immunological and various medical and neurological causes.

8.4.1 TYPICAL INDICATIONS FOR ANXIOLYTICS

About one-third of all adults suffer at some time in their lives from states of anxiety and tension that can considerably impair their quality of life (Lader, 1981). The majority of these individuals seek medical help sooner or later, about half of them within a year after the outbreak of the symptoms. Statistics from the UK show that some 10% of these patients are referred to a psychiatrist. Psychiatrists consequently only see a small proportion of patients suffering from states of anxiety, generally the rather severe, chronic, neurotic, perhaps socially decompensated cases. The remaining 90% of patients mostly turn to their general practitioner; they are predominantly persons who react to burdensome circumstances with acute anxiety or stress symptoms. States of this nature are generally known to wane after some 6 weeks, although this remission can be facilitated by taking a tranquillizer.

Most of these patients' disease states belong to DSM-IV categories such as acute stress disorder, post-traumatic stress disorder (PTSD) or generalized anxiety disorder (GAD). Clinically, intensive or apparently exaggerated anxiety and worries about the existing circumstances of life are most prominent, and the patients often also have physically experienced tension and stress, vegetative disturbances of all types, hypervigilance and irritability. These patients almost always respond rapidly to benzodiazepine agents with marked improvement of symptoms (Shader and Greenblatt, 1993). However, long-term response can be obtained with SSRIs and serotonin–norepinephrine reuptake inhibitors (SNRIs) such as paroxetine, citalopram and venlafaxine.

Panic disorders are sudden attacks of severe anxiety accompanied or even dominated by physical symptoms such as heart palpitations, difficulty in breathing and a constrictive feeling in the chest, which can intensify the anxiety attack and put the subject in fear of his life. Panic attacks often arise spontaneously without detectable cause or are associated with particular situations such as being in a crowd, in a small, enclosed space or on an exposed street. Both syndromes can be treated successfully with benzodiazepines. Alternatives to tranquillizers include certain antidepressants, e.g. SSRIs, and non-drug therapeutic procedures (see below).

Independently of these specific indications, the symptomatic efficacy of tranquillizers on mental and physical anxiety and tension symptoms has been demonstrated in hundreds of individual investigations. According to a survey by Freedman (1980), 80–90% of all controlled studies with tranquillizers show a clear superiority compared with placebo. The success rate appears to be independent of the nature of the functional symptoms.

8.4.2 ALTERNATIVES TO BENZODIAZEPINE ANXIOLYTICS

Beta-receptor Blockers

An alternative to the use of benzodiazepine anxiolytics is the administration of beta-receptor blockers, generally called beta-blockers for short, to control the vegetative concomitant symptoms of anxiety and tension states (Kelly, 1980; Suzman, 1981). Affective arousal is accompanied by an increased release of adrenaline and noradrenaline into the blood, which in turn produce physical signs such as palpitations, trembling, sweating and irregular breathing. These individually variable vegetative changes are noticed by the subject and may potentiate the excitement; they can thus become detached from their original cause and become a problem as such. With beta-blockers, i.e. substances that occupy a subgroup of adrenergic receptors and protect them against the action of released catecholamines, the vegetative arousal is reduced so that a state of excitement can lose much of its severity.

Experiments with ski jumpers and parachutists have shown that beta-blockers dampen the emotional tachycardia that arises before a jump. Public speakers and singers can overcome their stage fright during public appearances by the use of these substances. Although vegetative symptoms of stress can be eliminated or attenuated with beta-blockers, mental clarity or artistic performance are not adversely affected (Neftel *et al.*, 1982). In controlled trials, students with examination nerves achieved better results with beta-blockers than with diazepam and placebo because, although they still felt the mental tension of the examination, they were not additionally disturbed by palpitations, tremor and other symptoms. Beta-blockers are generally well tolerated, but contraindications include asthma, bronchospasm and certain cardiac arrhythmias.

Benzodiazepines, Antidepressants and Other Agents

Treatment of GAD can be undertaken using a number of pharmacological agents. Benzodiazepines have been found to be superior to placebo in several studies and all benzodiazepines appear to be equally effective. However, side effects include sedation, psychomotor impairment, amnesia and tolerance (Chapter 1). Recent clinical data indicate that SSRIs and SNRIs are effective in the treatment of acute GAD symptoms. Venlafaxine, paroxetine and imipramine have been shown to be effective antianxiety medications in placebo-controlled studies. Case studies also indicate the usefulness of clomipramine, nefazodone, mirtazapine, fluoxetine and fluvoxamine in GAD. Buspirone, a 5-HT1a receptor partial agonist, has been shown to be effective in several placebo-controlled, double-blind trials (Roy-Byrne and Cowley, 2002). Buspirone has a later onset of action than both benzodiazepines and SSRIs but with the advantage of being non-addictive and non-sedating.

A larger set of placebo-controlled studies show conclusively that imipramine is also effective for the treatment of panic disorders. Other agents shown to be effective in panic disorders include the SSRIs paroxetine, sertraline, fluvoxamine, fluoxetine and citalopram. Generally, initial treatment of moderate to severe panic disorders may require the initiation of a short course of benzodiazepines e.g. clonazepam (0.5–1 mg twice daily), and an SSRI. The patient will obtain immediate relief from panic attacks with the benzodiazepine whereas the SSRI may take 1–6 weeks to become effective. Once a patient is relieved of initial panic attacks, clonazepam should be tapered and discontinued over several weeks and SSRI therapy continued thereafter. There are no pharmacological treatments available for specific phobias, however controlled trials have shown efficacy for several agents, e.g. phenelzine, moclobemide, clonazepam, alprazolam, fluvoxamine, sertraline and paroxetine in the treatment of social phobia (Roy-Byrne and Cowley, 2002).

Psychotherapy and/or DrugTherapy?

According to older surveys by Luborsky *et al.* (1975) and Freedman (1980), drug treatments with anxiolytics are more effective overall than psychotherapy in anxiety and tension states. However, the comparative studies considered here were mostly of short duration and thereby favored the drug therapy. It is also interesting that combined drug therapy and psychotherapy in these older studies usually produced higher success rates than treatment with anxiolytics alone, and that there were no reports of adverse interactions, e.g. no adverse effect of drug therapy on the psychotherapeutic process. An analysis by Wardle (1990), which was directed particularly to the question of whether benzo-diazepines could have an adverse effect on the results of behavioral therapy (e.g. as a result of state-dependent learning within the context of flooding or exposure techniques), came to a very similar conclusion as the older authors. In four of six studies considered, the results with combined behavioral and anxiolytic treatment were better than with behavioral therapy alone, in one study there was no difference and in only one study (in which barbiturate infusions had been used, not an anxiolytic) was there evidence of a superior action of behavioral therapy without concomitant drug therapy.

In the meantime, both the psychotherapeutic approaches and the possible drug therapies for the treatment of anxiety and obsessional syndromes have been refined and several models were developed for the interplay of the two approaches that initially appeared so different (see Hersen, 1986; Coryell and Winokur, 1991). A review of several meta-analyses of non-drug treatment studies shows that in many indications, including the anxiety syndromes of interest here, psychotherapeutic procedures of various types can be expected to produce therapeutic effects of the same magnitude as with psychopharmaceu-ticals (Lipsey and Wilson, 1993). Behavioral therapy, cognitively orientated therapies and many combinations and variants of these procedures produce satisfactory results that open up alternatives to drug therapy for patients and their doctors or psychotherapists (see also Gelernter *et al.*, 1991; Cox *et al.*, 1993).

A study by Welkowitz *et al.* (1991) shows that positive therapeutic results with non-drug procedures can also be obtained in institutions and by therapists who initially are less familiar with psychotherapeutic techniques. In a psychiatric center traditionally orientated towards drug therapy in New York, several psychiatrists, nurses and psychologists were introduced to a cognitively orientated behavioral therapy (CBT) technique on the basis of instruction books and videotapes and then treated a group of 24 patients with panic disorders. These were patients, mainly women, who had previously responded insufficiently to drugs or who desired a non-drug therapy. After concluding the program of 12 sessions that were highly structured in time and content, 14 of the 24 patients were assessed as being asymptomatic and another three had far fewer panic attacks than before, or even none at all. As the authors admit, the favorable therapeutic result may be attributable partly to the positive motivation of the 'experimental therapists' and the special selection of patients, but the study also shows that non-drug methods of treatment can be learned quickly and practiced successfully in indications for which anxiolytics conventionally tend to be used.

In contrast to some of the above, a review and critical analysis by Westra and Stewart (1998), who compared the effects of CBT and pharmacotherapy and of combining both in anxiety disorders, concluded that these two treatment modalities often fail to operate in a complementary fashion. According to the authors, high-potency anxiolytics (e.g. alprazolam) may actually impact negatively on the effects of CBT, whereas low-potency benzodiazepines such as diazepam and antidepressants generally have a negligible effect, i.e. no clear enhancement of CBT effects in patients. Although it is conceded that short-term use of anxiolytic drugs is likely to produce symptomatic relief, the durability of treatment gains with these drugs is said to be doubtful, as manifested by the reappearance of symptoms after drug discontinuation. Westra and Stewart discuss several hypothetical mechanisms underlying the pharmacological and psychotherapeutic treatment approaches and their differential effects in anxiety disorders; they also provide some practical suggestions as to how patients' expectations from drug treatment and its eventual discontinuation should be managed.

8.4.3 RECOMMENDED TREATMENTS

It is generally recommended that benzodiazepine anxiolytics be prescribed for not more than 6–12 weeks for states of anxiety, unrest and tension not arising within the context of psychosis (Rickels and Schweizer, 1987). One advantage of these drugs is their rapid onset of action. On the other hand, alternative drugs (Ninan *et al.*, 1998) or a non-drug treatment should be introduced whenever possible in the case of more prolonged disturbances. Practically all leading authors stress the need to adapt drug therapy, psychotherapy and combined therapies to match the individual symptoms and requirements of each patient and not to approach the individual case with a predetermined regimen (Roy-Byrne *et al.*, 1993b). Nevertheless, some general recommendations shown in Table 8.2, based on a scheme by Freedman (1980), can be given.

8.5 PSYCHOSTIMULANTS AND THE TREATMENT OF ATTENTION DEFICIT HYPERACTIVITY DISORDER

The most important clinical use of amphetamine-like stimulants is for attention deficit hyperactivity disorder (ADHD) in children. Methylphenidate, the drug

Table 8.2 Preferred forms of therapy for anxiety syndromes (the individual therapy must be guided by the symptoms and responses of the patient, as well as the means available in practice)

	Severity of physical symptoms	
	Severe	Mild
Syndromes with strong 'cognitive' component	*Panic disorder* Combination of low-dose anxiolytic such as clonazepam with SSRI or SNRI initially (1–2 months) and later SSRI or SNRI only Psychotherapy if indicated	*Generalized anxiety disorder* SSRI, SNRI or low-dose anxiolytic or buspirone
Syndromes with weak 'cognitive' component	*Social phobia* SSRI or beta-blocker (propranolol) or anxiolytic or psychotherapy	*Transient states of unrest* Advice, calming

most prescribed today in ADHD, leads to a significant improvement of symptoms in about 70% of cases, whereas 20–30% of children show no significant change on psychostimulants or may even deteriorate on these drugs. Several slow-release forms of methylphenidate and of mixed amphetamines are currently available; these preparations allow once-a-day drug administration and thus avoid the embarassment and risks involved if stimulant medication has to be handed out by a nurse to the child at school or carried by the child while away from home. Caffeine, a psychostimulant with a mechanism of action different from that of amphetamines, has no beneficial effect in ADHD.

8.5.1 QUESTIONS OF LONG-TERM MEDICATION

Because ADHD represents a severe disorder usually lasting for years, in many cases well into adulthood (Faraone *et al.*, 2000) and making prolonged treatment necessary, questions arise about the long-term action and safety of psychostimulants used in this indication. The therapeutic action of amphetamines and methylphenidate is thought to be maintained for years in the vast majority of patients, and there is no need to increase the dose to a relevant degree (Safer and Allen, 1989). Controlled studies reported in Chapter 7 (Gilberg *et al.*, 1997; MTA Cooperative Group 1999) confirm that stimulant drugs maintain their efficacy well beyond 1 year of treatment. Discontinuation studies have shown that a proportion of children can do without psychostimulants temporarily or entirely. Because of this, it is advisable to withdraw the medication from time to time so that the patient does not continue to take a product that is no longer effective or no longer necessary (Dulcan, 1997).

Amphetamines and methylphenidate inhibit appetite and modify various endocrine processes, so that the question arises as to whether the physical development and growth of patients treated long term with these drugs will run a normal course. Children undergoing long-term treatment with methylphenidate grow somewhat slower but make up the deficit during adolescence and achieve normal stature in adulthood. As Gittelman Klein (1987) commented, this observation applies to children whose treatment was discontinued during adolescence.

There have been only a few studies dealing with the question of the positive long-term impact of stimulants in ADHD. After weighing up the available clinical evidence, Gittelman Klein (1987) concluded that treatment with psychostimulants is certainly effective during prolonged periods of time, but it cannot be said with certainty whether the ultimate outcome is modified to a significant degree. This rather cautious evaluation contrasts with some positive results of long-term observations of drug-treated ADHD children as published by Weiss and Hechtman (1986).

8.5.2 DRUG THERAPY AND PSYCHOTHERAPY OF ADHD

In her review, Gittelman Klein (1987) considered nine studies published between 1977 and 1985 dealing with combined drug therapy and psychotherapy of ADHD children. The non-drug treatments included cognitive training (five studies), various forms of behavioral therapy (five studies) and parent training (one study), and more than one method was used in some studies. The results are unanimous and surprising in that not one of the studies showed a clearly detectable advantage of combined treatment over drug therapy with stimulants alone in everyday or school behavior.

This conclusion stands in contrast to the statements made in an earlier review (Kauffmann and Hallahan, 1979) that behavioral therapeutic techniques have an important role to play in ADHD, and partly contradicts the results of some more recent studies. As summarized in Chapter 7 (p. 250 f.), the US MTA study did not detect any significant difference between combined treatments and treatment with methylphenidate alone with regard to their effects on ADHD symptoms; however combined treatments had some advantage over drug alone on features such as anxiety disorders, social skills, consumer (mainly parent) satisfaction and possibly academic achievement (Pelham *et al.*, 2000). Additional statistical analysis of the MTA study by responders and in terms of composite outcome measures also revealed additional benefit of combined treatments over drug therapy alone (Jensen *et al.*, 2001).

8.6 CONCLUDING COMMENTS

An attempt has been made to discuss the position of drug therapy of various types of mental disorders within a wider perspective, and especially to clarify the relationship between drug therapy and non-drug treatments. It was necessary to deal separately with the various classes of psychopharmaceuticals and the disorders treated with them, and for our purposes it was also sensible to refer as far as possible to controlled, i.e. comparative, studies. The drawback of this 'evidence-based' approach is obvious: comparative studies of therapeutic procedures almost necessarily favor one of the compared treatments because they can never be carried out with completely identical preconditions for all treatments (Elkin *et al.*, 1988). Indeed, as discussed by Klein (2000), various meta-analytical studies comparing psychotherapy with pharmacotherapy were scrutinized and discovered to include studies that were not entirely blind, random, controlled or of high quality, leading to inaccurate conclusions. Thus, meta-analyses based on flawed studies are clearly inadequate for the establishment of treatment guidelines (Klein, 2000). On the other hand, the value of an admittedly incomplete summary such as presented here is that results obtained in different places by different authors with different preconditions can be critically compared and related one to the other.

As Karasu (1982) has stated some time ago, the relative positions of drug therapy and psychotherapy have changed several times over recent decades. In the 1950s most psychiatrists and psychotherapists were chiefly interested in psychoanalytically orientated psychotherapy of predominantly neurotic disorders. "Drug treatment was considered as inhibitory or, at best, superfluous." Some of the critical arguments represented in the upper-right panel of Fig. 8.2 therefore derive from this period. Over the following decade neuroleptics became established as the therapy of choice for schizophrenic psychoses, whereas psychotherapy, mainly in the form of group therapy or social measures, initially proved to be a not very effective adjuvant in these patients. A certain arrogance on the part of drug therapists, expressed by statements such as those in the lower-right panel of Fig. 8.2, also derived from that period. During the 1970s the advantages of a combined approach to therapy were recognized, initially in the treatment of affective disorders, and thoughts of synergistic effects arose, at least for some indications. This positive aspect is summarized on the left-hand side of Fig. 8.2, even though it is accepted that additive or even supra-additive actions of drug therapy and psychotherapy have not been demonstrated in all indications.

In the course of the treatment of schizophrenia, depressive and various anxiety syndromes, it has been found repeatedly that psychopharmaceuticals and psychotherapies are likely to modify different types of symptoms and

Effects of drug therapy on psychotherapy

Positive

1. The symptomatic improvement (calming, reduction of anxiety) makes patients more accessible to therapy

2. Autonomous ego functions such as attention, speech and memory are strengthened, especially in psychotics

3. Drugs have a symbolic significance: "The doctor has given me something, he is helping me"

4. Drugs are part of the usual interaction between doctor and patient; a mental illness is no different in this respect

Negative

1. The rapid symptomatic improvement inhibits confrontation with problems and conflicts

2. The patient believes that nothing can be done any more without drugs, and he becomes dependent on them

3. The undesirable dependency on the doctor is strengthened; an authoritarian attitude is encouraged

4. The patient's feeling of being ill is intensified

Effects of psychotherapy on drug therapy

1. The patient receives the impression of being perceived as a person and not just as a patient

2. Owing to the improved relationship between doctor and patient, the latter takes his medicine reliably

1. Psychotherapeutic efforts (which are useless) signify for the patient an undesirable intrusion into his privacy

2. Psychotherapy induces anxiety and conflict, and hazards a painfully restored balance

Figure 8.2 Arguments for and against combined drug therapy and psychotherapy (Pfefferbaum, 1977; Weissman, 1978; Karasu, 1982)

stages of illness, which in fact could – to simplify matters very considerably and possibly overoptimistically – pave the way to the more efficient use of therapy. Of practical significance is a statement made by DiMascio *et al.* (1979) and echoed by more recent authors (e.g. Kupfer and Frank, 2001) that, in the course of the treatment of depression, patients having different expectations and practical possibilities of therapy *can today be offered various forms of treatment with good prospects of success*, without the therapist having to work within the framework of a specific psychotherapeutic or pharmacotherapeutic school of thought.

Have all the fears and critical questions raised at the beginning of this chapter been reassuringly and satisfactorily answered? Within the scope of empirical and quantitatively orientated studies the answer is presumably yes – but it is not possible to go any further. Some of the negative interactions sketched in Fig. 8.2 originate from practical experience, i.e. from therapeutic failures incurred by many doctors and psychotherapists (see Westra and Stewart, 1998). They can, however, be exemplified only by means of a qualitative analysis of individual cases and are lost in the global success figures typical for large comparative investigations. In other words, even if the left-hand side of Fig. 8.2 appears to be largely supported by the statistical data put forward, this does not definitively refute the right-hand side thereof.

Psychopharmaceuticals can – if used incorrectly or at the wrong moment (or if not used at all!) – impede or wreck the psychotherapeutic process, and the same applies to psychotherapeutic intervention introduced at the wrong moment or in a substantially incorrect manner in the context of psychopharmacotherapies. Although the possible synergy between the two forms of therapy, which has been demonstrated in several indications, does increase the prospects of success from a statistical point of view, it is by no means a guarantee of success in the individual case.

9

Psychopharmacology and Health Economics

By
ED SNYDER

9.1 INTRODUCTION

Today the cost of healthcare is higher than ever before and, in most of the world's economies, rising faster than any other sector. These rising costs are absorbing a rapidly growing share of nations' economic resources. Part of the task of healthcare policy-makers, who are responsible for the management of the healthcare system, is to encourage the use of cost-effective therapies and limit the use of those therapies that are not as cost-effective as their alternatives. The field of health economics uses economic techniques to demonstrate the value of various therapeutic approaches available in healthcare. Several introductory texts are available that present the basics of an economic evaluation of healthcare, such as those by Drummond *et al.* (1997) and Gold *et al.* (1996). In recent years the level of sophistication in using such economic techniques has evolved to the extent that there are now distinct subfields in health economics. When these economic techniques are used to demonstrate the value of pharmaceuticals, for example, the field is referred to as pharmacoeconomics.

The demonstration of the value of pharmaceuticals, such as psychopharmaceuticals, always involves a comparative analysis of alternative courses of action, such as the use of two psychopharmaceuticals or the use of a psychopharmaceutical and psychotherapy, or one of the courses of action can

Psychopharmacology, Fourth Edition. By R. Spiegel
© 2003 John Wiley & Sons, Ltd: ISBN 0 471 56039 1: 0 470 84691 7 (PB)

be a choice to do nothing at all. The difference in the cost of the two alternatives is then compared with their relative effectiveness. The effectiveness of the therapies may incorporate clinical as well as patient-reported outcomes, such as the quality of life of the patient receiving the therapy.

The demonstration of the value of a pharmaceutical is part of a larger process of demonstrating the efficacy, safety, quality of manufacture and cost-effectiveness of the drug. Establishing the efficacy, safety and quality of manufacture of a drug is the traditional method of screening new therapies by health policy-makers, such as national health authorities, but in recent years health policy-makers in many countries have also requested a demonstration of the value of a drug's effectiveness, its impact on the quality of life of the patients and the effect on the healthcare system's budget. This is the role of pharmacoeconomics. Even for a drug of proven efficacy, healthcare policy-makers may require a demonstration of the impact of the drug on the healthcare system budget if, for example, the disease for which it is used has a high prevalence or because the disease is chronic in nature and treatment is expected to last for a long time. In many healthcare markets, this high prevalence or chronic nature of the disease combined with the cost of a given drug may affect the system's budget in such a way as to drain it of resources that could be used to treat other conditions. The demonstration of the impact of the cost of the drug on the healthcare system budget also considers the current costs incurred by the healthcare system in treating the disease with current therapies, and how those costs may be lowered or raised by the use of this new therapy. In most healthcare systems, these concerns can be addressed by the demonstration of the economic and quality-of-life impact of the drug.

9.2 PHARMACOECONOMICS DEMONSTRATES A DRUG'S VALUE

Pharmacoeconomics demonstrates a drug's value to the patient, policy-maker and society. The purpose of pharmacoeconomics is to demonstrate a drug's effect on the quality of life of the patient, as well as the drug's economic effect on the healthcare systems, the effect on payors (such as managed-care organizations or health insurance groups who usually pay the direct medical costs) and the effect on patients and caregivers (who are mostly interested in the out-of-pocket costs, or the hours of caregiving required).

Today's healthcare policy-makers, including government officials, health insurance companies and managed-care organizations, are faced with the reality of limited resources for healthcare and the knowledge that much medical care is of uncertain value. The value of vitamin E therapy in Alzheimer's disease, for example, is still unclear, but some physicians have recommended it for years without any real measures of its effect on the disease.

There is also evidence that there is significant variation in medical practice patterns both between and within countries. Research by Wennberg (1984) found a high variation in the use of medical procedures for specific conditions in the USA that were not explained by population morbidity or mortality figures.

These realities of the current state of healthcare have caused healthcare policy-makers to use several methods to regulate the supply and demand of health services and thereby control the cost of those services. Attempts to reduce the supply of services include a reduction in the reimbursement for services or a reduction in the number of physicians and specialists. These approaches may contain the growth of healthcare costs but a reduction in the capacity of the healthcare system also limits the patient access to services, resulting in longer waits for non-emergency services. Attempts to reduce the demand for services include:

- Raising barriers to the access of services. Such barriers may include paperwork and approval processes that discourage providers and patients from seeking the service.
- Delays to the entry of services into the healthcare system, such as a separate approval process for the reimbursement of a pharmaceutical by the healthcare system after the approval of the safety, efficacy and quality of manufacture.

Therefore, when new psychopharmaceuticals are developed the demonstration of their value to both the patient and the healthcare system is essential to ensure that patients have practical access to the therapy. Clinical efficacy evaluations (Chapter 5) demonstrate clinical effects to such health authorities as the Food and Drug Administration (FDA) in the USA, and the European Medicine Evaluation Agency (EMEA) in Europe. After the clinical effect has been established, the pharmacoeconomic evaluation demonstrates the value of the clinical effect to country-specific reimbursement bodies that are responsible for supporting the healthcare budget. These include the National Institute for Clinical Excellence (NICE) in the UK and Pharmacy and Therapeutics Committees (P&T Committees) for managed-care organizations in the USA. Most European countries have healthcare policy bodies that review this evidence too. The purpose of these reviews is to determine the impact on the healthcare budget when the use of the drug or device is paid from the budget. These bodies conduct economic evaluations to determine the value of the clinical effect and review the evidence produced by academics and pharmaceutical companies. Both the cost of the therapy and the effectiveness of the therapy determine the value of a drug or device. The costs of the therapy include the cost of the drug, the cost of administration, the cost of managing side effects and the cost of switching therapies. Also considered in the total cost are any savings resulting from reduced resource use due to the therapy. The effectiveness of the therapy is expressed as the improvement in clinical parameters as reported by clinicians in clinical trials or other supportive evidence, or it can be expressed from the patient's point of view, such as improvements in the quality of life.

9.2.1 THE PERSPECTIVE OF THE ANALYSIS

Every economic analysis of the value of a psychopharmaceutical is not the same. One analysis can vary considerably from the next, depending on the costs and outcomes included in the analysis. The outcome of the therapy on the patient's quality of life or the costs of the therapy in terms of the number of hours of a caregiver's time consumed with patient care will be given different weight depending on the perspective from which the analysis is done. The payor (or the body responsible for managing the healthcare budget) may not be interested in some of the specific effects of the therapy, such as the number of hours of patient care that will be required by family and friends. Payors may be interested only in the costs that directly affect their budgets and not the larger economic issues for which they are not directly responsible. For example, managed-care organizations in the USA are responsible for the costs directly associated with the delivery of healthcare but not for covering the cost of an increase or decrease in the number of hours a spouse caregiver must spend in caring for the patient.

In contrast, the patient and the patient's family may be very interested in the outcome that this therapy has on the caregiving burden; on the other hand, they may not be interested in the direct costs of the therapy for which they are not directly responsible. Most national regulatory bodies, such as the NICE in the UK, prefer a comprehensive, societal perspective on a drug's value because such a perspective incorporates all these variables. This broader perspective examines direct costs, caregiving costs and indirect costs.

The costs associated with the treatment of a disease are categorized as direct costs and indirect costs. Those who are responsible for the payment of healthcare services are usually most interested in *direct costs*, or costs that are incurred directly as a result of the care of the patient's condition. These costs include hospitalization, physician visits, drugs, laboratory tests and procedures. They also include the treatment of drug-related side effects, the treatment of unfavorable drug–drug interactions and the costs of switching from the current therapy to a new therapy. Direct costs may also include savings due to costs that are avoided: inpatient days, outpatient visits, procedures and laboratory tests that do not occur.

Those not formally employed, such as a spouse caregiver, also incur costs in the care of a patient at home. This is called 'informal' caregiving because it is usually provided free of charge by a family member or friend. The *costs of informal caregiving* include expenditures incurred to accommodate the patient's current condition at home, including modifications to the home, such as the installation of wheelchair ramps, the widening of doorways, changes in plumbing and bathroom fixtures and the purchase of special furniture, such as a hospital bed, and medical equipment. The hours of care provided by the caregiver also may be used to estimate the value of the costs of this informal caregiving. Some researchers calculate the cost of these hours of care by using the hourly rate of a professional caregiver performing similar tasks, whereas others measure the opportunity costs of a caregiver whose hours are now devoted to caring for the patient. Opportunity costs are determined by the wages given up by the caregiver to care for the patient, or the value of leisure time forgone because of the care that is necessary for the patient. In economic analysis, the cost of informal caregiving is usually reported separately because payors and policy-makers are not particularly interested in these kinds of costs. The cost of informal caregiving is considered relevant for government policy-makers and others who adapt a societal perspective on the economic analysis, as well as, of course, the patients and caregivers.

Indirect costs, sometimes called productivity costs, are incurred as a consequence of the patient's condition and the patient's experience of the condition and not as a direct result of the treatment of the patient's condition. For those gainfully employed, this includes disability, absenteeism and lost productivity. These measures are quantifiable and the total indirect costs can be a substantial portion of the total societal costs of the treatment of the patient's condition. For example, the costs of schizophrenia in Canada are over Can\$2.3 billion in direct healthcare costs and an additional Can\$2 billion in indirect costs annually (Procyshyn *et al.*, 2000). The societal cost of the disease is almost as much as the direct cost of treating the disease.

9.2.2 QUALITY OF LIFE AS AN OUTCOME IN PHARMACOECONOMIC ANALYSIS

Because the principal focus of pharmacoeconomics is to incorporate outcomes in the demonstration of the value of a therapy, the quality of life that results from a therapy has received a great deal of attention in recent years. Most frequently, quality of life is measured using standardized instruments to collect patient-reported quality of life. These instruments are traditionally developed using patient or expert interviews to establish the areas of inquiry or 'domains' of the instrument. The use of these instruments in pharmacoeconomics is heavily dependent on the demonstrated psychometric properties of the instrument, such as its reliability, validity and responsiveness, or on sensitivity to the changes in the disease to be studied.

A psychopharmaceutical can be safe and efficacious when used in a clinical trial but what is its effectiveness when it is used in real life conditions? If a patient has a bad experience with a drug, there is likelihood that persistency and compliance with the therapeutic regimen will be compromised. This, of course, makes the drug less effective than originally estimated. For example, patient assessments of their quality of life are directly related to the therapeutic compliance that is to be expected. In cases for which antipsychotic medications with extrapyramidal symptoms and poor control of negative symptoms and other serious side effects result in impaired quality of life, poor adherence with the medication regimen may result. Measuring the subjective experiences of patients with schizophrenia along with clinical endpoints provides a comprehensive picture of both the impact of the condition and the impact of its treatment (Awad *et al.*, 1995).

Therefore, an economic analysis must measure the quality of life of the patient to ensure that the value of the drug incorporates the patient's perspective. Quality of life is a concept that usually incorporates the physical, mental and social well-being of the patient. Initial doubts concerning the ability of schizophrenic patients to provide reliable and valid reports of their own quality of life led to the use of proxies for patient interviews. Caregivers and clinicians were consulted most often. However, recent research has shown that the use of proxies can produce very different results to those derived directly from the patient's responses. In addition, research now indicates that schizophrenic patients are able to provide stable, reliable and valid self-reports of their psychological well-being, health status and subjective evaluation of drug therapies (Awad *et al.*, 1995).

In measuring the quality of life to demonstrate a drug's value, selection of the instrument, such as a questionnaire, depends on several factors. Instruments that have been designed to be particularly sensitive to the effect of a given disease and the drug therapy on the patient are called disease-specific instruments. One good example of this is the Quality of Life in Schizophrenia instrument, or QLS. The QLS is a quality-of-life scale developed to measure significant impairment in patients' intrapsychic, interpersonal and instrumental functioning due to the deficit symptoms of schizophrenia. The QLS has been validated in several schizophrenic patient populations and has been used in clinical trials of novel antipsychotic medications (Meltzer *et al.*, 1993; Rosenheck *et al.*, 1997; Hamilton *et al.*, 1998).

Like other assessment instruments, the QLS was developed using patient interviews and factor analysis to derive those dimensions and questions that are most relevant to the patient's experience (Heinrichs *et al.*, 1984). The QLS scale contains 21 items and is intended to be administered as a semi-structured interview. Each item consists of three parts: a brief statement is provided to help the interviewee understand and focus on the parameter to be assessed; a number of suggested questions are provided that may help the interviewer begin his exploration with the subject; and a seven-point scale is provided for each item, with a brief description at four points to help the interviewee make his judgement and mark the appropriate point on the scale. The QLS provides a total scale score and four subscale scores in the areas of Intrapsychic Foundations, Interpersonal Relations, Instrumental Role and Common Objects and Activities.

Besides disease-specific instruments such as the QLS, more generic instruments such as the EQ-5D (EuroQol Group, 1990) are available. The EQ-5D was developed to measure the quality of life of the general population. This instrument has five dimensions or areas of focus: mobility, self-care, usual activity, pain/discomfort and anxiety/depression. Patients are asked to respond to questions about these dimensions by checking the level that best describes their current experience. Responses are "no problem", "some problem" or "extreme problem". As with another generic instrument commonly used in most disease states, the SF-36 (Ware, 1993), these responses can be compared with those of other disease states and therefore are more useful to the health authorities in determining the worth of the therapy. The EQ-5D is self-administered and was developed initially in Dutch, English, Finnish, Norwegian and Swedish at the same time. It is now available in many languages.

In summary, disease-specific instruments are the most sensitive to changes in the patient's experience, whereas findings collected using generic instruments are more easily compared with population values for other therapies.

9.3 METHODS OF CALCULATING THE VALUE OF PSYCHOPHARMACEUTICALS

The evidence of a drug's value can be as simple as demonstrating efficacy and safety that is equal to but less costly than a readily available therapy. Or, the pharmacoeconomic evidence of value can be expressed as highly technical mathematical models using several sources of data to demonstrate the cost per quality-adjusted life-years gained (QALYs gained) by the new therapy instead of the current therapies. Common elements of the demonstration of the value of pharmaceuticals, such as psychopharmaceuticals, include an assessment of the costs and the outcomes of therapy. An assessment of costs includes the costs of delivering the therapy and the costs avoided because of the therapy. The cost of delivering the therapy includes physician office visits for drug titration monitoring or the cost of treating side effects. Side-effect treatment costs can be relatively low (nausea, vomiting, headache) or more costly, such as treatment for agranulocytosis (a rare but serious side effect of some antipsychotic and antidepressant medication). The costs avoided because of the therapy can include reductions in the rates of hospitalizations, outpatient visits or costly procedures. An assessment of the outcomes of therapy can include such measures as a reduction in the relapse rate for epileptics or an

Table 9.1 Health economic analyses

Type of study	Valuation of costs in both alternatives	Identification of consequences	Valuation of consequences
Cost-effectiveness analysis	Currency, such as dollars, euros or francs	Single effect of interest common to both alternatives but achieved to different degrees	Natural units (e.g. life-years gained, disability-days saved, points of blood pressure reduction, etc.)
Cost-utility analysis	Currency, such as dollars, euros or francs	Single or multiple effects not necessarily common to both alternatives	Healthy years or (more often) quality-adjusted life-years
Cost-minimization analysis	Currency, such as dollars, euros or francs	Identical in all relevant respects	None
Cost–benefit analysis	Currency, such as dollars, euros or francs	Single or multiple effects not necessarily common to both alternatives	Currency, such as dollars, euros or francs

Adapted from Drummond *et al.* (1997).

increase in the quality of life of the bipolar patient. In all cases, the costs considered are those related to the outcome being measured. Health economists express this relationship between costs and a unit of clinical or patient-reported outcomes as a cost-effectiveness ratio. This ratio is used to estimate the value of the drug to the patient, to the healthcare system and to society as a whole.

Common methods used to demonstrate the value of a pharmaceutical are presented in Table 9.1, and discussed below. Table 9.1 refers to alternative therapies used to treat the same condition.

9.3.1 COST-EFFECTIVENESS ANALYSIS: COSTS PER COMMON UNIT OF OUTCOME

Cost-effectiveness is an economic evaluation in which both the costs and the consequences of treatments are examined. The denominator of the cost-effectiveness ratio can be an intermediate outcome, such as a delay in the progression of a disease, or a final outcome, such as life-years saved. Once the outcome is measured, the costs associated with attaining this outcome form the numerator of the ratio. For example, suppose our interest is determining the relative value of drug therapy for epilepsy versus epilepsy surgery. The outcome of interest is seizure-free days, which is common to both therapies. The therapies have a different degree of success in this outcome, as well as different costs. We would not automatically choose the lowest cost option without first evaluating the differences in the outcome as well. So, we calculate the number of seizure-free days and compare the cost of seizure-free days for each therapy. This analysis, in which costs are related to a single, common effect that may differ in magnitude between alternative programs, is the substance of a cost-effectiveness analysis. The results of this analysis are expressed in terms of cost per seizure-free day. The outcome of interest is any outcome common to both therapies, and can include life-years gained, QALYs gained or costs per hospitalization days avoided.

9.3.2 COST-UTILITY ANALYSIS: COSTS PER QALY

A cost-effectiveness ratio is specific to the outcome measured, such as costs per additional life-years gained or costs per hospital days avoided. What some health authorities want to determine with regard to a drug's value is a single measure that incorporates all the outcomes as well as all the costs of the drug treatment. Such a broad-based measure captures how much improved the patient's life becomes as the result of treatment and at what cost. Each drug can have its unique effect on a combination of factors that determines the drug's value overall. These factors may include increases in the life expectancy of a patient as well as factors reflecting preferences for the experience of life during that increased number of years.

These preferences for the different disease states, expressed as numbers, are called utilities, and are used to quality-adjust or to weight the additional years of survival. The result is a quality-adjusted life-year (QALY) gained. Quality-adjusted life-years gained are also used frequently as the denominator of a cost-effectiveness ratio, as in costs per QALYs gained.

Utilities are assessed using methods such as clinical judgement, standard gamble techniques or time trade-off techniques. (For more information on these techniques see Drummond et al., 1997, because a description of these techniques is beyond the scope of this text.) However, a helpful illustration of how these utilities could be calculated is provided by the example of using a visual analog scale (Fig. 9.1). When presented with such a scale, with death as the zero point on the scale and perfect health as the value of 1 at the other end of the scale, patients are asked, "How would you rate your experience while on treatment A (or treatment B)?" Patients on treatment B rate their experience as higher (better) than those on treatment A. This expressed preference for a treatment takes into consideration all aspects of each of these treatments from the patient's perspective. From this information, the two treatments can be compared with each other by calculating the costs per QALY gained for each treatment.

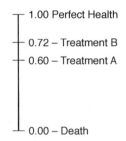

Figure 9.1 Visual analog scale for cost-utility analysis

Table 9.2 Comparison of two treatments using cost-utility analysis

Intervention	Cost ($)	Effectiveness (life expectancy)	Health state (utility)	QALYs
Treatment A	20 000	4.5	0.60	2.7
Treatment B	10 000	3.5	0.72	2.5

The following example is meant to provide an understanding of the concept of costs per QALYs gained. Suppose we have two treatments: treatment A and treatment B. The costs and the outcomes of these therapies are presented in Table 9.2. At first glance, it appears that an additional year of life resulting from treatment A will cost $10 000 ($10 000 more than treatment B for one more year of life). However, the utilities for each of these treatments reflect the quality of life during those years, and treatment A is not rated as highly as treatment B when it comes to the patient's perspective (health state). When the life expectancy on the drug is weighted by the utility of that time (life expectancy multiplied by health state), we have QALYs that differ by only 0.2 years, or about 2.4 months, instead of 12 unadjusted months.

Thus, the concept of utility is a general concept for measuring the value that individuals attach to the consequences of various actions, in this case the consequences of different treatment options (Lane, 1987). The goal of this measurement technique is to obtain a numerical value that represents the strength of the general public's preferences for a particular outcome (Torrance and Feeny, 1989). An important point about this technique is that these preferences can be developed using patient-reports or using a representative sample of a healthcare system's population. The reason why the public's preferences are used more commonly than those of patients who actually experience the disease stages being rated is the issue of rationing healthcare. Because most national healthcare systems have limited budgets, health authorities tend to use the perception of the general public to ration needed

Table 9.3 Analysis of the costs per QALYs for two treatments

Intervention	Cost ($)	Effectiveness (life expectancy)	Health state (utility)	QALYs
Treatment A	20 000	4.5	0.60	2.7
Treatment B	10 000	3.5	0.72	2.5

$$\text{Incremental cost effectiveness ratio} = \frac{\$20\,000 - \$10\,000}{4.5\,\text{y} - 3.5\,\text{y}} = \$10\,000 \text{ per life-year gained}$$

$$\text{Incremental cost-utility ratio} = \frac{\$20\,000 - \$10\,000}{2.7 - 2.5\,\text{QALYs}} = \$50\,000 \text{ per QALY gained}$$

Source: Bootman, J. L. *et al.*, *Principles of Pharmacoeconomics*, Harvey Whitney Books, Co., 1996, p. 120. Reproduced with permission.

services. Using the public's preferences in comparing QALYs gained from many differing therapies gives these health authorities a more accurate picture of the relative merits of these differing therapies.

Usually utilities are presented as a single unit value for a defined disease state. They reflect the physical, mental and social aspects of the disease. The intent is to come up with a single number that reflects the person's experience of a disease state. Generally defined disease states are descriptions of normal (unimpaired), mild, moderate or severely impaired states of a disease or symptom. The utilities attached to them can represent specific aspects of the disease experiences. For example, utilities can be measured for a specific drug-induced side effect.

Returning to our example, we can now examine the costs per QALYs for treatment A and treatment B. Table 9.3 illustrates these calculations. As the table shows, when calculating the incremental cost per effect (cost-effectiveness ratio) using unadjusted life-years gained, treatment A costs $10 000 for that additional year of life. But when we use the QALYs gained we see that this additional QALY actually costs $50 000.

This example illustrates the concept of utilities and their use in comparing two therapies, but utilities can be compared between disease states as well as comparing two therapies for the same disease. Table 9.4 lists the utilities for selected disease states from the literature.

When presenting a cost per QALY gained figure, it is important to put it in perspective. At what point does the cost for an additional QALY become too high? For this answer, the cost of a QALY can be compared to the cost of QALYs in other treatments. Examples of cost per QALY ratios (in 1999 US dollars) include estrogen therapy for postmenopausal women ($67 165), coronary artery bypass graft for single-vessel disease with moderate to severe

Table 9.4 Utilities for selected disease states

Health state	Utility
Full health (reference state)	1.00
Side effects of antihypertensive medication	0.95–0.99
Mild angina	0.90
Hypertension	0.88
Kidney transplantation	0.84
Moderate angina	0.70
Home dialysis	0.64
Severe angina	0.50
Hospitalized with AIDS	0.33
Major depression	0.31
Dead (reference state)	0.00

Sources: Torrance *et al.*, 1989; Rutten-van Molken *et al.*, 1995.

angina ($89 030) (Hatziandreu *et al.*, 1994) and the use of cholestyramine in treating high blood cholesterol ($277 378) (Kinosian and Eisenberg, 1988). These costs per QALY ratios represent the cost to society to offer these services. When introducing a new therapy, the cost/QALY ratio can be compared with other, currently accepted therapies to determine the relative merit of the new therapy to the population.

9.3.3 COST-MINIMIZATION ANALYSIS: COMPARISON OF PROGRAMS WITH EQUAL OUTCOMES

When it is assumed that the effectiveness of two therapies is equal, the effectiveness part of the cost-effectiveness ratio can be dropped from the analysis. In this situation, only the cost differences between the two therapies are examined. Usually this includes the cost of the drug, costs of administration, the treatment of side effects or adverse reactions and the incidence and prevalence of the condition. For example, Fenton *et al.* (1982) compared the costs of home versus hospital treatment of psychiatric patients when the outcomes of each were considered not to differ in any respect except that one requires a hospital stay and the other does not. The cost-minimization analysis simply looked at the differences in costs of the two treatments. The result is, not unexpectedly, that hospitalization was 64% more expensive than home-based treatment.

9.3.4 COST–BENEFIT ANALYSIS: COMPARISON OF PROGRAMS WITH DIFFERENT OUTCOMES

The term *cost–benefit* refers to the comparison of incremental program costs with incremental program benefits, and both are expressed in monetary terms. The results of the analysis are expressed in the form of a ratio of costs (expressed in local currency) of the therapies to the value (expressed in the same local currency) of benefits resulting from the therapy. This enables an examination of whether or not each of the programs' benefits exceeds its costs, indicating that there is a net social benefit and the programs are worthwhile. This analysis also allows the comparison of programs with outcomes across different clinical indications, such as a comparison of programs for schizophrenia and epilepsy, where the outcomes might be hospital days avoided and seizure-free days, respectively. Because all costs and benefits are measured in monetary terms, it is possible to compare a program's benefits with other healthcare programs and to make informed resource allocation decisions both within and between sectors of the economy. For example, Weisbrod *et al.* (1980) quantified and valued a wide range of costs and benefits on conventional hospital-oriented versus community-based programs for mental illness. Generally speaking, they found that the community-based programs were more costly, but they produced a higher value of benefits because the patients are able to gain employment while being treated as outpatients.

9.3.5 MODELING AS A TOOL FOR ECONOMIC ANALYSIS

Modeling is an analytical tool that can be used to extrapolate shorter term clinical results, such as days of improved symptoms in Parkinson's disease patients in a study over 6 months, to longer time periods. A model was developed to extrapolate the results of a 6-month trial in which patients received either levodopa alone or levodopa plus the catechol-*o*-methyltransferase (COMT) inhibitor entacapone. Comtan® (entacapone) is designed to reduce the metabolism of levodopa in peripheral tissue and vessels so that more of the drug is available in the brain at a more constant rate than is seen with levodopa alone. The 6-month clinical trial produced clinical results that allow us to establish entacapone's effect on the 'OFF' time associated with levodopa therapy. 'OFF' time refers to a re-emergence of symptoms prior to the next scheduled levodopa dose. Entacapone reduces the 'OFF' time and increases the 'ON' time of levodopa therapy.

Figure 9.2 illustrates the various inputs and outputs of a model built to demonstrate the 5-year results of therapy with entacapone (Comtan®), which represents a novel pharmacological principle used in combination with levodopa therapy. The inputs list the data fed into the model. The clinical effects of the therapy are taken from the clinical trials. The costs by disease stage are defined as costs for >25% 'OFF' time per day (severe stage) and costs for <25% 'OFF' time per day (less severe) and are taken from literature sources. Patient preference data (used to calculate QALYs) for these two disease stages are taken from a separate study of patient preferences. The outputs of the model list some of the more common uses of the model:

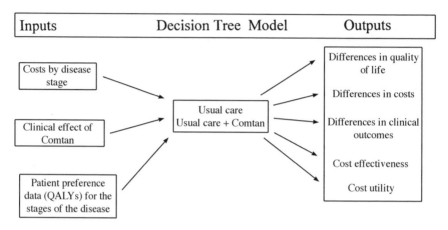

Figure 9.2 Model used to show the 5-year results of therapy with entacapone (Comtan®)

differences in the quality of life of the two therapy alternatives (usual care vs. usual care plus entacapone), differences in the costs of these two therapies, differences in the 5-year clinical outcomes based on the 6-month results of the clinical trial and the cost utility (or costs/QALY).

Presented in Fig. 9.3 is an example of a model used to extrapolate the 6-month trial results of a COMT inhibitor (entacapone) used in combination with levodopa versus levodopa alone in the treatment of Parkinson's disease. This particular model is an example of a Markov model.

A Markov process model describes several discrete health states in which a person can exist at time t, as well as the health states into which the person may move at time $t+1$. A person can reside in just one health state at any given time. The progression from time t to time $t+1$ is known as a cycle. All clinically important events are modeled as transitions in which a person moves from one health state to another. The probabilities associated with each change between health states are known as transition probabilities. Each transition probability is a function of the health state and the treatment.

The Markov model uses the clinical data to calculate the probability of transitioning from a severe disease state ('OFF' time >25% of the day), to a less severe disease state ('OFF' time <25% of the day) for entacapone therapy. This enables a calculation of the total amount of time a cohort of patients will

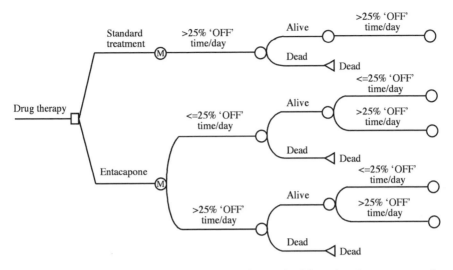

Figure 9.3 Markov model used to extrapolate 6-month trial results of entacapone plus levodopa versus lovodopa alone (standard treatment) (From Nuijten *et al.*, 2001). Reprinted with permission of Blackwell Publishing

spend in the less severe state, versus placebo, after extrapolating the clinical trial results from 6 months to 5 years. The difference in the time spent in these two disease states is reflected in the differences between the costs of managing patients in these two disease states, with costs being higher for the more severe state. The difference in those costs over the 5-year period equals the incremental cost effectiveness of entacapone, expressed as incremental costs per years in <25% 'OFF' time per day.

The results of the application of this model are, among others, that: differences in clinical outcomes exist between levodopa alone and entacapone plus levodopa; entacapone substantially improved the amount of time spent with <25% 'OFF' time; living with <25% 'OFF' time per day was increased by 0.63 years (or 7.6 months) over the 5-year time period; and the costs per QALY gained were $9221 and $20 986 for total and direct medical costs, respectively.

Models are also useful in strategic project planning to compare the costs and benefits of competing therapies, such as the current standard therapy for schizophrenia and a theoretical drug profile of an antipsychotic designed to improve the therapeutic effect for schizophrenia patients. The costs and benefits can be compared to determine the optimal profile (one that would produce the best possible results) as well as the minimal profile (the properties that a compound must demonstrate to show a clinically meaningful improvement over the standard therapy).

9.4 SUMMARY

The field of health economics uses economic techniques to demonstrate the value of therapeutic approaches and technological advances available in healthcare. When these economic techniques are used to demonstrate the value of pharmaceuticals, the field is referred to as pharmacoeconomics. The demonstration of the value of a pharmaceutical is part of a larger process of demonstrating the efficacy, safety, quality of manufacture and cost-effectiveness of the drug. Establishing the efficacy, safety and quality of manufacture of a drug is the traditional method of screening new therapies by health policy-makers but in recent years health policy-makers in many countries have also requested a demonstration of the value of the drug's effectiveness, its impact on the quality of life of the patients and the effect on the healthcare system's budget. Because of the pressure on health authorities to keep the cost of healthcare under control, when new psychopharmaceuticals are developed the demonstration of their value to both the patient and the healthcare system is essential to ensure that patients have practical access to the therapy. The perspective of the pharmacoeconomic analysis can differ, either by incorporating only direct medical costs or by using a societal perspective that incorporates all costs, including indirect medical costs, productivity costs and costs of caregiving by family or friends.

The quality of life of the patient while on therapy is an important determinant of the effectiveness of the therapy. If a patient has a bad experience with a drug, there is a likelihood that persistency and compliance with the therapeutic regimen will be compromised. This, of course, makes the drug less effective than originally valued. Therefore, an economic analysis must measure the quality of life of the patient to ensure that the value of the drug incorporates the patient's perspective. Quality of life is a concept that usually incorporates the physical, mental and social well-being of the patient. An example of a disease-specific instrument, the QLS, is designed to be sensitive to changes in this specific disease. Although the data collected using the QLS are useful to compare the quality of life of patients, e.g. in the two arms of a clinical trial, these results cannot be generalized to other populations outside of the trial cohort. This problem with disease-specific instruments is not the case with more generic instruments such as the EQ-5D.

Establishing the value of a new pharmaceutical can be done through a cost-effectiveness ratio, where the costs are compared with currently accepted therapy and the effect is expressed in natural units such as life-years gained or disability-free days. A cost-utility analysis uses QALYs as the expression of the drug's effect, which is a measure that incorporates all the outcomes as well as all the costs of the drug treatment. Such a broad-based measure captures how much improved the patient's life becomes as a result of the treatment and at what cost. Quality-adjusted life-years can be viewed as life-years gained, weighted by the patient's experience of the treatment and its effects during those additional life-years. Costs per QALYs can be compared between diseases and their treatment to optimize the healthcare budget expenditure. Cost minimization is used to compare therapies with a similar outcome but differing costs. Cost–benefit analyses are used when the effect of competing therapies can be expressed in monetary terms.

Economic modeling is used to extrapolate surrogate endpoints (Chapter 5) from clinical trials into longer term outcomes for a more comprehensive analysis of the long-term treatment effects of a therapy. Various data sources reporting the costs of treating the different disease stages, the clinical effect of the drug and the patient's experience of each of those disease stages are used to demonstrate long-term treatment effects and costs.

Epilogue

Modern psychopharmacology is about 50 years old. Few doctors and nurses survive to relate how clinical and ambulatory psychiatry looked and felt before the first neuroleptic and antidepressant medications became available. Drug treatment is routine in today's psychiatric practice, and even some of the most severe mental disorders are no longer fatal. In view of the dramatic therapeutic advances brought about by psychopharmaceuticals it is of interest to ask how the introduction of these drugs has affected psychiatry as a science and what impact psychopharmacology has had on psychology.

Effect of Psychopharmacology on Psychiatry

Pathophysiology and Nosology

Speaking in very general terms, the therapeutic effectiveness of psychopharmaceuticals promoted the view that some of the mental illnesses are treatable and that even healing can be obtained or facilitated with medicines, i.e. by material and scientifically comprehensible means. Previously, views on the pathogenesis of mental disturbances had been largely psychodynamic and in this sense immaterial: life history and social factors were considered decisive for the pathogenesis and course of schizophrenic psychoses, affective disorder and so-called neuroses, whereas the biological side of psychiatric pathophysiology was viewed as inaccessible. A rapid change occurred with the discovery of neuroleptic and antidepressant drugs: the biological substrate of mental disorders returned to center-stage and *biological psychiatry* increased in significance. Klerman (1987) spoke of a paradigm shift to highlight the return from psychodynamically accentuated thinking to biologically orientated views in psychiatry, and to the nosological categories introduced by Kraepelin and Bleuler early in the twentieth century: because neuroleptics were found to be

Psychopharmacology, Fourth Edition. By R. Spiegel
© 2003 John Wiley & Sons, Ltd: ISBN 0 471 56039 1: 0 470 84691 7 (PB)

specifically effective in schizophrenic psychoses and antidepressants act on depressions and because they have different pharmacological activities, different biological mechanisms must also underlie schizophrenias and affective psychoses. This new view signified a rejection of the tendency, detectable until about 1955, to consider neuroses, depressions and schizophrenias as vaguely delimited sections on a psychopathological continuum and not as separate nosological categories.

Research in Psychiatry

The new orientation of psychiatry also had consequences for its research methodology: study design and the statistical evaluation of clinical trials, use of standardized methods for the clinical evaluation of patients, application of electrophysiological, biochemical, neuroendocrinological and, more recently, imaging procedures to study brain structures and processes are among the everyday matters of biological psychiatry. Research activity is multidisciplinary and psychiatrists nowadays must be able to interact with chemists, endocrinologists, psychologists, statisticians and even physicists and engineers. However, criticism of this technological form of psychiatry and research is not lacking even among biologically orientated authors: Goodwin and Roy Byrne (1987) complained of a "decline in scholarship" and by this they mean the tendency of many researchers to carry out expansive studies with the widest possible range of modern equipment and procedures in the hope that something useful will emerge in any case. They urge the execution of studies that either derive from and are planned on the basis of reasoned and formulated hypotheses or are characterized as exploratory and, in the service of finding hypotheses, are interpreted as such.

Criticism of the 'Medical Model'

The opinion is sometimes heard or read that the advent of psychopharmaceuticals has brought back psychiatric thinking to the medical model. Mental disorders, it is said, are again considered to be due to one or perhaps a few biological causes that can be corrected by suitable means. A multifactorial way of thinking (the view that genetic, historical, social, familial and individual life history factors interact in a complex way until a mental disorder arises) is said to be hindered, if not made impossible, by the medical model. A typical example of this monocausal and, in the final analysis, materialistic way of thinking was the dopamine hypothesis of schizophrenia, which places the emphasis on a single neurotransmitter and neglects other important elements, so that in turn it is discordant even with biological reality (in this case the interaction between different neurotransmitter systems). Here is not the place to discuss further or even refute this fundamental criticism of biologically orientated psychiatry; however it should be understood that the emphasis on and the scientific study of one or a few hypothetical pathogenetic factors of a disease do not necessarily imply that other factors are ignored or denied.

Impact of Psychopharmacology on Psychology

Opportunities for Psychologists

With the rise of psychopharmacology, new opportunities arose for psychologists to do research work in mental hospitals and university-affiliated and private industry departments. Experimental studies and clinical trials with psychotropic substances provide attractive settings for psychologists to apply fruitfully their knowledge of study design and methodology and play an important part in the mostly multidisciplinary research teams. Examples include the study of new psychopharmaceuticals in healthy subjects (Chapter 3) and patients (Chapter 5), conducting studies of drug effects on cognitive processes (Chapter 7) as well as studying the effects of pharmacological and non-drug interventions in psychiatric patients (Chapter 8).

Psychologists as Prescribers of Psychopharmaceuticals?

Psychotherapists without medical background are not licensed to prescribe medicines, so their therapeutic means were not immediately enhanced by the introduction of modern psychopharmaceuticals. On the contrary, owing to the possibility of choosing between or combining psychopharmaceuticals and non-drug therapies, medically qualified therapists had gained an advantage that led many psychologists to a violent rejection of drug therapies and combined treatments. Historically, however, the number of patients accessible to psychotherapy, and who requested non-drug treatment, increased as a result of the de-institutionalization of psychiatry, so that the demand for the services of non-medical psychotherapists also increased.

In the USA a discussion of whether psychologists should be granted 'prescription privileges' for psychopharmaceuticals and whether training in psychopharmacology needed to be part of the psychology curriculum was launched some time ago. Wiggins (1994) pointed out that the number of practicing psychologists exceeded that of psychiatrists, and that psychologists make a decisive contribution to public health. As a consequence, he and others urged that non-medical psychotherapists be granted prescription authority, putting forward the following arguments (DeLeon and Wiggins, 1996; Pachman, 1996):

- Psychologists are highly trained mental health professionals. Their professional activities overlap by more than 90% with those of psychiatrists, except for the prescription of medication. In the interest of public mental health, and given the importance of psychopharmaceuticals in today's therapy, it should be ascertained that these effective therapeutic means become available to the largest group of mental health providers.

- The example of other health workers in the USA – nurse practitioners, physician assistants and optometrists – demonstrates that non-medical professionals can be trained to adequately prescribe drugs within their area of expertise. Pilot projects, e.g. in the state of California, with psychologists prescribing psychopharmaceuticals with appropriate training and supervision were successful in that "both the patients and supervising physicians were comfortable with the clinical performance of the trainees" (De Leon and Wiggins, 1996, p. 226).
- More than 80% of all psychiatric drugs are prescribed in the USA by non-psychiatrists, i.e. by physicians usually lacking the necessary training and expertise regarding mental functioning and disorders. Licensed psychologists would be more qualified to diagnose and treat mental disorders, including prescribing and monitoring the effects of psychotropic medication.

Other arguments put forward in the discussion deal with the symbolic meaning of medication as part of the relationship between therapists and clients (Pachman, 1996) and with the difficulty of splitting responsibilities for treatment between separate providers of pharmacological and psychotherapy. However, not all psychologists support the initiative to extend prescribing authority to non-medical psychotherapists (see Lavoie and Fleet, 2002, for review). Opponents generally pursue two separate lines of argument, one dealing with the basic difference between pharmaco- and psychotherapy (see also Westra and Stewart, 1998), and the other with the professional identity and image of psychologists:

- Although psychological and behavioral interventions may require more time and effort than drug prescribing, these approaches are effective and often more lasting than the use of medication. Drugs provide short-term relief and symptomatic improvement; however, their effect is said to be transient and there is evidence that medication can interfere with the patient acquiring more adaptive thinking and behavioral patterns. Furthermore, with drug treatment the patients "tend to attribute help as coming from outside of themselves, rather than seeing improvement as the product of their own effort" (DeNelsky, 1996, p. 207).
- The authority to prescribe drugs necessitates extensive and thorough training in areas such as pharmacodynamics, pharmacokinetics, metabolism and drug interactions. This entails the risk that psychologists spend more time studying medicine and less time learning psychology, i.e. to acquire less competence in the domains where their knowledge and experience must excel that of other mental health professionals. In exchange they may earn

the reputation of "junior psychiatrists" and "psychology would likely be increasingly perceived as those 'other guys' who can prescribe psychoactive medications – the ones who can write prescriptions without having gone to medical school." (DeNelsky, 1996, p. 209).

As a psychologist who has spent most of his professional life doing research and teaching in psychopharmacology I will not attempt to determine which group owns the better arguments. I am convinced, however, that thorough knowledge of psychotropic drugs, especially psychopharmaceuticals, is a necessity for mental health professionals who are in contact with patients and clients who are, have been or will be taking one of these drugs. Counseling and clinical psychologists, psychotherapists as well as community and social workers will deal with these individuals and solid knowledge of psychopharmaceuticals is indispensable – also when talking to physicians who are in medical charge of shared patients.

Psychotropic Drugs and Psychology as a Science

A question of interest is whether psychology as a science has been influenced by psychopharmacology, e.g. in what areas and to what extent could psychological theory profit from modern psychopharmacology. From the history of psychology it is known that great figures like Freud and William James experimented to various degrees with psychotropic drugs, but it is probably difficult to demonstrate direct relationships between these authors' experiments and theories. Ornstein (1972) expressed the view that the preoccupation with hallucinogenic drugs such as LSD and marihuana, the so-called drug culture of the 1960s, has contributed to the reawakening of interest in questions of the psychology of consciousness. More specifically, in the early years of modern psychopharmacology, authors such as Eysenck (1962), Lienert (1964) and Janke (1964) performed pharmacopsychological experiments primarily with theoretical objectives. Drugs were applied because they made it possible to induce reproducible, qualitatively different and quantitatively graded modifications of the mental state in healthy volunteers. Manipulations of this kind can hardly be performed in ethical ways by other means, e.g. sleep deprivation or frustration and other challenging situations. Eysenck (1962) tested specific predictions of his personality theory by modifying the drive level of healthy subjects using stimulant and sedative substances. Lienert (1964) hoped to clarify some ontogenetic aspects of the development of intelligence by using LSD. Seen from today's perspective, the theoretical yield of these experiments was modest and they were subsequently virtually abandoned.

On the other hand, pharmacopsychology has brought some practical benefit to applied psychology. From experiments with drugs we now know the sensitivities of various methods for measuring modifications of arousal and mood (Chapter 3) and the methodological experience gained in these studies can be transferred to other fields such as occupational and traffic psychology as well as therapeutic research.

However, in my own opinion the primary relevance of psychopharmacology to psychology lies in the recognition that psychological theories and practice are incomplete and not appropriate to their subject unless they consider the biological substrate underlying all mental processes (mood, affect, arousal, cognition, actions and reflection). It is biological processes, controlled and influenced partly internally and partly externally, that underlie our mental life. Some of these processes and their biological carriers are accessible today by technical means: we study cells, cell constituents, synapses; and we measure concentrations of neurotransmitters, enzyme activities and intracellular messengers in the living organism. Electroencephalogram and evoked potential recordings give an overview on the electrical correlates of mental processes, and techniques such as single-photon-emission computed tomography (SPECT), positron emission tomography (PET) and functional magnetic resonance imaging (fMRI) provide surprisingly detailed information on processes occurring in different brain areas while we listen, observe, imagine, decide, etc. Tomorrow there will be other, still better measurement methods, other targets to measure and novel concepts of brain function. An essential and particularly exciting element of these activities is the oscillation between various levels of study and measurement, all covering a part of reality, and in this way the interdisciplinary approach to working and thinking also answers the old question of the primacy of material and spirit: there is no primacy, we are and we need both.

World Medical Association Declaration of Helsinki

Ethical Principles for Medical Research Involving Human Subjects

Adopted by the 18th WMA General Assembly
Helsinki, Finland, June 1964

and amended by the
29th WMA General Assembly, Tokyo, Japan, October 1975
35th WMA General Assembly, Venice, Italy, October 1983
41st WMA General Assembly, Hong Kong, September 1989
48th WMA General Assembly, Somerset West, Republic of South Africa,
    October 1996
52nd WMA General Assembly, Edinburgh, Scotland, October 2000

Introduction

(1) The World Medical Association has developed the Declaration of Helsinki as a statement of ethical principles to provide guidance to physicians and other participants in medical research involving human subjects. Medical research involving human subjects includes research on identifiable human material or identifiable data.

(2) It is the duty of the physician to promote and safeguard the health of the people. The physician's knowledge and conscience are dedicated to the fulfilment of this duty.

(3) The Declaration of Geneva of the World Medical Association binds the physician with the words, "The health of my patient will be my first consideration", and the International Code of Medical Ethics declares that, "A physician shall act only in the patient's interest when providing

Psychopharmacology, Fourth Edition. By R. Spiegel
© 2003 John Wiley & Sons, Ltd: ISBN 0 471 56039 1: 0 470 84691 7 (PB)

medical care which might have the effect of weakening the physical and mental condition of the patient".

(4) Medical progress is based on research that ultimately must rest in part on experimentation involving human subjects.

(5) In medical research on human subjects, considerations related to the well-being of the human subject should take precedence over the interests of science and society.

(6) The primary purpose of medical research involving human subjects is to improve prophylactic, diagnostic and therapeutic procedures and the understanding of the etiology and pathogenesis of disease. Even the best proven prophylactic, diagnostic and therapeutic methods must be challenged continuously through research for their effectiveness, efficiency, accessibility and quality.

(7) In current medical practice and in medical research, most prophylactic, diagnostic and therapeutic procedures involve risks and burdens.

(8) Medical research is subject to ethical standards that promote respect for all human beings and protect their health and rights. Some research populations are vulnerable and need special protection. The particular needs of the economically and medically disadvantaged must be recognized. Special attention is also required for those who cannot give or refuse consent for themselves, for those who may be subject to giving consent under duress, for those who will not benefit personally from the research and for those for whom the research is combined with care.

(9) Research investigators should be aware of the ethical, legal and regulatory requirements for research on human subjects in their own countries as well as applicable international requirements. No national ethical, legal or regulatory requirement should be allowed to reduce or eliminate any of the protections for human subjects set forth in this Declaration.

Basic Principles for All Medical Research

(10) It is the duty of the physician in medical research to protect the life, health, privacy and dignity of the human subject.

(11) Medical research involving human subjects must conform to generally accepted scientific principles and be based on a thorough knowledge of the scientific literature, other relevant sources of information and adequate laboratory and, where appropriate, animal experimentation.

(12) Appropriate caution must be exercised in the conduct of research that may affect the environment, and the welfare of animals used for research must be respected.

(13) The design and performance of each experimental procedure involving human subjects should be formulated clearly in an experimental protocol. This protocol should be submitted for consideration, comment, guidance

and, where appropriate, approval to a specially appointed ethical review committee, which must be independent of the investigator, the sponsor or any other kind of undue influence. This independent committee should be in conformity with the laws and regulations of the country in which the research experiment is performed. The committee has the right to monitor ongoing trials. The researcher has the obligation to provide monitoring information to the committee, especially any serious adverse events. The researcher should also submit to the committee, for review, information regarding funding, sponsors, institutional affiliations, other potential conflicts of interest and incentives for subjects.

(14) The research protocol should always contain a statement of the ethical considerations involved and should indicate that there is compliance with the principles enunciated in this Declaration.

(15) Medical research involving human subjects should be conducted only by scientifically qualified persons and under the supervision of a clinically competent medical person. The responsibility for the human subject must always rest with a medically qualified person and never rest on the subject of the research, even though the subject has given consent.

(16) Every medical research project involving human subjects should be preceded by careful assessment of predictable risks and burdens in comparison with foreseeable benefits to the subject or to others. This does not preclude the participation of healthy volunteers in medical research. The design of all studies should be publicly available.

(17) Physicians should abstain from engaging in research projects involving human subjects unless they are confident that the risks involved have been assessed adequately and can be managed satisfactorily. Physicians should cease any investigation if the risks are found to outweigh the potential benefits or if there is conclusive proof of positive and beneficial results.

(18) Medical research involving human subjects should be conducted only if the importance of the objective outweighs the inherent risks and burdens to the subject. This is especially important when the human subjects are healthy volunteers.

(19) Medical research is only justified if there is a reasonable likelihood that the populations in which the research is carried out stand to benefit from the results of the research.

(20) The subjects must be volunteers and informed participants in the research project.

(21) The right of research subjects to safeguard their integrity must always be respected. Every precaution should be taken to respect the privacy of the subject, the confidentiality of the patient's information and to minimize the impact of the study on the subject's physical and mental integrity and on the personality of the subject.

(22) In any research on human beings, each potential subject must be adequately informed of the aims, methods, sources of funding, any possible conflicts of interest, institutional affiliations of the researcher, the anticipated benefits and potential risks of the study and the discomfort it may entail. The subject should be informed of the right to abstain from participation in the study or to withdraw consent to participate at any time without reprisal. After ensuring that the subject has understood the information, the physician should then obtain the subject's freely-given informed consent, preferably in writing. If the consent cannot be obtained in writing, the non-written consent must be formally documented and witnessed.

(23) When obtaining informed consent for the research project the physician should be particularly cautious if the subject is in a dependent relationship with the physician or may consent under duress. In that case the informed consent should be obtained by a well-informed physician who is not engaged in the investigation and who is completely independent of this relationship.

(24) For a research subject who is legally incompetent, physically or mentally incapable of giving consent or is a legally incompetent minor, the investigator must obtain informed consent from the legally authorized representative in accordance with applicable law. These groups should not be included in research unless the research is necessary to promote the health of the population represented and this research cannot instead be performed on legally competent persons.

(25) When a subject deemed legally incompetent, such as a minor child, is able to give assent to decisions about participation in research, the investigator must obtain that assent in addition to the consent of the legally authorized representative.

(26) Research on individuals from whom it is not possible to obtain consent, including proxy or advance consent, should be done only if the physical/ mental condition that prevents obtaining informed consent is a necessary characteristic of the research population. The specific reasons for involving research subjects with a condition that renders them unable to give informed consent should be stated in the experimental protocol for consideration and approval of the review committee. The protocol should state that consent to remain in the research should be obtained as soon as possible from the individual or a legally authorized surrogate.

(27) Both authors and publishers have ethical obligations. In publication of the results of research, the investigators are obliged to preserve the accuracy of the results. Negative as well as positive results should be published or otherwise publicly available. Sources of funding, institutional affiliations and any possible conflicts of interest should be declared in the publication. Reports of experimentation not in accordance

with the principles laid down in this Declaration should not be accepted for publication.

(28) The physician may combine medical research with medical care only to the extent that the research is justified by its potential prophylactic, diagnostic or therapeutic value. When medical research is combined with medical care, additional standards apply to protect the patients who are research subjects.

(29) The benefits, risks, burdens and effectiveness of a new method should be tested against those of the best current prophylactic, diagnostic and therapeutic methods. This does not exclude the use of placebo, or no treatment, in studies where no proven prophylactic, diagnostic or therapeutic method exists.

To clarify further the WMA position on the use of placebo-controlled trials, the WMA Council issued, during October 2001, a note of clarification on Paragraph 29 readable at the end of this list.

(30) At the conclusion of the study, every patient entered into the study should be assured of access to the best proven prophylactic, diagnostic and therapeutic methods identified by the study.

(31) The physician should fully inform the patient which aspects of the care are related to the research. The refusal of a patient to participate in a study must never interfere with the patient–physician relationship.

(32) In the treatment of a patient, where proven prophylactic, diagnostic and therapeutic methods do not exist or have been ineffective, the physician, with informed consent from the patient, must be free to use unproven or new prophylactic, diagnostic and therapeutic measures if, in the physician's judgment, it offers hope of saving life, re-establishing health or alleviating suffering. Where possible, these measures should be made the object of research, designed to evaluate their safety and efficacy. In all cases, new information should be recorded and, where appropriate, published. The other relevant guidelines of this Declaration should be followed.

Note of Clarification on Paragraph 29 of the Declaration

The WMA is concerned that Paragraph 29 of the revised Declaration of Helsinki (October 2000) has led to diverse interpretations and possible confusion. It hereby reaffirms its position that extreme care must be taken in making use of a placebo-controlled trial and that in general this methodology should be used only in the absence of existing proven therapy. However, a placebo-controlled trial may be ethically acceptable, even if proven therapy is available, under the following circumstances:

- Where, for compelling and scientifically sound methodological reasons, its use is necessary to determine the efficacy or safety of a prophylactic, diagnostic or therapeutic method.
- Where a prophylactic, diagnostic or therapeutic method is being investigated for a minor condition and the patients who receive placebo will not be subject to any additional risk of serious or irreversible harm.

All other provisions of the Declaration of Helsinki must be adhered to, especially the need for appropriate ethical and scientific review.

References

Ackerknecht, E.H.: *Kurze Geschichte der Psychiatrie*. Enke, Stuttgart, 1967.

Addington, D., Addington, J., Maticka-Tyndale, E.: Assessing depression in schizophrenia: the Calgary Depression Scale. *Br. J. Psychiatry* **163** (Suppl. 22), 39–44, 1993.

Akunne, H.C., Zoski, K.T., Whetzel, S.Z., Cordon, J.J.: Neuropharmacological profile of a selective sigma ligand, igmesine: a potential antidepressant and anti-stress actions. *Neuropharmacology* **41**, 138–149, 2001.

Alanen, Y.O., Räkköläinen, V., Laakso, J., Rasimus, R., Kaljonen, A.: *Towards Need-specific Treatment of Schizophrenic Psychoses*. Springer, New York, 1986.

Aldrich, M.S.: Narcolepsy. *N. Engl. J. Med.* **323**, 389–394, 1990.

Allgulander, C.: History and current status of sedative–hypnotic drug use and abuse. *Acta Psychiatr. Scand.* **73**, 465–478, 1986.

Anderson I.M.: Meta-analytical studies on new antidepressants. *Br. Med. Bull.* **57**, 161–178, 2001.

Anderson, I.M., Clark, L., Elliot, R.: 5HT2C receptor activation by m-chlorophenylpiperazine detected in humans with fMRI. *Neuroreport* **13**(12), 1547–1551, 2002.

Angrist, B., Peselow, E., Rubinstein, M., Corwin, J., Rotrosen, J.: Partial improvement in negative schizophrenic symptoms after amphetamine. *Psychopharmacology* **78**, 128–130, 1982.

Aoki, C., Go, C.G., Venkatesan, C., Kurose, H.: Perikaryal and synaptic localization of alpha 2A-adrenergic receptor-like immunoreactivity. *Brain Res.* **650**(2), 181–204, 1994.

APA (American Psychiatric Association): *Diagnostic and Statistical Manual of Mental Disorders (DSM-III-R)*, 3rd edn, revised. Washington, DC, 1987.

APA (American Psychiatric Association): *Diagnostic and Statistical Manual of Mental Disorders (DSM-IV)*, 4th edn. Washington, DC, 1994.

Arborelius, L., Owens, M.J., Plotsky, P.M., Nemeroff, C.B.: The role of corticotropin-releasing factor in depression and anxiety disorders. *J. Endocrinol.* **160**, 1–12, 1999.

Arthurs, O.J., Boniface, S.: How well do we understand the neural origins of the fMRI BOLD signal? *Trends Neurosci.* **25**(1), 27–31, 2002.

Asberg, M., Thoren, P., Trasknan, L.: 'Serotonin depression': a biochemical subgroup within the affective disorders? *Science* **191**, 478–480, 1976.

Psychopharmacology, Fourth Edition. By R. Spiegel
© 2003 John Wiley & Sons, Ltd: ISBN 0 471 56039 1: 0 470 84691 7 (PB)

Asheikh, J.I., Londborg, P., Clay, C.M., *et al.*: The efficacy of sertraline in panic disorder: combined results from two fixed-dose studies. *Int. Clin. Psychopharm.* **15**, 335–342, 2000.

Austin, M.-P., Mitchell, Ph., Goodwin, G.M.: Cognitive deficits in depression. *Br. J. Psychiatry* **178**, 200–206, 2001.

Awad, A.G., Hogan, T.P., Voruganti, L.N.P., *et al.*: Patients' subjective experience with antipsychotic medications: implication for outcome and quality of life. *Int. Clin. Psychopharmacol.* **10** (Suppl. 3), 123–132, 1995.

Azcona, A., Roth, S., Spiegel, R.: Effects of the muscarinic agonist RS 86 in healthy volunteers. *Pharmacopsychiatry* **19**, 323–325, 1986.

Baddeley, A.D.: *Working Memory.* Clarendon Press, Oxford, 1986.

Baldessarini, R.J.: *Chemotherapy in Psychiatry: Principles and Practice.* Harvard University Press, Cambridge, MA, 1985.

Baldessarini, R.J., Davis, J.M.: What is the best maintenance dose of neuroleptics in schizophrenia? *Psychiatry Res.* **3**, 115–122, 1980.

Baldessarini, R.J., Cohen, B.M., Teicher, M.H.: Significance of neuroleptics dose and plasma level in the pharmacological treatment of psychoses. *Arch. Gen. Psychiatry* **45**, 79–91, 1988.

Baldessarini, R.J., Tondo, L., Hennen, J.: Effects of lithium treatment and its discontinuation on suicidal behavior in bipolar manic–depressive disorders. *J. Clin. Psychiatry* **60** (Suppl. 2), 77–84, 111–116, 1999.

Ban, T.A.: *Psychopharmacology.* Williams & Wilkins, Baltimore, 1969.

Bartus, R.T., Dean, R.L., Beer, B., Lippa, A.S.: The cholinergic hypothesis of geriatric memory dysfunction. *Science* **217**, 408–417, 1982.

Bauer, M., Whybrow, P.C., Angst, J., *et al.*: Worlds Federation of Societies of Biological Psychiatry (WFSBP) guidelines for biological treatment of unipolar depressive disorders. Part 1: Acute and continuation treatment of major depressive disorder. *World J. Biol. Psychiatry* **3**, 5–43, 2002.

Bech, P., Bolwig, T.G., Kramp, P., *et al.*: The Bech–Rafaelsen Mania Scale and the Hamilton Depression Scale. *Acta Psychiatr. Scand.* **59**(4), 420–430, 1979.

Bech, P., Allerup, P., Reisby, N., *et al.*: Assessment of symptom change from improvement curves on the Hamilton Depression Scale in trials with antidepressants. *Psychopharmacology (Berlin)* **84**, 276–281, 1984.

Beck, A.T.: Cognitive therapy, a 30-year restrospective. *Am. Psychol.* **46**, 368–375, 1991.

Beck, A.T., Hollon, S.D., Young, J.E., Bedrosian, R.C., Budenz, D.: Treatment of depression with cognitive therapy and amitriptyline. *Arch. Gen. Psychiatry* **42**, 142–148, 1985.

Beck, A.T., Steer, R.A., Garbing, M.G.: Psychometric properties of the Beck Depression Inventory: twenty-five years of evaluation. *Clin. Psychol. Rev.* **8**, 77–100, 1988.

Becker, R.E., Giacobini, E.: Mechanisms of cholinesterase inhibition in senile dementia of the Alzheimer type: clinical, pharmacological and therapeutic aspects. *Drug Dev. Res.* **12**, 163–195, 1988.

Beckmann, N., Gentsch, C., Baumann, D., *et al.*: Non-invasive, quantitative assessment of the anatomical phenotype of corticotropin-releasing factor-overexpressing mice by MRI. *NMR Biomed.* **14**, 210–216, 2001.

Beigel, A., Murphy, D.L., Bunney, W.E. Jr.: The manic state rating scale: scale construction, reliability and validity. *Arch. Gen. Psychiatry* **25**, 256–262, 1971.

Belanoff, J.K., Gross, K., Yager, A., Schatzberg, A.F.: Corticosteroids and cognition. *J. Psychiatr. Res.* **35**, 127–145, 2001.

Bell, C., Forshall, S., Adrover, M., et al.: Does 5-HT restrain panic ? A tryptophan depletion study in panic disorder patients recovered on paroxetine. J. Psychopharmacol. **16**(1), 5–14, 2002.

Bellack, A.S., Hersen, M., Himmelhoch, J.: Social skills training compared with pharmacotherapy and psychotherapy in the treatment of unipolar depression. Am. J. Psychiatry **138**, 1562–1567, 1981.

Belliveau, J.W., Kennedy, D.N., Jr., McKinstry, R.C., et al.: Functional mapping of the human visual cortex by magnetic resonance imaging. Science **254**(5032), 716–719, 1991.

Benkert, O., Hippius, H.: Psychiatrische Pharmakotherapie. Springer, Berlin, 1980.

Bente, D.: Elektroencephalographische Gesichtspunkte zur Klassifikation neuro- und thymoleptischer Pharmaka, 1. Teil. Med. Exp. **5**, 337–346, 1961.

Bergen, J., Kitchin, R., Berry, G.: Predictors of the course of tardive dyskinesia in patients receiving neuroleptics. Biol. Psychiatry **32**, 580–594, 1992.

Berger, F.M.: Anxiety and the discovery of the tranquillizers. In: Ayd, F.J., Blackwell, B. (eds): Discoveries in Biological Psychiatry. Lippincott, Philadelphia, 1970, pp. 115–129.

Berger, H.: Über das Elektrenkephalogramm des Menschen. 3 Mitteilung. Arch. Psychiatr. Nervenkr. **94**, 16–60, 1931.

Bergstrom, M., Fasth, K.J., Kilpatrick, G., et al.: Brain uptake and receptor binding of two [11C] labeled selective high affinity NK1-antagonists, GR203040 and GR205171 – PET studies in rhesus monkey. Neuropharmacology **39**(4), 664–670, 2000.

Berk, J.P., Ichim, M., Brook, S.: Olanzapine compared to lithium in mania: a double-blind randomized controlled trial. Int. J. Clin. Psychopharmacol. **14**, 339–343, 1999.

Berkowitz, A., Sutton, L., Janowsky, D.S., Gillin, J.C.: Pilocarpine, an orally active muscarinic cholinergic agonist, induces REM sleep and reduces delta sleep in normal volunteers. Psychiatry Res. **33**, 112–119, 1990.

Berman, R.M., Narasimhan, M., Sanacora, G., et al.: A randomized clinical trial of repetitive transcranial magnetic stimulation in the treatment of major depression. Biol. Psychiatry **47**, 332–337, 2000.

Berman, T., Douglas, V.I., Barr, R.G.: Effects of methylphenidate on complex cognitive processing in attention-deficit hyperactivity disorder. J. Abnorm. Psychol. **108**, 90–105, 1999.

Bernard, H.R.: Research Methods in Anthropology. Qualitative and Quantitative Approaches. Altamira Press, Walnut Creek, CA, 1995.

Beuzen, J.N., Taylor, N., Wesnes, K., Wood, A.: A comparison of the effects of olanzapine, haloperidol and placebo on cognitive and psychomotor functions in healthy elderly volunteers. J. Psychopharmacol. **13**, 152–158, 1999.

Biederman, J.: Attention deficit hyperactivity disorder (ADHD). Ann. Clin. Psychiatry **3**, 9–22, 1991.

Bilder, R.M., Goldman, R.S., Robinson, D., et al.: Neuropsychology of first episode schizophrenia: initial characterization and clinical correlates. Am. J. Psychiatry **157**, 549–559, 2000.

Bilder, R.M., Goldman, R.S., Volavka, J., et al.: Neurocognitive effects of clozapine, olanzapine, risperidone, and haloperidol in patients with chronic schizophrenia or schizoaffective disorder. Am. J. Psychiatry **159**, 1018–1028, 2002.

Blackburn, I.M., Bishop, S., Glen, A.I.M., Whalley, L.J., Christie, J.E.: The efficacy of cognitive therapy in depression: a treatment trial using cognitive therapy and pharmacotherapy, each alone and in combination. Br. J. Psychiatry **139**, 181–189, 1981.

Blake, D.D., Weathers, F.W., Nagy, L.M., *et al.*: A clinician rating scale for assessing current and lifetime PTSD: the CAPS-1. *Behav. Ther.* **13**, 187–188, 1990.

Blake, D.D., Weathers, F.W., Nagy, L.M., *et al.*: The development of a clinician administered PTSD scale. *J. Trauma Stress* **8**, 75–90, 1995.

Bleuler, E.: *Dementia praecox oder Gruppe der Schizophrenia.* Deuticke, Leipzig, 1911.

Bleuler, E.: *Lehrbuch der Psychiatrie.* Springer, Berlin 1916 (15th Ed 1983).

Bleuler, M.: Psychiatrische Intümer in der Serotonin-Forschung. *Dtsch. Med. Wochenschr.* **81**, 1078–1081, 1956.

Bloom, A.S., Hoffmann, R.G., Fuller, S.A., *et al.*: Determination of drug-induced changes in functional MRI signal using a pharmacokinetic model. *Hum. Brain Mapp.* **8**, 235–244, 1999.

Bond, A., Lader, M.: The use of analog scales in rating subjective feelings. *Br. J. Med. Psychol.* **47**, 211–218, 1974.

Bondareff, W., Alpert, M., Friedhoff, A.J., *et al.*: Comparison of sertraline and nortriptyline in the treatment of major depressive disorder in late life. *Am. J. Psychiatry* **157**, 729–736, 2000.

Bowden, C.L., Brugger, A.M., Swann, A.C., *et al.*: Efficacy of divalproex sodium vs lithium and placebo in the treatment of mania. *J. Am. Med. Assoc.* **271**, 918–924, 1994.

Bowden, C.L., Calabrese, J.R., Wallis, B., *et al.*: Who enters therapeutic trials? Illness characteristics of patients in clinical drug studies of mania. *Psychopharmacol. Bull.* **31**, 103–109, 1995.

Bowen, D.M., Smith, C.B., White, P., Davison, A.N.: Neurotransmitter-related enzymes and indices of hypoxia in senile dementia and other abiotrophies. *Brain* **99**, 459–496, 1976.

Bradford, D., Stroup, S., Lieberman, J.: Pharmacological treatments for schizophrenia. In: Nathan, P., Gorman, J.M. (eds): *A Guide to Treatments that Work*, 2nd edn. Oxford University Press, Oxford, 2002, pp. 169–199.

Braff, D.L., Swerdlow, N.R., Geyer, M.A.: Symptom correlates of prepulse inhibition deficits in male schizophrenic patients. *Am. J. Psychiatry* **156**, 596–602, 1999.

Branconnier, R.J., Harto, N.E., Dessain, E.C., *et al.*: Speech blockage, memory impairment, and age: a prospective comparison of amitriptyline and maprotiline. *Psychopharmacol. Bull.* **23**, 230–234, 1987.

Brauer, L.H., de Wit, H.: Subjective responses to *d*-amphetamine alone and after pimozide pretreatment in normal, healthy volunteers. *Biol. Psychiatry* **39**, 26–32, 1996.

Brauer, L.H., Rukstalis, M.R., de Wit, H.: Acute subjective responses to paroxetine in normal volunteers. *Drug Alcohol Depend* **39**, 223–230, 1995.

Brazo, P., Marié, R.M., Halbecq, I., *et al.*: Cognitive patterns in subtypes of schizophrenia. *Eur. Psychiatry* **17**, 155–162, 2002.

Breggin, P.R.: Psychostimulants in the treatment of children diagnosed with ADHD. I: Acute risks and psychological effects. *Eth. Hum. Sci. Serv.* **1**, 13–33, 1999.

Breiter, H.C., Gollub, R.L., Weisskoff, R.M., *et al.*: Acute effects of cocaine on human brain activity and emotion. *Neuron* **19**(3), 591–611, 1997.

Breitner, J.C.S., Zandi, P.P.: Do nonsteroidal antiinflammatory drugs reduce the risk of Alzheimer's disease? *New Engl. J. Med.* **345**, 1567–1568, 2001.

Briere, J.: *Psychological Assessment of Adult Posttraumatic Stress Disorder.* American Psychological Association, Washington, DC, 1997.

Broadhurst, A.D.: The discovery of imipramine from a personal viewpoint. In: Ban, T.A., Healy, D., Shorter, E. (eds): *The Rise of Psychopharmacology and the Story of CINP.* Animula Publishing, Budapest, 1998, pp. 69–75.

Brooks, D.J.: Monitoring neuroprotection and restorative therapies in Parkinson's disease with PET. *J. Neural Transm. Suppl.* **60**, 125–137, 2000.

Burns, A., Spiegel, R., Quarg, P.: Benefits of rivastigmine in patients with severe Alzheimer's Disease (AD). Poster presented at the *Annual Meeting of the American College for Neuro-Psychopharmacology*, San Juan, Puerto Rico, 6–10 December, 2002.

Burns, H.D., Gibson, R.E., Dannals, R.F.: *Nuclear Imaging in Drug Discovery, Development, and Approval*. Springer Verlag, Berlin, 1993, pp. 11–31.

Bustillo, J.R., Lauriello, J., Horan, W.P., Keith, S.J.: The psychosocial treatment of schizophrenia: an update. *Am. J. Psychiatry* **158**, 163–175, 2001.

Busto, U., Sellers, E.M., Naranjo, C.A., et al.: Withdrawal reaction after long-term therapeutic use of benzodiazepines. *N. Engl. J. Med.* **315**, 854–859, 1986.

Butters, M.A., Becker, J.T., Nebes, R.D., et al.: Changes in cognitive functioning following treatment of late-life depression. *Am. J. Psychiatry* **157**, 1949–1954, 2000.

Buxton, R.B.: *Introduction to Functional Magnetic Resonance Imaging: Principles and Techniques*. Cambridge University Press, 2002.

Bye, C., Munro-Faure, A.D., Peck, A.W., Young, P.A.: A comparison of the effects of *l*-benzylpiperazine and dexamphetamine on human performance tests. *Eur. J. Clin. Pharmacol.* **6**, 163–169, 1973.

Bye, C., Clubley, M., Peck, A.W.: Drowsiness, impaired performance and tricyclic antidepressant drugs. *Br. J. Clin. Pharmacol.* **6**, 155–161, 1978.

Cade, J.F.J.: The story of lithium. In: Ayd, F.J., Blackwell, B. (eds): *Discoveries in Biological Psychiatry*. Lippincott, Philadelphia, 1970, pp. 218–229.

Cadenhead, K.S., Swerdlow, N.R., Shafer, K.M., et al.: Modulation of the startle response and startle laterality in relatives of schizophrenic patients and in subjects with schizotypal personality disorder: evidence of inhibitory deficits. *Am. J. Psychiatry* **157**, 1660–1668, 2000.

Calabrese, J.R., Markovitz, P.J., Kimmel, S.E., et al.: Spectrum of efficacy of valproate in 78 rapid cycling bipolar patients. *J. Clin. Psychopharm.* **12**(S), 53–56, 1992.

Calabrese, J.R., Bowden, C.L., Sachs, G.S., et al.: A double-blind placebo-controlled study of lamotrigine monotherapy in patients with bipolar I depression. *J. Clin. Psychiatry* **60**, 79–88, 1999.

Calabrese, J.R., Suppes, T, Bowden, C.L. et al.: A double blind, placebo controlled, prophylaxis study of lamortigine in rapid cycling bipolar disorder. *J. Clin. Psychiatry* **61**, 841–850, 2000.

Calabrese, J.R., Bowden, C.L., Fieve, R., et al.: Lamotrigine or lithium in the maintenance treatment of bipolar I disorder. *Eur. Neuropsychopharmacol.* **12** (Suppl. 3), S217, 2002.

Caldwell, A.E.: *Origins of Psychopharmacology: from CPZ to LSD*. Thomas, Springfield, IL, 1970.

Caldwell, A.E.: History of psychopharmacology. In: Clark, W.G., del Giudice, J. (eds): *Principles of Psychopharmacology*. Academic Press, New York, 1978, pp. 9–40.

Caldwell, J.A., Caldwell, J.L., Smythe, N.K., Hall, K.K.: A double-blind, placebo-controlled investigation of the efficacy of modafinil for sustaining the alertness and performance of aviators: a helicopter simulator study. *Psychopharmacology* **150**, 272–282, 2000.

Camargo, E.E., Szabo, Z., Links, J.M., et al. The influence of biological and technical factors on the variability of global and regional brain metabolism of 2-[18F]fluoro-2-deoxy-D-glucose. *J. Cerebr. Blood Flow Metab.* **12**(2), 281–290, 1992.

Cantwell, D.P.: Attention deficit disorder: a review of the past 10 years. *J. Am. Acad. Child Adolesc. Psychiatry* **35**, 978–987, 1996.

Carlsson, A.: Perspectives on the discovery of central monoaminergic neurotranmission. *Annu. Rev. Neurosci.* **10**, 19–40, 1987.

Carlsson, A.: Neuropharmacology. In: Ban, T.A., Healy, E., Shorter, E. (eds): *The Rise of Psychopharmacology and the Story of CINP*. Animula Publishing, Budapest, 1998, pp. 124–128.

Carlsson, A., Lindquist, M.: Effect of chlorpromazine or haloperidol on formation of 3-methoxytryptamine and normetanephrine. *Acta Pharmacol. (Kobenhavn)* **20**, 140–144, 1963.

Carpenter, W.T., Buchanan, R.W.: Schizophrenia. *N. Engl. J. Med.* **330**, 681–690, 1994.

Carson, R., Daube-Witherspoon, M., Herscovitch, P.: *Quantitative Functional Brain Imaging With Positron Emission Tomography*. Academic Press, New York, 1998.

Cascalenda, N., Perry, J.C., Looper, K.: Remission in major depressive disorder: a comparison of pharmacotherapy, psychotherapy and control conditions. *Am. J. Psychiatry* **189**, 1354–1360, 2002.

Cassano, G.B., Jori, M.C., on behalf of the AMIMAJOR investigators: Efficacy and safety of amisulpride 50 mg versus paroxetine 20 mg in major depression: a randomized, double-blind, parallel group study. *Int. Clin. Psychopharmacol.* **17**, 27–32, 2002.

Cassens, G., Inglis, A.K., Appelbaum, P.S., Gutheil, T.G.: Neuroleptics: effects on neuropsychological function in chronic schizophrenic patients. *Schizophr. Bull.* **16**, 477–499, 1990.

Charney, D.S., Woods, S.W., Heninger, G.R.: Noradrenergic function in generalized anxiety disorder: effects of yohimbine in healthy subjects and patients with generalized anxiety disorder. *Psychiatry Res.* **27**(2), 173–182, 1989.

Cheeta, S., Tucci, S., Sandhu, J., *et al.*: Anxiolytic actions of the substance P (NK1) receptor antagonist L-760735 and the 5-HT1A agonist 8-OH-DPAT in the social interaction test in gerbils. *Brain Res.* **915**, 170–175, 2001.

Chen, Y., Lader, M.: Long-term benzodiazepine treatment: is it ever justified? *Hum. Psychopharmacol.* **5**, 301–312, 1990.

Chouinard, G., Jones, B., Remington, G., *et al.*: A Canadian multi-center placebo controlled study of fixed doses of risperidone and haloperidol in the treatment of chronic schizophrenic patients. *J. Clin. Psychopharmacol.* **13**, 25–40, 1993.

Cigánek, L.: The EEG response (evoked potential) to light stimulus in man. *Electroencephalogr. Clin. Neurophysiol.* **13**, 165–172, 1961.

CINP Task Force: Impact of neuropharmacology in the 1990s: strategies for the therapy of depressive illness. *Eur. Neuropsychopharmacol.* **3**, 153–156, 1993.

CIPS: *Internationale Skalen für Psychiatrie*. Collegium internationale scalarum, dritte Auflage. Beltz, Weinheim, 1986.

Claridge, G.S.: *Personality and Arousal: a Psychophysiological Study of Psychiatric Disorder*. Pergamon Press, Oxford, 1967.

Clerc, G.E., Ruimy, P., Verdeau-Pailles, J., *et al.*: A double-blind comparison of venlafaxine and fluoxetine in patients hospitalized for major depression and melancholia. *Int. Clin. Psychopharmacol.* **9**, 139–143, 1994.

Clubley, M., Bye, C., Henson, T.A., Peck, A.W., Riddington, C.J.: Effects of caffeine and cyclizine and in combination on human performance, subjective effects and EEG activity. *Br. J. Clin. Pharmacol.* **7**, 157–163, 1979.

Clyde, D.J.: *Manual for the Clyde Mood Scale*. Biometric Lab., University of Miami, Coral Gables, FL, 1963.

Coenders, C.J., Kerbusch, S.M., Vossen, J.M., Cools, A.R.: Problem-solving behaviour in apomorphine-susceptible and unsusceptible rats. *Physiol. Behav.* **52**, 321–326, 1992.

Cohen, I.M.: The benzodiazepines. In: Ayd, F.J., Blackwell, B. (eds): *Discoveries in Biological Psychiatry*. Lippincott, Philadelphia, 1970, pp. 130–141.

Cohen, L.S., Friedman, J.M., Jefferson, J.W., *et al.*: A re-evaluation of risk of *in utero* exposure to lithium. *J. Am. Med. Assoc.* **271**(2), 146–150, 1994.

Cohen, R.M., Nordahl, T.E., Semple, W.E., Pickar, D.: The brain metabolic patterns of clozapine- and fluphenazine-treated female patients with schizophrenia: evidence of a sex effect. *Neuropsychopharmacology* **21**(5), 632–640, 1999.

Comité Lyonnais de Recherches Thérapeutiques en Psychiatrie (Paul Brouillot, Paul Broussolle, Jacques Greffe, Jean Guyotat, Pierre Lambert, Patrick Lemoine, Isabelle Soares-Boucaud): The birth of psychopharmacotherapy: explorations in a new world – 1952–1968. In: *The Psychopharmacologists III*. Interviews by David Healy. Arnold, London, 2000, pp. 1–53.

Conners, C.K.: *Conners Rating Scales Manual, Conners Teacher Rating Scales, Conners Parent Rating Scales: Instruments for Use with Children and Adolescents*. Multihealth Systems, North Tonawanda, NY, 1990.

Cook, E.H., Jr., Metz, J., Leventhal, B.L., *et al.*: Fluoxetine effects on cerebral glucose metabolism. *NeuroReport* **5**(14), 1745–1748, 1994.

Cook, M.R., Graham, Ch., Sastre, A., Gerkovich, M.M.: Physiological and performance effects of pyridostigmine bromide in healthy volunteers: a dose–response study. *Psychopharmacology* **162**, 186–192, 2002.

Coper, H., Kanowski, S.: Nootropika-Grundlagen und Therapie. In: Langer, G., Heimann, H. (eds): *Psychopharmaka. Grundlagen und Therapie*. Springer, Vienna, 1983, pp. 409–433.

Coper, H., Heimann, H., Kanowski, S., Künkel, H.: *Hirnorganische Psychosyndrome im Alter III*: Methoden zum klinischen Wirksamkeitsnachweis von Nootropika. Springer, Berlin, 1987.

Coppen, A.: Biochemistry of affective disorders. *Br. J. Psychiatry* **113**, 1237–1264, 1967.

Cornblatt, B.A.: The New York high risk project to the Hillside recognition and prevention (RAP) program. *Am. J. Med. Genet.* **114**(8), 956–966, 2002.

Corr, P.J., Kumari, V.: Individual differences in mood reactions to *d*-amphetamine: a test of three personality factors. *J. Psychopharmacol.* **14**, 371–377, 2000.

Coryell, W., Winokur, G.: *The Clinical Management of Anxiety Disorders*. Oxford University Press, New York, 1991.

Coupland, N.J., Bell, C., Potokar, J.P., *et al.*: Flumazenil challenge in social phobia. *Depress. Anxiety* **11**(1), 27–30, 2000.

Covi, L., Lipman, R.S., Derogatis, L.R., Smith, J.E., Pattison, J.: Drugs and group psychotherapy in neurotic depression. *Am. J. Psychiatry* **131**, 191–198, 1974.

Cox, B.J., Swinson, R.P., Morrison, B., Lee, P.S.: Clomipramine, fluoxetine, and behavior therapy in the treatment of obsessive–compulsive disorder: a meta-analysis. *J. Behav. Ther. Exp. Psychiatry* **24**, 149–153, 1993.

Cox, J., Holden, J., Sagovsky, R.: Detection of postnatal depression. Development of the 10-item EPDS. *Br. J. Psychiatry* **150**, 782–786, 1987.

Craik, F.I.M., Salthouse, T.A.: *The Handbook of Aging and Cognition*, L. Erlbaum, Hillsdale, NJ, 1992.

Creese, I., Burt, D.R., Snyder, S.H.: Dopamine receptor binding predicts clinical and pharmacological potencies of antischizophrenic drugs. *Science* **192**, 481–483, 1976.

Crisby, M., Carlson, L.A., Winblad, B.: Statins in the prevention and treatment of Alzheimer disease. *Alzheim. Dis. Assoc. Disord.* **16**, 131–136, 2002.

Crook, Th., Ferris, S., Bartus, R.: *Assessment in Geriatric Psychopharmacology*. Mark Powley Assoc., New Canaan, CT, 1983.

Crosbie, J., Schachar, R.: Deficient inhibition as a marker for familial ADHD. *Am. J. Psychiatry* **158**, 1884–1890, 2001.

Crow, T.J.: The biology of schizophrenia. *Experientia* **38**, 1275–1282, 1982.

Cryan, J.F., Markou, A., Lucki, I.: Assessing antidepressant activity in rodents: recent developments and future needs. *Trends Pharmacol. Sci.* **23**, 238–245, 2002.

Csernansky, J.G., Mahmoud, R., Breener, R.: A comparison of risperidone and haloperidol for the prevention of relapse in patients with schizophrenia. *N. Engl. J. Med.* **346**, 16–22, 2002.

Cummings, J.L., Cole, G.: Alzheimer disease. *J. Am. Med. Assoc.* **287**, 2335–2338, 2002.

Curran, H.V.: Benzodiazepines, memory and mood: a review. *Psychopharmacology* **105**, 1–8, 1991.

Curran, H.V.: Antidepressant drugs, cognitive function and human performance. In: Smith, A., Jones, D. (eds): *Handbook of Human Performance*, Vol. 2. Academic Press, New York, 1992a, pp. 319–336.

Curran, H.V.: Memory functions, alertness and mood of long-term benzodiazepine users: a preliminary investigation of the effects of a normal daily dose. *J. Psychopharmacol.* **6**, 69–75, 1992b.

Curran, H.V., Lader, M.: The psychopharmacological effects of repeated doses of fluvoxamine, mianserin and placebo in healthy subjects. *Eur. J. Clin. Pharmacol.* **29**, 601–607, 1986.

Curran, H.V., Sakulsripong, M., Lader, M.: Antidepressants and human memory: an investigation of four drugs with different sedative and anticholinergic profiles. *Psychopharmacology* **95**, 520–527, 1988.

Curran, S., Wattis, J.P.: Critical Flicker Fusion threshold: a useful research tool in patients with Alzheimer's disease. *Hum. Psychopharmacol.* **13**, 337–355, 1998.

Curran, H.V., Pooviboonsuk, P., Dalton, J.A., Lader, M.H.: Differentiating the effects of centrally acting drugs on arousal and memory: an event-related potential study of scopolamine, lorazepam and diphenhydramine. *Psychopharmacology* **135**, 27–36, 1998.

Danion, J.-M., Mulemans, T., Kaufmann-Muller, F., Vermaat, H.: Intact implicit learning in schizophrenia. *Am. J. Psychiatry* **158**, 944–948, 2001.

Davidson, J.R., Colket, J.T.: The eight-item treatment-outcome post-traumatic stress disorder scale: a brief measure to assess treatment outcome in post-traumatic stress disorder. *Int. Clin. Psychopharmacol.* **12**(1), 41–45, 1997.

Davidson, J.R., Book, S.W., Colket, J.T., *et al.*: Assessment of a new self-rating scale for post-traumatic stress disorder. *Psychol. Med.* **27**(1), 153–160, 1997.

Davies, A.P., Maloney, A.J.F.: Selective loss of cholinergic neurons in Alzheimer's disease. *Lancet ii*, 1403–1404, 1976.

Davis, J. M.: A two-factor theory of schizophrenia. *J. Psychiatr. Res.* **11**, 25–29, 1974.

Davis, J.M., Casper, R.C.: General principles of the clinical use of neuroleptics. In: Clark, W.G., Del Giudice, J. (eds): *Principles of Psychopharmacology*. Academic Press, New York, 1978, pp. 511–536.

Davis, J.M., Wang, Z., Janicak, Ph.G.: A quantitative analysis of clinical drug trials for the treatment of affective disorders. *Psychopharmacol. Bull.* **29**, 175–181, 1993.

Davis, K.L., Kahn, R.S., Ko, G., Davidson, M.: Dopamine in schizophrenia: a review and reconceptualization. *Am. J. Psychiatry* **148**, 1474–1486, 1991.

Davis, K.L., Thal, L.J., Gamzu, E.R., *et al.*: A double-blind, placebo-controlled, multicenter study of tacrine for Alzheimer's disease. *N. Engl. J. Med.* **327**, 1253–1259, 1992.

Davis, K.L., Mohs, R.C., Marin, D., *et al.*: Cholinergic markers in elderly patients with early signs of Alzheimer disease. *J. Am. Geriatr. Assoc.* **281**, 1401–1406, 1999.

De Visser, S.J., van der Post, J., Pieters, M.S.M., *et al.*: Biomarkers for the effects of antipsychotic drugs in healthy volunteers. *Br. J. Clin. Pharmacol.* **51**, 119–132, 2001.

Debus, G., Janke, W.: Algemeine und differentielle Wirkungen von Tranquillantien bei gesunden Personen in Hinblick auf Angstreduktion. In: Jenke, W., Netter, P. (eds): *Angst und Psychopharmaka*. Kohlhammer, Stuttgart, 1986, pp. 135–149.

Degkwitz, R.: *Leitfaden der Psychopharmakologie*. Wissenschaftliche Verlagsgesellschaft, Stuttgart, 1967.

Delay, J., Deniker, P.: Les neuroplégiques en thérapeutique psychiatrique. *Therapie* **8**, 347–364, 1953.

Delay, J., Deniker, P., Harl, J.-M.: Utilisation en thérapeutique psychiatrique d'une phénothiazine d'action centrale élective (4560 RP). *Ann. Med.-Psychol.* **110**, 112–117, 1952.

Delay, J., Pichot, P., Nicolas-Charles, P., Perse, J.: Etude psychométrique des effets de l'amobarbital (amytal) et de la chlorpromazine sur des sujets normaux. *Psychopharmacologia* **1**, 48–58, 1959.

DeLeon, P.H., Wiggins, J.G.: Prescription privileges for psychologists. *Am. Psychol.* **51**, 225–229, 1996.

Delgado, P.L., Charney, D.S., Price, L.H., *et al.*: Serotonin function and the mechanism of antidepressant action. Reversal of antidepressant-induced remission by rapid depletion of plasma tryptophan. *Arch. Gen. Psychiatry* **47**, 411–418, 1990.

DeNelsky, G.Y.: The case against prescription privileges for psychologists. *Am. Psychol.* **51**, 207–212, 1996.

Deniker, P.: Die Geschichte der Neuroleptika. In: Linde, O.K. (ed.): *Pharmakopsychiatrie im Wandel der Zeit*. Tilia-Verlag, Klingenmünster, Germany, 1988, pp. 119–133.

Deptula, D., Pomara, N.: Effects of antidepressants on human performance: a review. *J. Clin. Psychopharmacol.* **10**, 105–111, 1990.

Derogatis, LR., *SCL-90-R. Administration, Scoring and Procedures, Manual II*. Clinical Psychometric Research, Baltimore, 1983.

Detre, J.A., Leigh, J.S., Williams, D.S.: Perfusion imaging. *Magn. Reson. Med.* **23**, 37–45, 1998.

Deutsch Lezak, M.: *Neuropsychological Assessment*, 3rd edn. Oxford University Press, Oxford, 1995.

Dielenberg, R.A., McGregor, I.S.: Defensive behavior in rats towards predatory odors: a review. *Neurosci. Biobehav. Rev.* **25**, 597–609, 2001.

Dietmaier, O., Laux, G.: Übersichtstabellen [Antidepressives]. In: Riederer, P., Laux, G., Pöldinger, W. (eds): *Neuro-Psychopharmaka, Bd.3: Antidepressiva und Phasenprophylaktika*. Springer, Vienna, 1993, pp. 579–600.

DiMascio, A., Haven, L.L., Klerman, G.L.: The psychopharmacology of phenothiazine compounds: a comparative study of the effects of chlorpromazine in normal males. *J. Nerv. Ment. Dis.* **136**, 15–28, 168–186, 1963.

DiMascio, A., Weissman, M.M., Prusoff, B.A., *et al.*: Differential symptom reduction by drugs and psychotherapy in acute depression. *Arch. Gen. Psychiatry* **36**, 1450–1456, 1979.

Dingemanse, J., Wood, N., Guentert, T., *et al.*: Clinical pharmacology of moclobemide during chronic administration of high doses to healthy subjects. *Psychopharmacology* **140**, 164–172, 1998.

Doody, R.S., Stevens, J.C., Beck, C., *et al.*: Practice parameter: management of dementia (an evidence-based review). *Neurology* **56**, 1154–1166, 2001.

Doraiswamy, P.M., Krishnan, K.R.R., Anand, R., *et al.*: Long-term effects of rivastigmine in moderately severe Alzheimer's disease: does early initiation of therapy offer sustained benefits? *Prog. Neuro-Psychopharmacol. Biol. Psychiatry* **26**, 705–712, 2002.

Dörner, K.: *Bürger und Irre. Zur Sozialgeschichte und Wissenschaftssoziologie der Psychiatrie.* Fischer, Frankfurt, 1975.

Doudet, D.J.: Monitoring disease progression in Parkinson's disease. *J. Clin. Pharmacol.* **41**(99), 72S–80S, 2001.

Doudet, D.J., Miyake, H., McLellan, C.A., *et al.*: 6-[18F]-L-Dopa imaging of the dopamine neostriatal system in normal and clinically normal MPTP-treated rhesus monkeys. *Exp. Brain Res.* **78**, 69–80, 1989.

Drummond, M.F., O'Brien, B., Stoddart, G.L., Torrance, G.W.: *Methods of the Economic Evaluation of Health Care Programmes*, 2nd edn. Oxford University Press, Oxford, 1997.

Druss, B.G., Hoff, R.A., Rosenheck, R.A.: Underuse of antidepressants in major depression: prevalence and correlates in a national sample of young adults. *J. Clin. Psychiatry* **61**, 234–237, 2000.

Duara, R., Gross-Glenn, K., Barker, W.W., *et al.*: Behavioral activation and the variability of cerebral glucose metabolic measurments. *J. Cereb. Blood Flow Metab.* **7**, 266–271, 1987.

Duerr, H. P.: *Traumzeit: über die Grenze zwischen Wildnis und Zivilisation.* Syndikat, Frankfurt, 1979.

Duffy, A.: Toward effective early intervention and prevention strategies for major affective disorders: a review of antecedents and risk factors. *Can. J. Psychiatry* **45**(4), 340–348, 2000.

Dugan, L., Fenton, M., Dardennes, R.M., El-Dosoky, A., Indran, S.: Olanzapine for schizophrenia (Cochrane Review). *Cochrane Library*, Issue 2. Update Software, Oxford, 2001.

Dulcan, M.: AACAP Guidelines: Practice parameters for the assessment and treatment of children, adolescents and adults with attention-deficit/hyperactivity disorder. *J. Am. Acad. Child Adolesc. Psychiatry* **36**, 85S–121S, 1997.

Dunner, D.L., Vijayalakshmy, P., Fieve, R.R.: Rapid cycling in manic depressive patients. *Comp. Psychiatry* **18**, 561–566, 1977.

ECDEU Assessment Manual. Guy, W., Bonato, R.B. (eds): US Department of Health, Education, and Welfare: National Institute of Mental Health. US Government Printing Office, 1976.

Egan, M.F., Goldberg, T.E., Gscheidle, T., *et al.*: Relative risk for cognitive impairments in siblings of patients with schizophrenia. *Biol. Psychiatry* **50**, 98–107, 2001.

Elia, J., Ambrosini, P.J., Rapoport, J.L.: Treatment of attention-deficit-hyperactivity disorder. *N. Engl. J. Med.* **340**, 780–788, 1999.

Elkin, I., Pilkonis, P.A., Docherty, J.P., Sotsky, S.M.: Conceptual and methodological issues in comparative studies of psychotherapy and pharmacotherapy. I: Active ingredients and mechanisms of change. *Am. J. Psychiatry* **145**, 909–917, 1988.

Elkin, I., Shea, T., Watkins, J.T., *et al.*: National Institute of Mental Health Treatment of Depression Collaborative Research Program. *Arch. Gen. Psychiatry* **46**, 971–982, 1989.

Elkin, I., Shea, T., Watkins, J.T., *et al.*: Initial severity and different treatment outcome in the National Institute of Mental Health treatment of depression collaborative research program. *J. Consult. Clin. Psychol.* **63**, 841–847, 1995.

Ellenbroek, B.A., Geyer, M.A., Cools, A.R.: The behavior of APO-SUS rats in animal models with construct validity for schizophrenia. *J. Neurosci.* **15**, 7604–7611, 1995.

Elomaa, A.: Long-term 'treatment' of schizophrenics with typical neuroleptics: a crime against humanity? *Med. Hypoth.* **41**, 434, 1993.

Engelsmann, F., Katz, J., Ghadirian, M., Schachter, D.: Lithium and memory: a long-term follow-up study. *J. Clin. Psychopharmacol.* **8**, 207–212, 1988.

Enz, A., Boddeke, H., Gray, J., Spiegel, R.: Pharmacologic and clinico-pharmacologic properties of SDZ ENA 713, a centrally selective acetylcholinesterase inhibitor. *Ann. NY Acad. Sci.* **640**, 272–275, 1991.

Ernst, M., Zametkin. A.J., Matochik, J., *et al.*: Intravenous dextroamphetamine and brain glucose metabolism. *Neuropsychopharmacology* **17**(6), 391–401, 1997.

Esquirol, J.E.D.: *Des maladies mentales*, 3 vols. Baillière, Paris, 1838.

EuroQol Group: EuroQol – a new facility for the measurement of health-related quality of life. *Healthy Policy* **16**(3), 199–208, 1990.

Eysenck, H.J.: *Experiments with Drugs*. Pergamon, Oxford, 1962.

Fairweather, D.B., Ashford, J., Hindmarch, I.: Effects of fluvoxamine and dothiepin on psychomotor abilities in healthy volunteers. *Pharmacol. Biochem. Behav.* **53**, 265–269, 1996.

Fairweather, D.B., Dal Pozzo, C., Kerr, J.S., *et al.*: Citalopram compared to dothiepin and placebo: effects on cognitive function and psychomotor performance. *Hum. Psychopharmacol.* **12**, 119–126, 1997.

Faraone, S.V., Biederman, J., Spencer, T., *et al.*: Attention-deficit/hyperactivity disorder in adults: an overview. *Biol. Psychiatry* **48**, 9–20, 2000.

Farde, L.: Brain imaging of schizophrenia – the dopamine hypothesis. *Schizophr. Res.* **28**(2/3), 157–162, 1997.

Farde, L., Suhara, T., Halldin, C., *et al.*: PET study of the M1-agonists [11C]xanomeline and [11C]butylthio-TZTP in monkey and man. *Dementia* **7**(4), 187–195, 1996.

Faries, D.E., Heiligenstein, J.H., Tollefson, G.D., Potter, W.B.: The double blind variable placebo lead-in period: results from two double blind placebo controlled trials. *J. Clin. Psychopharmacol.* **21**(6), 561–568, 2002.

Farlow, M., Gracon, S.I., Hershey, L.A., *et al.*: A controlled trial of tacrine in Alzheimer's disease. *J. Am. Med. Assoc.* **268**, 2523–2528, 1992.

Farmer, A.E., Blewett, A.: Drug treatment of resistant schizophrenia. *Drugs* **45**, 374–383, 1993.

Fatemi, S.H., Meltzer, H.Y., Roth, B.L.: Atypical antipsychotic drugs: clinical and preclinical studies. In: Csernansky, J.G. (ed.): *Experimental Handbook of Pharmacology, 'Antipsychotics'*. Springer Verlag, Berlin, 1996, pp. 77–115.

Fatemi, S.H., Rapport, D.J., Calabrese, J.R., Thuras, P.: Lamotrigine in rapid-cycling bipolar disorder. *J. Clin. Psychiatry* **58**, 522–527, 1997.

Fatemi, S.H., Emamian, E.S., Kist, D.: Venlafaxine and bupropion combination therapy in a case of treatment-resistant depression. *Ann. Pharmacother.* **33**, 701–703, 1999.

Fava, G.A., Kellner, R.: Prodromal symptoms in affective disorders. *Am. J. Psychiatry* **148**, 823–830, 1991.

Feighner, J.P., Overo, K.: Multicenter, placebo-controlled, fixed-dose study of citalopram in moderate-to-severe depression. *J. Clin. Psychiatry* **60**: 824–830, 1999.

Feldman, B., Wand, E., Willan, A., Szalai, J.P.: The randomized placebo-phase design for clinical trials. *J. Epidemiol.* **54**, 550–557, 2001.

Feltner, D.R., Kobal, K., Crockatt, J., *et al.*: Interactive voice response (IVR) for patients screening of anxiety in a clinical drug trial. NCDEU Poster Abstracts, www.nimh.nih.gov/ncdeu/abstracts2001.

Fenton, F.R., Tessier, L., Contrandriopoulos, A.P., Nguyer, H., Struening, E.L.: A comparative trial of home and hospital psychiatric treatment: financial costs. *Can. J. Psychiatry* **26**(3), 177–187, 1982.

Ferkarny, J.W.: Receptor binding. In: Enna, S.J., *et al.* (eds): *Current Protocols in Pharmacology*. Wiley, New York, 1998.

File, S.E.: The use of social interaction as a method for detecting anxiolytic activity of chlordiazepoxide-like drugs. *J. Neurosci. Methods* **2**: 219–238, 1980.

File, S.E.: Animal models for predicting clinical efficacy of anxiolytic drugs: social behaviour. *Neuropsychobiology* **13**, 55–62, 1985.

File, S.E.: Anxiolytic action of a neurokinin-1 receptor antagonist in the social interaction test. *Pharmacol. Biochem. Behav.* **58**, 747–752, 1997.

File, S.E.: NKP608, an NK1 receptor antagonist, has an anxiolytic action in the social interaction test in rats. *Psychopharmacology* **152**, 105–109, 2000.

Finger, S.: *Origins of Neuroscience: a History of Explorations into the Brain*. Oxford University Press, Oxford, 1994.

Fink, M.: Classification of psychoactive drugs: quantitative EEG analysis in man. In: Van Praag, H.M., *et al.* (eds): *Handbook of Biological Psychiatry*, Part VI. Marcel Dekker, New York, 1981, pp. 309–326.

First, M.B., Spitzer, R.L., Gibbon, M., Williams, J.B.W.: *Structured Clinical Interview for DSM-IV Axis I Disorders*. American Psychiatric Press, Washington, DC, 1997.

Fischer, A., Heldman, E., Gurwitz, D., *et al.*: M1 agonist for the treatment of Alzheimer's disease: novel properties and clinical update. *Ann. NY Acad. Sci.* **77**, 189–196, 1996.

Fleming, T.R., DeMets, D.L.: Surrogate end points in clinical trials: are we being misled? *Ann. Intern. Med.* **125**, 605–613, 1996.

Folstein, M.F., Folstein, S.E., McHugh, P.R.: Mini-Mental State: a practical method for grading the cognitive state of patients for the clinician. *J. Psychiatr. Res.* **12**, 189–201, 1975.

Foucault, M.: *Wahnsinn und Gesellschaft*, 3rd edn. Suhrkamp, Frankfurt, 1978.

Fowler, J.S., Volkow, N.D., Wang, G.J., *et al.*: Brain monoamine oxidase A inhibition in cigarette smokers. *Proc. Natl. Acad. Sci. USA* **93**(24), 14065–14069, 1996.

Fowler, J.S., Volkow, N.D., Wang, G.J., *et al.*: Visualization of monoamine oxidase in human brain. *Adv. Pharmacol.* **42**, 304–307, 1998.

Fowler, J.S., Volkow, N.D., Wang, G.-J., *et al.*: PET and drug research and development. *J. Nucl. Med.* **40**, 1154–1163, 1999.

Fox, N.C., Freeborough, P.A.: Brain atrophy progression measured from registered serial MRI: validation and application to Alzheimer's disease. *J. Magn. Res. Imag.* **7**, 1069–1075, 1997.

Fox, P.T., Miezin, F.M., Allman, J.M., *et al.*: Retinotopic organization of human visual cortex mapped with positron-emission tomography. *J. Neurosci.* **7**, 913–922, 1987.

Foy, A., O'Connell, D., Henry, D., *et al.*: Benzodiazepine use as a cause of cognitive impairment in elderly hospital inpatients. *J. Gerontol. Ser.* **50A**, M99–106, 1995.

Frankenburg, F.R.: History of the development of antipsychotic medication. *Psychiatr. Clin. North Am.* **17**, 531–546, 1994.

Freedman, A.M.: Psychopharmacology and psychotherapy in the treatment of anxiety. *Pharmakopsychiatrie* **13**, 277–289, 1980.

Freedman, B.: Equipoise and the ethics of clinical research. *N. Engl. J. Med.* **317**(3), 141–145, 1987.

Fresco, D.M., Coles, M.E., Heimberg, R.G., *et al.*: The Liebowitz Social Anxiety Scale: a comparison of the psychometric properties of self-report and clinician administered formats. *Psychol. Med.* **31**(6), 1025–1035, 2001.

Friedman, A.S.: Interaction of drug therapy with marital therapy in depressive patients. *Arch. Gen. Psychiatry* **32**, 619–637, 1975.

Frye, M., Ketter, T.A., Kimbrell, J.A., *et al*.: A placebo controlled study of lamotrigine and gabapentin monotherapy in refractory mood disorder. *J. Clin. Psychopharmacol.* **20**, 607–614, 2000.

Fujishiro, J., Imanishi, T., Baba, J., Kosaka, K.: Comparison of noradrenergic and serotonergic antidepressants in reducing immobility time in the tail suspension test. *Jap. J. Pharmacol.* **85**(3), 327–330, 2001.

Furlan, P.M., Kallan, M.J., Ten Have, T., *et al*.: Cognitive and psychomotor effects of paroxetine and sertraline on healthy elderly volunteers. *Am. J. Geriatr. Psychiatry* **9**, 429–438, 2001.

Gaertner, I., Gilot, C., Heidrich, P., Gaertner, H.J.: A case control study on psychopharmacotherapy before suicide committed by 61 psychiatric inpatients. *Pharmacopsychiatry* **35**(2), 37–43, 2002.

Gardos, G., Cole, J.O.: Maintenance antipsychotic therapy. For whom and how long? In: Lipton, M.A., Di Mascio, A., Killam, K.F. (eds): *Psychopharmacology: a Generation of Progress*. Raven, New York, 1978, pp. 1169–1178.

Garnett, E.S., Firnau, G., Chan, P.K., *et al*.: [18F]Fluoro-dopa an analogue of dopa, and its use in direct external measurements of storage, degradation, and turnover of intracerebral dopamine. *Proc. Natl. Acad. Sci. USA* **75**, 464–467, 1978.

Gastpar, M., Rimpel, J.: Klinik [der Beta-Rezeptoren-Blocker]. In: Riederer, P., Laux, G., Pöldinger, W. (eds): *Neuro-Psychopharmaka, Bd.6: Notfalltherapie, Antiepileptika, Beta-Rezeptoren-Blocker und sonstige Psychopharmaka*. Springer, Vienna, 1993, pp. 111–124.

Gauthier, S.: Long-term efficacy of cholinesterase inhibitors. *Brain Aging* **2**, 19–22, 2002.

Geddes, J., Freemantle, N., Harrison, P., Bebbington, P.: Atypical antipsychotics in the treatment of schizophrenia: systematic overview and meta-regression analysis. *Br. Med. J.* **321**, 1371–1376, 2000.

Geerlings, M.I., Schoevers, R.A., Beekman, A.T.F., *et al*.: Depression and the risk of cognitive decline and Alzheimer's disease. *Br. J. Psychiatry* **176**, 568–575, 2000.

Gefvert, O., Bergstrom, M., Langstrom, B., *et al*.: Time course of central nervous dopamine-D2 and 5-HT2 receptor blockade and plasma concentrations after discontinuation of quetiapine (Seroquel) in patients with schizophrenia. *Psychopharmacology* **135**, 119–126, 1998.

Gelernter, Ch.Sh., Uhde, T.W., Cimbolic, P., *et al*.: Cognitive–behavioral and pharmacological treatments of social phobia. *Arch. Gen. Psychiatry* **48**, 938–945, 1991.

Gelfin, Y., Gorfine, M., Lerer, B.: Effect of clinical doses of fluoxetine on psychological variables in healthy volunteers. *Am. J. Psychiatry* **155**, 290–292, 1998.

Genton, P., Gelisse, Ph.: Valproic acid – adverse effects. In: Levy, R.H., Mattson, R.H., Meldrum, B.S., Perucca, E. (eds): *Antiepileptic Drugs*, 5th edn. Lippincott Williams & Wilkins, Philadelphia, 2002, pp. 837–854.

Gentsch, C., Lichtsteiner, M., Feer, H.: Locomotor activity, defecation score and corticosterone levels during an openfield exposure: a comparison among individually and group-housed rats, and genetically selected rat lines. *Physiol. Behav.* **27**, 183–186, 1981.

Gentsch, C., Lichtsteiner, M., Feer, H.: Genetic and environmental influences on behavioral and neurochemical aspects of emotionality in rats. *Experientia* **44**, 482–490, 1988.

Gentsch, C., Cutler, M., Vassout, A., *et al.*: Anxiolytic effect of NKP608, a NK1-receptor antagonist, in the social investigation test in gerbils. *Behav. Brain Res.* **133**, 363–368, 2002.

George, K.A., Dundee, J.W.: Relative amnesic actions of diazepam, flunitrazepam and lorazepam in man. *Br. J. Clin. Pharmacol.* **4**, 45–50, 1977.

Ghoneim, M.M.: The reversal of benzodiazepine-induced amnesia by flumazenil: a review. *Curr. Ther. Res.* **52**, 757–767, 1992.

Ghoneim, M.M., Mewaldt, S.P.: Benzodiazepines and human memory: a review. *Anesthesiology* **72**, 926–938, 1990.

Ghoneim, M.M., Hinrichs, J.V., Mewaldt, S.P.: Dose–response analysis of the behavioral effects of diazepam: I. Learning and memory. *Psychopharmacology* **82**, 291–295, 1984a.

Ghoneim, M.M., Mewaldt, S.P., Hinrichs, J.V.: Dose–response analysis of the behavioral effects of diazepam: II. Psychomotor performance, cognition and mood. *Psychopharmacology* **82**, 296–300, 1984b.

Giacobini, E.: Cholinesterase inhibitor therapy stabilizes symptoms of Alzheimer disease. *Alzheimer Dis. Assoc. Disord.* **14** (Suppl. 1), S3–S10, 2000.

Gibbons, R.D., Clark, D.C., Kupfer, D.J.: Exactly what does the Hamilton Depression Rating Scale measure? *J. Psychiatr. Res.* **27**, 259–273, 1993.

Gilbert, P.L., Harris, M.J., McAdams, L.A., Jeste, D.V.: Neuroleptic withdrawal in schizophrenic patients. *Arch. Gen. Psychiatry* **52**, 173–187, 1995.

Gillberg, Ch., Melander, H., von Knorring, A.-L., *et al.*: Long-term stimulant treatment of children with attention-deficit hyperactivity symptoms. *Arch. Gen. Psychiatry* **54**, 857–864, 1997.

Gillin, J.Ch., Sitaram, N.: Rapid eye movement (REM) sleep: cholinergic mechanisms. *Psychol. Med.* **14**, 501–506, 1984.

Gittelman Klein, R.: Pharmacotherapy of childhood hyperactivity: an update. In: Meltzer, H.Y. (ed.): *Psychopharmacology: the Third Generation of Progress*. Raven, New York, 1987, pp. 1215–1224.

Goddard, A.W., Woods, S.W., Money, R., *et al.*: Effects of the CCK(B) antagonist CI-988 on responses to mCPP in generalized anxiety disorder. *Psychiatry Res.* **85**(3), 225–240, 1999.

Gold, M.R., Siegel, J.E., Russell, L.B., Weinstein, M.C.: *Cost-effectiveness in Health and Medicine*, Oxford University Press, New York, 1996.

Goldstein, D.J., Mallickrodt, C., Lu, Y., Demitrack, M.A.: Duloxetine in the treatment of major depressive disorder: a double blind clinical trial. *J. Clin Psychiatry* **63**, 225–231, 2002.

Golombok, S., Moodley, P. Lader, M.: Cognitive impairment in long-term benzodiaepine users. *Psychol. Med.* **18**, 365–374, 1988.

Goodmann, W.K., Price, L.D., Rasmussen, S.A., *et al.*: The Yale–Brown Obsessive Compulsive Scale: I. Development, use and reliability. *Arch. Gen. Psychiatry* **46**(11), 1006–1011, 1989.

Goodwin, F.K., Roy-Byrne, P.P.: Future directions in biological psychiatry. In: Meltzer, H.Y. (ed.): *Psychopharmacology: the Third Generation of Progress*. Raven, New York, 1987, pp. 1691–1698.

Gray, J.R., Kagan, J.: The challenge of predicting which children with attention deficit-hyperactivity disorder will respond positively to methylphenidate. *J. Appl. Dev. Psychol.* **21**, 471–489, 2000.

Green, M.F.: Recent studies on the neurocognitive effects of second-generation antipsychotic medications. *Curr. Opin. Psychiatry* **15**, 25–29, 2002.

Green, M.F., Marder, S.R., Glynn, S.M., *et al.*: The neurocognitive effects of low-dose haloperidol: a two-year comparison with risperidone. *Biol. Psychiatry* **51**, 972–978, 2002.

Greenblatt, D.J., Harmatz, J.S., Gouthro, T.A., *et al.*: Distinguishing a benzodiazepine agonist (triazolam) from a nonagonist anxiolytic (buspirone) by electroencephalography: kinetic-dynamic studies. *Clin. Pharmacol. Ther.* **56**, 100–111, 1994.

Greenblatt, D.J., Patki, K.C., Von Moltke, L.L., Shader, R.I.: Drug interactions with grapefruit juice: an update. *J. Clin. Psychopharmacol.* **21**, 357–359, 2001.

Greenhill, L.L., Halperin, J.M., Abikoff, H.: Stimulant medications. *J. Am. Acad. Child Adolesc. Psychiatry* **38**, 503–512, 1999.

Greil, W., Van Calker, D.: Lithium: Grundlagen und Therapie. In: Langer, G., Heimann, H. (eds): *Psychopharmaka. Grundlagen und Therapie.* Springer, Vienna, 1983, pp. 161–202.

Griesinger, W.: *Die Pathologie and Therapie der psychischen Krankheiten,* Zweite Auflage, Stuttgart, 1861.

Griffiths, R.R., Sannerud, Ch.A.: Abuse of and dependence on benzodiazepines and other anxiolytic sedative drugs. In: Meltzer, H.Y. (ed.): *Psychopharmacology: the Third Generation of Progress.* Raven, New York, 1987, pp. 1535–1541.

Gross, H., Langner, E.: Das Wirkungsprofil eines chemisch neuartigen Breitband-Neuroleptikums der Dibenzodiazepingruppe. *Wien. Med. Wochenschr.* **116**, 614–621, 1966.

Grunder, G., Yokoi, F., Offord, S.J., *et al.*: Time course of 5-HT2A receptor occupancy in the human brain after a single oral dose of the putative antipsychotic drug MDL 100,907 measured by positron emission tomography. [erratum appears in *Neuropsychopharmacology* **19**(2), 161, 1998]. *Neuropsychopharmacology* **17**(3), 175–185, 1997.

Hamilton, M.: The assessment of anxiety states by rating. *Br. J. Med. Psychol.* **32**, 50–55, 1959.

Hamilton, S.H., Revicki, D.A., Genduso, L.A., *et al.*: Olanzapine versus placebo and haloperidol: quality of life and efficacy results of the North American double-blind trial. *Neuropsychopharmacology* **18**, 41–49, 1998.

Hamon, J., Paraire, J., Velluz, J.: Remarques sur l'action du 4560 RP sur l'agitation maniaque. *Ann. Med. Psychol.* **110**, 331–335, 1952.

Hanano, M., Matsuoka, K., Tomotake, M., *et al.*: The acute effects of antidepressants on the human SEP (somatosensory evoked potential) and EEG. *Shikoku Acta Med.* **53**, 83–90, 1997.

Hanlon, J.T., Horner, R.D., Schmader, K.E., *et al.*: Benzodiazepine use and cognitive function among community-dwelling elderly. *Clin. Pharmacol. Ther.* **64**, 684–692, 1998.

Hanyu, H., Tanaka, Y., Sakurai, H., Takasaki, M., Abe, K.: Atrophy of the substantia innominata on magnetic resonance imaging and response to donepezil treatment in Alzheimer's disease. *Neurosci. Lett.* **319**(1), 33–36, 2002.

Hardy, J., Selkoe, D.J.: The amyloid hypothesis of Alzheimer's disease: progress and problems on the road to therapeutics. *Science* **297**, 353–356, 2002.

Harmer, C.J., Bhagwagar, Z., Cowen, P.J., Goodwin, G.M.: Acute administration of citalopram facilitates memory consolidation in healthy volunteers. *Psychopharmacology* **163**, 106–110, 2002.

Harvey, P.D., Keefe, R.S.E.: Studies of cognitive change in patients with schizophrenia following novel antipsychotic treatment. *Am. J. Psychiatry* **158**, 176–184, 2001.

Hatziandreu, E.J., Brown, R.E., Revicki, D.A., et al.: Cost utility of maintenance treatment of recurrent depression with sertraline versus episodic treatment with dothiepin. Pharmacoeconomics 5, 249–268, 1994.

Healy, D.: The Psychopharmacologists III. Arnold, London, 2000, pp. xiii–xxiii.

Heaton, R.K., Gladsjo, J.A., Palmer, B.W., et al.: Stability and course of neuropsychological deficits in schizophrenia. Arch. Gen. Psychiatry 58, 24–32, 2001.

Hegerl, U., Herrmann, W.M., Ulrich, G., Müller-Oerlinghausen, B.: Effects of lithium on auditory evoked potentials in healthy subjects. Biol. Psychiatry 27, 552–555, 1990.

Heiberg, J.L.: Geisteskrankheiten im klassischen Altertum. De Gruyter, Berlin, 1927.

Heimberg, R.G., Horner, K.J., Safren, S.A., et al.: Psychometric properties of the Liebowitz Social Anxiety Scale. Psychol. Med. 29(1), 199–212, 1999.

Heinrich, K.: Psychopharmaka in Klinik und Praxis. Thieme, Stuttgart, 1976.

Heinrichs, D.W., Hanlon, T.E., Carpenter, W.T.: The Quality of Life Scale: an instrument for rating the schizophrenic deficit syndrome. Schizophr. Bull. 10, 388–398, 1984.

Helsinki Declaration: Declaration of Helsinki recommendations guiding doctors in clinical research. Fed. Reg. 40(69), 16056, 1975.

Henderson, A.S.: Epidemiology of mental illness. In: Häfner, L., Moschel, G., Sartorius, N. (eds): Mental Health in the Elderly. Springer, Berlin, 1986, pp. 29–34.

Henry, M.E., Moore, C.M., Kaufman, M.J., et al.: Brain kinetics of paroxetine and fluoxetine on the third day of placebo substitution: a fluorine MRS study. Am. J. Psychiatry 157(9), 1506–1508, 2000.

Henry, M.E., Kaufman, M.J., Lange, N., et al.: Test–retest reliability of DSC MRI CBV mapping in healthy volunteers. NeuroReport 12(8), 1567–1569, 2001.

Heresco-Lewy, U., Javitt, D.C., Ermilov, M., et al.: Double-blind, placebo-controlled, crossover trial of glycine adjuvant therapy for treatment-resistant schizophrenia. Br. J. Psychiatry 169, 610–617, 1996.

Hersen, M.: Pharmacological and behavioral treatment: an Integrative Approach. Wiley, New York, 1986.

Herz, M.I., Melville, Ch.: Relapse in schizophrenia. Am. J. Psychiatry 137, 801–805, 1980.

Heyman, A., Fillenbaum, G., Nash, F.: Consortium to establish a registry for Alzheimer's disease. Neurology 49 (Suppl. 3), S1–S23, 1997.

Hillyard, S.A., Kutas, M.: Electrophysiology of cognitive processing. Annu. Rev. Psychol. 34, 33–61, 1983.

Hindmarch, I.: Cognition and anxiety: the cognitive effects of anti-anxiety medication. Acta Psychiatr. Scand. 98 (Suppl. 393), 89–94, 1998.

Hindmarch, I., Coleston, D.M., Kerr, J.S.: Psychopharmacological effects of pyritinol in normal volunteers. Neuropsychobiology 24, 159–164, 1990.

Hinterhuber, H., Haring, Ch.: Unerwünschte Wirkungen, Kontraindikationen, Überdosierungen, Intoxikationen [von Neuroleptika]. In: Riederer, P., Laux, G., Pöldinger, W. (eds): Neuro-Psychopharmaka, Bd. 4: Neuroleptika. Springer, Vienna, 1992, pp. 102–121.

Ho, P.C., Saville, D.J.: Inhibition of human CYP3A4 activity by grapefruit flavenoids, furanocoumarins and related compounds. J. Pharm. Pharmaceut. Sci. 4, 217–227, 2001.

Hogarty, G., Goldberg, S.: Drug and sociotherapy in the aftercare of schizophrenic patients: one year relapse rates. Arch. Gen. Psychiatry 28, 54–64, 1973.

Hogarty, G.E., Ulrich, R., Goldberg, S., Schooler, N.: Sociotherapy and the prevention of relapse among schizophrenic patients: an artifact of drug? In: Spitzer, R.I., Klein,

D.F. (eds): *Evaluation of Psychological Therapies.* Johns Hopkins University Press, Baltimore, 1976, pp. 285–293.

Hohagen, F., Riemann, D., Spiegel, R., *et al.*: Influence of the cholinergic agonist SDZ 210-086 on sleep in healthy subjects. *Neuropsychopharmacology* **9**, 225–232, 1993.

Hohol, M.J., Guttmann, C.R.G., Orav, J., *et al.*: Serial neuropsychological assessment and MRI analysis in multiple sclerosis. *Arch. Neurol.* **54**, 1018–1025, 1997.

Hollister, L.E.: Tricyclic antidepressants (second of two parts). *N. Engl. J. Med.* **299**, 1168–1172, 1978.

Hollister, L.E., Jones, J.K., Fisher, S.: Post-marketing surveillance of drugs. In: Prien, R.F., Robinson, D.S. (eds): *Clinical Evaluation of Psychotropic Drugs.* Raven Press, New York, 1994, pp. 217–235.

Hollon, St.D., Shelton, R.C., Loosen, P.T.: Cognitive therapy and pharmacotherapy for depression. *J. Consult. Clin. Psychol.* **59**, 88–99, 1991.

Hollon, St.D., DeRubeis, R.J., Evans, M.D., *et al.*: Cognitive therapy and pharmacotherapy for depression. *Arch. Gen. Psychiatry* **49**, 774–781, 1992.

Holmes, A.: Targeted gene mutation approaches to the study of anxiety-like behavior in mice. *Neurosci. Biobehav. Rev.* **25**, 261–273, 2001.

Holsboer, F.: The corticosteroid receptor hypothesis of depression. *Neuropsychopharmacology* **23**, 477–501, 2000.

Holsboer-Trachsler, E., Hatzinger, M., Stohler, R., *et al.*: Effects of the novel acetylcholinesterase inhibitor SDZ ENA 713 on sleep in man. *Neuropsychopharmacology* **8**, 87–92, 1993.

Holttum, J.R., Gershon, S.: The cholinergic model of dementia, Alzheimer type: progression from the unitary transmitter concept. *Dementia* **3**, 174–185, 1992.

Hoozemans, J.J.M., Veerhuis, R., Rozemuller, A.J.M., Eikelenboom, P.: The pathological cascade of Alzheimer's disease: the role of inflammation and its therapeutic implications. *Drugs Today* **38**, 429–443, 2002.

Hordern, A.: Psychopharmacology: some historical considerations. In: Joyce, C.R.B. (ed.): *Psychopharmacology: Dimensions and Perspectives.* Tavistock, London, 1968, pp. 95–148.

Huang, S.C., Phelps, M.E.: Principles of tracer kinetic modeling in positron emission tomography and autoradiography. In: Phelps, M.E., Mazziota, J., Schelbert, H. (eds): *Positron Emission Tomography and Autoradiography: Principles and Applications for the Brain and Heart.* Raven Press, New York, 1986.

Hypericum Depression Trial Study Group: Effect of *Hypericum perforatum* (St John's wort) in major depresssive disorder. *J. Am. Med. Assoc.* **287**, 1807–1814, 2002.

Ichim, L., Berk, M., Brook, S.: Lamotrigine compared with lithium in mania: a double-blind randomized controlled trial. *Am. J. Clin. Psychiatry* **12**, 5–10, 2000.

In't Veld, B.A., Ruitenberg, A., Hofman, A., *et al.*: Nonsteroidal antiinflammatory drugs and the risk of Alzheimer's disease. *N. Engl. J. Med.* **345**, 1515–1521, 2001.

Isacsson, G., Boëthius, G., Bergman, U.: Low level of antidepressant prescription for people who later commit suicide: 15 years of experience from a population-based drug database in Sweden. *Acta Psychiatr. Scand.* **85**, 444–448, 1992.

Itil, T.M.: The discovery of psychotropic drugs by computer-analyzed cerebral bioelectrical potentials (CEEG). *Drug Dev. Res.* **1**, 373–407, 1981.

Jablensky, A.: Prediction of the course and outcome of depression. *Psychol. Med.* **17**, 1–9, 1987.

Jacobs, B.L., van Praag, H., Gage, F.H.: Adult brain neurogenesis and psychiatry: a novel theory of depression. *Mol. Psychiatry* **5**, 262–269, 2000.

Jacobsen, J.S.: Alzheimer's disease: an overview of current and emerging therapeutic strategies. *Curr. Top. Med. Chem.* **2**, 343–352, 2002.

Janicak, Ph.G., Davis, J.M., Preskorn, S.H., Ayd, F.J.: *Principles and Practice of Psychopharmacotherapy*. Williams & Wilkins, Baltimore, 1993.

Janicak, P.G., Davis, J.M., Preskorn, S.H., Ayd, F.J., Jr.: *Principles and Practice of Psychopharmacotherapy*, 3rd edn. Lippincot, Williams & Wilkins, Philadelphia, 2001.

Janke, W.: *Experimentelle Untersuchungen zur Abhängigkeit der Wirkungen psychotroper Substanzen von Persönlichkeitsmerkmalen*. Akad. Verlagsgesellschaft, Frankfurt, 1964.

Janke, W., Debus, G.: Experimental studies on antianxiety agents with normal subjects: methodological considerations and review of the main effects. In: Efron, D.H., Cole, J.O., Levine, J.R., Wittenborn, J.R. (eds): *Psychopharmacology: a Review of Progress 1957–1967*. US Public Health Service Publication No. 1836. US Government Printing Office, Washington, DC, 1968, pp. 205–230.

Janke, W., Erdmann, G.: Pharmakopsychiatrie. In: Riederer, P., Laux, G., Pöldinger, W. (eds): *Neuro-Psychopharmaka*, Vol. I. Springer, Vienna, 1992, pp. 109–130.

Jann, M.W., Shirley, K.L., Small, G.W.: Clinical pharmacokinetics and pharmacodynamics of cholinesterase inhibitors. *Clin. Pharmacokin.* **41**, 719–739, 2002.

Jensen, P.S., Hinshaw, S.P., Swanson, J.M., *et al.*: Findings from the NIMH Multimodal Treatment study of ADHD (MTA): implications and applications for primary care providers. *J. Dev. Behav. Pediatr.* **22**, 60–73, 2001.

Jeste, D.V., Gillin, Ch., Wyatt, R.J.: Serendipity in biological psychiatry: a myth? *Arch. Gen. Psychiatry* **36**, 1173–1178, 1979.

Jetty, P.V., Cahrney, D.S., Goddard, A.W.: Neurobiology of generalized anxiety disorder. *Psychiatr. Clin. North Am.* **24**(1), 75–97, 2001.

Joffe, R.T., MacDonald, C., Kutcher, S.P.: Lack of differential cognitive effects of lithium and carbamazepine in bipolar affective disorder. *J. Clin. Psychopharmacol.* **8**, 425–428, 1988.

John, E.R., Prichep, L.S., Alper, K.L., *et al.*: Quantitative electrophysiological characteristics and subtyping of schizophrenia. *Biol. Psychiatry* **36**, 801–826, 1994.

Jonkman, L.M., Kemner, C., Verbaten, M.N., *et al.*: Attentional capacity, a probe ERP study: differences between children with attention-deficit hyperactivity disorder and normal control children and effects of methylphenidate. *Psychophysiology* **37**, 334–346, 2000.

Jorgensen, P.: Early signs of psychotic relapse in schizophrenia. *Br. J. Psychiatry* **172**, 327–330, 1998.

Judd, L.L., Squire, L.R., Butters, N., Salmon, D.P., Paller, K.A.: Effects of psychotropic drugs on cognition and memory in normal humans and animals. In: Meltzer, H. (ed.): *Psychopharmacology: the Third Generation of Progress*. Raven, New York, 1987, pp. 1467–1475.

Kane, J.M., Smith, J.M.: Tardive dyskinesia. *Arch. Gen. Psychiatry* **39**, 473–481, 1982.

Kane, J.M., Lieberman, J.A.: Maintenance therapy in schizophrenia. In: Meltzer, H.Y. (ed.): *Psychopharmacology: the Third Generation of Progress*. Raven, New York, 1987, pp. 1103–1109.

Kane, J. M., Honigfeld, G., Singer, J., Meltzer, H.: Clozapine for the treatment-resistant schizophrenic: a double-blind comparison with chlorpromazine. *Arch. Gen. Psychiatry* **45**, 789–796, 1988.

Kapur, S., McClelland, R.A., VanderSpek, S.C., *et al.*: *NeuroReport* **13**, 831–834, 2002.

Karasu, T.B.: Psychotherapy and pharmacotherapy: toward an integrative model. *Am. J. Psychiatry* **139**, 1102–1113, 1982.

Karoum, F., Karson, C. N., Bigelov, L.B., Lawson, W.B., Wyatt, R.J.: Preliminary evidence of reduced combined output of dopamine and its metabolites in chronic schizophrenia. *Arch. Gen. Psychiatry* **44**, 604–607, 1987.

Katzman, R.: Alzheimer's disease. *N. Engl. J. Med.* **314**, 964–973, 1986.

Kauffmann, J.M., Hallahan, D.P.: Learning disability and hyperactivity (with comments on minimal brain dysfunction). In: Lahey, B.B., Kazoin, A.E. (eds): *Advances in Clinical Child Psychology*, Vol. 2. Plenum, New York, 1979, pp. 71–105.

Kaufman, M.J., Levin, J.M., Maas, L.C., et al. Cocaine decreases relative cerebral blood volume in humans: a dynamic susceptibility contrast magnetic resonance imaging study. *Psychopharmacology* **138**(1), 76–81, 1998.

Kay, S.R., Sandyk, R.: Experimental models of schizophrenia. *Int. J. Neurosci.* **58**(1/2), 69–82, 1991.

Kay, S.R., Opler, L.A., Fiszbein, A.: Significance of positive and negative syndromes in chronic schizophrenia. *Br. J. Psychiatry* **149**, 439–448, 1986.

Kay, S.R., Fiszbein, A., Opler, L.A.: The positive and negative syndrome scale (PANSS) for schizophrenia. *Schizophr. Bull.* **13**, 261–276, 1987.

Keck, P.E., McElroy, S.L.: Pharmacologic treatments for bipolar disorder. In: Nathan, P.E., Gorman, J.M. (eds): *A Guide to Treatments that Work*. Oxford University Press, New York, 2002, pp. 277–299.

Keck, P.E., Cohen, B.M., Baldessarini, R.J., McElroy, S.L.: Time course of antipsychotic effects of neuroleptic drugs. *Am. J. Psychiatry* **146**, 1289–1292, 1989.

Keck, P.E., McElroy, S.L., Nemeroff, C.B.: Anticonvulsants in the treatment of bipolar disorder. *J. Neuropsychiatry Clin. Neurosci.* **4**, 595–605, 1992.

Keck, P.E., Welt, T., Wigger, A., et al.: The anxiolytic effect of the CRH1 receptor antagonist R121919 depends on innate emotionality in rats. *Eur. J. Neurosci.* **13**, 373–380, 2001.

Kegeles, L.S., Martinez, D., Kochan, L.D., et al.: NMDA antagonist effects on striatal dopamine release: positron emission tomography studies in humans. *Synapse* **43**(1), 19–29, 2002.

Kellam, A.M.P.: The (frequently) neuroleptic (potentially) malignant syndrome. *Br. J. Psychiatry* **157**, 169–173, 1990.

Keller, M.B., Klerman, G.L., Lavori, P.W., et al.: Treatment received by depressed patients. *J. Am. Med. Assoc.* **248**, 1848–1855, 1982.

Keller, M.B., McCullough, J.P., Klein, D.N., et al.: A comparison of nefazodone, the cognitive-behavioral-analysis system of psychotherapy and their combination for the treatment of chronic depression. *N. Engl. J. Med.* **342**, 1462–1470, 2000.

Kelly, D.: Clinical review of beta-blockers in anxiety. *Pharmakopsychiatrie* **13**, 259–266, 1980.

Kennedy, S.H., Evans, K.R., Kruger, S., et al.: Changes in regional brain glucose metabolism measured with positron emission tomography after paroxetine treatment of major depression. *Am. J. Psychiatry* **158**(6), 899–905, 2001.

Kennedy, S.H., McIntyre, R., Fallu, A., Lam, R.: Pharmacotherapy to sustain the fully remitted state. *J. Psychiatry Neurosci.* **27**, 269–280, 2002.

Keshavan, M.S., Rosenberg, D., Sweeney, J.A., Pettegrew, J.W.: Decreased caudate volume in neuroleptic naïve psychotic patients. *Am. J. Psychiatry* **155**, 774–778, 1998.

Kety, S.S., Schmidt, C.F.: The nitrous oxide method for the quantitative determination of cerebral blood flow in man: theory, procedure, and normal values. *J. Clin. Invest.* **27**, 476–483, 1948.

Khan, A., Khan, S., Brown, W.A.: Are placebo controls necessary to test new antidepressants and anxiolytics? *Int. J. Neuropsychopharmacol.* **5**(3), 193–197, 2002.

Kilts, C.D.: The changing roles and targets for animal models of schizophrenia. *Biol. Psychiatry* **50**, 845–855, 2001.

King, D.J.: Benzodiazepines, amnesia and sedation: theoretical and clinical issues and controversies. *Hum. Psychopharmacol.* **7**, 79–87, 1992.

King, D. J., Henry, G.: The affect of neuroleptics on cognitive and psychomotor function: a preliminary study in healthy volunteers. *Br. J. Psychiatry* **160**, 647–653, 1992.

King, D.J., Burke, M., Lucas, R.A.: Antipsychotic drug-induced dysphoria. *Br. J. Psychiatry* **167**, 480–482, 1995.

Kinosian, B.P., Eisenberg, J.M.: Cutting into cholesterol. Cost-effective alternatives for treating hypercholesterolemia. *J. Am. Med. Assoc.* **259**(15), 2249–2254, 1988.

Kirchhoff, Th.: Geschichte der Psychiatrie. In: Aschaffenburg, G. (ed.): *Handbuch der Psychiatrie*, Bd. I. Deuticke, Vienna, 1912.

Kissling, W.: The current unsatisfactory state of relapse prevention in schizophrenic psychoses: suggestions for improvement. *Clin. Neuropharmacol.* **14**, 33–44, 1991.

Klein, D.F.: False suffocation alarms, spontaneous panics, and related conditions. An integrative hypothesis. *Arch. Gen. Psychiatry* **50**, 306–317, 1993.

Klein, D.F.: Flawed meta-analyses comparing psychotherapy with pharmacotherapy. *Am. J. Psychiatry* **157**, 1204–1211, 2000.

Klerman, G.L.: Future prospects for clinical psychopharmacology. In: Meltzer, H.Y. (ed.): *Psychopharmacology: the Third Generation of Progress*. Raven, New York, 1987, pp. 1699–1705.

Klerman, G.L., Weissman, M.M.: The course, morbidity, and costs of depression. *Arch. Gen. Psychiatry* **49**, 831–834, 1992.

Klerman, G.L., DiMascio, A., Weissman, M., Prusoff, B., Paykel, E.S.: Treatment of depression by drugs and psychotherapy. *Am. J. Psychiatry* **131**, 186–191, 1974.

Klerman, G.L., Weissman, M.M., Prusoff, B.A.: RDC endogenous depression as a predictor of response to antidepressant drugs and psychotherapy. In: Costa, E., Racagni, G. (eds): *Typical and Atypical Antidepressants: Clinical Practice*. Raven, New York, 1982, pp. 165–174.

Klerman, G.L., Weissman, M.M., Rounsaville, B.J., Chevron, E.S.: *Interpersonal Psychotherapy of Depression*. Basic Books, New York, 1984.

Kline, N.S.: Monoamine oxydase inhibitors: an unfinished picaresque tale. In: Ayd, F.J., Blackwell, B. (eds): *Discoveries in Biological Psychiatry*. Lippincott, Philadelphia, 1970, pp. 194–204.

Klorman, R., Brumaghim, J.T., Fitzpatrick, P.A., *et al.*: Clinical and cognitive effects of methylphenidate on children with attention deficit disorder as a function of aggression/oppositionality and age. *J. Abnorm. Psychol.* **103**, 206–221, 1994.

Kobak, K.A., Greist, J.H., Jefferson, J.W., Katzelnick, D.J.: Fluoxetine in social phobia: a double-blind, placebo controlled pilot study. *J. Clin. Psychopharmacol.* **22**, 257–262, 2002.

Koelega, H.S.: Benzodiazepines and vigilance performance: a review. *Psychopharmacology* **98**, 145–156, 1989.

Koelega, H.S.: Stimulant drugs and vigilance performance: a review. *Psychopharmacology* **111**, 1–16, 1993.

Kohnen, R.: Über die Beeinflussung sozialer Verhaltensweisen durch Pharmaka. Bausteine einer Sozio-Pharmakopsychologie. In: Oldigs-Kerber, J., Leonard, J.P. (eds): *Pharmakopsychologie experimentelle und klinische Aspekte*. G. Fischer, Jena, 1992, pp. 201–215.

Kolbitsch, C., Lorenz, I.H., Hoermann, C., *et al.*: Sevoflurane and nitrous oxide increase regional blood-flow (rCBF) and regional cerebral blood volume (rCBV) in a drug-specific manner in human volunteers. *Magn. Reson. Imag.* **19**, 1253–1260, 2001.

Kovacs, M.: The efficacy of cognitive and behavior therapies for depression. *Am. J. Psychiatry* **137**, 1495–1501, 1980.

Kraemer, H.C.: Methodological and statistical progress in psychiatric clinical research: a statistician's perspective: In: Bloom, F.E., Kupfer, D.J.: *Psychopharmacology: the Fourth Generation of Progress.* Raven Press, New York, 1994, pp. 1849–1860.

Kraepelin, E.: *Über die Beeinflussung einfacher psychischer Vorgänge durch einige Arzneimittel.* John Ambrosius Barth, Jena, 1892.

Kraepelin, E.: *Psychiatrie.* Bd.I: Allgemeine Psychiatrie, sechste Auflage. Leipzig, 1899.

Kramer, M., Cutler, N., Feighner, J., *et al.*: Distinct mechanism for antidepressant activity by blockade of central substance P receptors. *Science* **281**, 1640–1645, 1998.

Krawiecka, M., Goldberg, A., Vaughan, M.: A standardized psychiatric assessment scale, for rating chronic psychiatric patients. *Acta Psychiatr. Scand.* **55**(4), 299–308, 1977.

Kuhn, R.: Über die Behandlung depressiver Zustände mit einem Iminodibenzylderivat (G22355). *Schweiz. Med. Wochenschr.* **87**, 1135–1140, 1957.

Kuhn, R.: The imipramine story. In: Ayd, P.J., Blackwell, B. (eds): *Discoveries in Biological Psychiatry.* Lippincott, Philadelphia, 1970, pp. 205–217.

Kunsman, G.W., Manno, J.E., Manno, B.R., Kunsman, C.M., Przekop, M.A.: The use of microcomputer-based psychomotor tests for the evaluation of benzodiazepine effects on human performance: a review with emphasis on temazepam. *Br. J. Clin. Pharmacol.* **34**, 289–301, 1992.

Kupfer, D.J., Frank, E.: The interaction of drug and psychotherapy in the long-term treatment of depression. *J. Affect. Disord.* **62**, 131–137, 2001.

Kupfer, D.J., Frank, E., Perel., J.M., *et al.*: Five-year outcome for maintenance therapies in recurrent depression. *Arch. Gen. Psychiatry* **49**, 769–773, 1992.

Labhardt, F.: Die Largactiltherapie bei Schizophrenien und anderen psychotischen Zuständen. *Schweiz. Arch. Neurol. Psychiatr.* **73**, 309–338, 1954.

Laborit, H., Huguenard, P., Alluaume, R.: Un nouveau stabilisateur végétatif (le 4560 R.P.). *Presse Med.* **60**, 206–208, 1952.

Lader, M.: Clinical anxiety and the benzodiazepines. In: Palmer, G.C. (ed.): *Neuropharmacology of Nervous System and Behavioural Disorders.* Academic Press, New York, 1981, pp. 225–241.

Lader, M.: Maintaining response to antidepressants. *Primary Care Psychiatry* **7**, 75–78, 2001.

Lader, M., Petursson, H.: Rational use of anxiolytic/sedative drugs. *Drugs* **25**, 514–528, 1983.

Lammertsma, A.A., Hume, S.P.: Simplified reference tissue model for PET receptor studies. *Neuroimage* **4**, 153–158, 1996.

Lane, D.A.: Utility, decision and quality of life. *J. Chron. Dis.* **40**(6), 585–591, 1987.

Lane, R., O'Hanlon, J.F.: Cognitive and psychomotor effects of antidepressants with emphasis on selective serotonin reuptake inhibitors and the depressed elderly patient. *Germ. J. Psychiatry* **2**, 1–28, 1999.

Latz, A.: Cognitive test performance of normal human adults under the influence of psychopharmacological agents: a brief review. In: Efron, D.H., Cole, J.O., Levine, J., Wittenborn, J.R. (eds): *Psychopharmacology: Review of Progress, 1957–1967*, US Public Health Service Publication No. 1836. US Government Printing Office, Washington, DC, 1968, pp. 83–90.

Laughren, T.P.: The scientific and ethical basis for placebo-controlled trials in depression and schizophrenia: an FDA perspective. *Eur. Psychiatry* **16**, 418–423, 2001.

Lavoie, K.L., Fleet, R.P.: Should psychologists be granted prescription privileges? A review of the prescription privilege debate for psychiatrists. *Can. J. Psychiatry* **47**, 443–449, 2002.

Leber, P.: Is there an alternative to the randomized controlled trial? *Psychopharmacol. Bull.*. **27**, 3–8, 1991.

Lecci, A., Borsini, F., Voltera, G., Meli, A.: Pharmacological validation of a novel model of anticipatory anxiety in mice. *Psychopharmacology* **101**, 255–261, 1990.

Leenders, K.L., Palmer, A.J., Quinn, N., Clark, J.C., Firnau, G., Garnett, E.S., Nahmias, C., Jones, T., Marsden, C.D.: Brain dopamine metabolism in patients with Parkinson's disease measured with positron emission tomography. *J. Neurol. Neurosurg. Psychiatry* **49**, 853–860, 1986.

Leff, J., Kuipers, L., Berkowitz, R., Eberlein-Vries, R., Sturgeon, D.: A controlled trial of social intervention in the families of schizophrenic patients. *Br. J. Psychiatry* **141**, 121–134, 1982.

Legangneux, E., McEwen, J., Wesnes, K., *et al.*: The acute effects of amisulpride (50 and 200 mg) and haloperidol (2 mg) on cognitive function in healthy elderly volunteers. *J. Psychopharmacol.* **14**, 164–171, 2000.

Lehmann, H.E., Ban, T.A.: The history of the psychopharmacology of schizophrenia. *Can. J. Psychiatry* **42**, 152–162, 1997.

Lenox, R.H., Manji, H.K.: Lithium. In: Schatzberg, A.F., Nemeroff, Ch.B. (eds): *Textbook of Psychopharmacology*, 2nd edn. American Psychiatric Press, Washington DC, 1998, pp. 379–429.

Lesko, L., Rowland, M., Peck, C., *et al.*: Optimizing the science of drug development: opportunities for better candidate selection and accelerated evaluation in humans. *Eur. J. Pharm. Sci.* **10**, iv–xiv, 2000.

Leverich, G.S., Post, R.M.: *The NIMH Life Chart Manual for Recurrent Affective Illness: the LCMS-S (Self Version)*. NIMH Monograph, Biological Psychiatry Branch, Bethesda, MD, 1993.

Levkovitz, Y., Caftori, R., Avital, A., Richter-Levin, G.: The SSRI drug fluoxetine, but not the noradrenergic tricyclic drug desipramine, improves memory performance during acute major depression. *Brain Res. Bull.* **58**, 345–350, 2002.

Lezak, M.D.: *Neuropsychological Assessment*. Oxford University Press, New York, 1983.

Lienert, G.A.: *Belastung und Regression – Versuch einer Theorie der systematischen Beeinträchtigung der intellektuellen Leistungsfähigkeit*. Anton Hain, Meisenheim, 1964.

Lipman, R.S.: Differentiating anxiety and depression in anxiety disorders: use of rating scales. *Psychopharmacol. Bull.* **18**(4), 69–77, 1982.

Lipsey, M.W., Wilson, D.B.: The efficacy of psychological, educational, and behavioral treatment. *Am. Psychologist* **48**, 1181–1209, 1993.

Lister, R.G.: The amnesic action of benzodiazepines in man. *Neurosci. Biobehav. Rev.* **9**, 87–94, 1985.

Llana, M.E., Crismon, M.L.: Methylphenidate: increased use or appropriate use? *J. Am. Pharm. Assoc.* **39**, 526–530, 1999.

Loiseau, P.: Carbamazepine – clinical efficacy and use in epilepsy. In: Levy, R.H., Mattson, R.H., Meldrum, B.S., Perucca, E. (eds): *Antiepileptic Drugs*, 5th edn. Lippincott Williams & Wilkins, Philadelphia, 2002, pp. 262–272.

London, E.D.: *Imaging Drug Action in the Brain*. CRC Press, Boca Raton, FL, 1993.

London, E.D., Cascella, N.G., Wong, D.F., *et al.*: Cocaine induced reduction of glucose utilization in human brain. *Arch. Gen. Psychiatry* **47**, 567–574, 1990.

Lourenco, C.M., Houle, S., Wilson, A.A., DaSilva, J.N.: Characterization of r-(11)C]rolipram for PET imaging of phosphodiesterase-4: in vitro binding, metabolism, and dosimetry studies in rats. *Nucl. Med. Biol.* **28**(4), 347–358, 2001.

Luborsky, L., Singer, B., Luborsky, L.: Comparative studies of psychotherapies. *Arch. Gen. Psychiatry* **32**, 995–1008, 1975.

Lucki, I., Rickels, K., Geller, A.M.: Chronic use of benzodiazepines and psychomotor and cognitive test performance. *Psychopharmacology* **88**, 426–433, 1986.

Lynch, G., King, D.J., Green, J.F., *et al.*: The effects of haloperidol on visual search, eye movements and psychomotor performance. *Psychopharmacology* **133**, 233–239, 1997.

Maas, J.W.: Biogenic amines and depression: biochemical and pharmacological separation of two types of depression. *Arch. Gen. Psychiatry* **32**, 1357–1361, 1975.

Mackworth, J.F.: The effect of amphetamine on the detectability of signals in a visual vigilance task. *Can. J. Psychol.* **19**, 104–109, 1965.

Maggini, C., Guazzelli, M., Ciapparelli, A., *et al.*: The effects of oxiracetam and *d*-amphetamine on all-night electronencephalogram sleep in young healthy subjects. *Curr. Ther. Res.* **43**, 979–990, 1988.

Mahmood, I., Balian, J.D.: The pharmacokinetic principles behind scaling from preclinical results to phase I protocols. *Clin. Pharmacokin.* **36**(1), 1–11, 1999.

Maier, W., Philipp, M., Heuser, I., *et al.*: Improving depression severity assessment – I. Reliability, internal validity and sensitivity to change of three observer depression scales. *J. Psychiatr. Res.* **22**, 3–12, 1988.

Malberg, J.E., Eisch, A.J., Nestler, E.J., Duman, R.S.: Chronic antidepressant treatment increases neurogenesis in adult rat hippocampus. *J. Neurosci.* **20**, 9104–9110, 2000.

Malla, A.K., Norman, R.M.G.: Prodromal symptoms in schizophrenia. *Br. J. Psychiatry* **164**, 487–493, 1994.

Malm, U.: The influence of group therapy on schizophrenia. *Acta Psychiatr. Scand.* **65**, (Suppl. 297), 1–65, 1982.

Marder, S.R., Meibach, R.C.: Risperidone in the treatment of schizophrenia. *Am. J. Psychiatry* **151**, 825–835, 1994.

Marin, D.B., Davis, K.L.: Cognitive enhancers. In: Schatzberg, A.F., Nemerof, Ch.B. (eds): *Textbook of Psychopharmacology*, 2nd edn. American Psychiatric Press, Washington, DC, 1998, pp. 473–486.

Marks, I.M., Mathews, A.M.: Brief standard self-rating for phobic patients. *Behav. Res. Ther.* **17**(3), 263–267, 1979.

Marks, J.: Techniques of benzodiazepine withdrawal in clinical practice. *Med. Toxicol.* **3**, 324–333, 1988.

Markstein, R.: Bedeutung neuer Dopaminrezeptoren für die Wirkung von Clozapin. In: Naber, D., Müller-Spahn, F. (eds): *Clozapin. Pharmakologie und Klinik einer atypischen Neuroleptikums*. Springer, Berlin, 1994, pp. 5–15.

Martényi, F., Brown, E.B., Zhang, H., Prakash, A., Koke, S.C.: Fluoxetine versus placebo in posttraumatic stress disorder. *J. Clin. Psychiatry* **63**(3), 199–206, 2002.

Mata, M., Fink, D.J., Gainer, H., *et al.*: Activity-dependent energy metabolism in rat posterior pituitary primarily reflects sodium pump activity. *J. Neurochem.* **34**, 213–215, 1980.

Matejcek, M.: Pharmaco-electroencephalography: the value of quantified EEG in psychopharmacology. *Pharmakopsychiatrie* **12**, 126–136, 1979.

Matochik, J.A., Nordahl, T.E., Gross, M., et al.: Effects of acute stimulant medication on cerebral metabolism in adults with hyperactivity. Neuropsychopharmacology 8(4), 377–386, 1993.

Matsuoka, K., Tomotake, M., Hanano, M., et al.: The acute effects of antidepressants on the human VEP and EEG. Shikoku Acta Med. 53, 91–99, 1997.

Matthew, E., Andreason, P., Pettigrew, K., et al.: Benzodiazepine receptors mediate regional blood flow changes in the living human brain. Proc. Natl. Acad. Sci. USA 92(7), 2775–2779, 1995.

Mattila, M.J.: Interactions of benzodiazepines on psychomotor skills. Br. J. Clin. Pharmacol. 18 (Suppl. 1), 215–265, 1984.

Mattis, S.: Mental state examination for organic mental syndromes in the elderly patient. In: Bellak, L., Karasu, T.B. (eds): Geriatric Psychiatry. Grune & Stratton, New York, 1976, pp. 77–121.

Mattson, R.H., Petroff, O., Rothman, D., Behar, K.: Vigabatrin: effects on human brain GABA levels by nuclear magnetic resonance spectroscopy. Epilepsia 35 (Suppl. 5), S29–S32, 1994.

Maxwell, C.: Sensitivity and accuracy of the visual analogue scale: a psycho-physical classroom experiment. Br. J. Clin. Pharmacol. 6, 15–24, 1978.

May, Ph.R.A.: Anti-psychotic drugs and other forms of therapy. In: Efron, D.H., Cole, J.O., Levine, J., Wittenborn, J.R. (eds): Psychopharmacology: a Review of Progress. US Government Printing Office, Washington, DC, PHS Publ. No. 1836, 1968, pp. 1155–1176.

May, Ph.R.A., Tuma, A.H., Yale, C., Potepan, P., Dixon, W.J.: Schizophrenia: a follow-up study of results of treatment. Arch. Gen. Psychiatry 33, 481–486, 1976.

McEvoy, J.P., Hogarty, G.E., Steingard, S.: Optimal dose of neuroleptic in acute schizophrenia. Arch. Gen. Psychiatry 48, 739–745, 1991.

McGorry, P.D., Yung, A.R., Phillips, L.J., et al.: Randomized controlled trial of interventions designed to reduce the risk of progression to first-episode psychosis in clinical sample with subthreshold symptoms. Arch. Gen. Psychiatry 59(10), 921–928, 2002.

McGuire, M.T., Raleigh, M.J., Brammer, G.L.: Sociopharmacology. Annu. Rev. Pharmacol. Toxicol. 22, 643–661, 1982.

McKeith, I.G., Burn, D.: Spectrum of Parkinson's disease, Parkinson's dementia, and Lewy body dementia. Neurol. Clin. 18, 865–883, 2000.

McKeith, I.G., Del Ser, T., Spano, P.F., et al.: Efficacy of rivastigmine in dementia with Lewy bodies: a randomised, double-blind, placebo controlled international study. Lancet 356, 2031–2036, 2000.

McKenna, P.J.: Pathology, phenomenology and the dopamine hypothesis of schizophrenia. Br. J. Psychiatry 151, 288–301, 1987.

McKenna, P.J., Bailey, P.E.: The strange story of clozapine. Br. J. Psychiatry 162, 32–37, 1993.

McKhann, G., Drachman, D., Folstein, M., et al.: Clinical diagnosis of Alzheimer's disease. Report of the NINCDS–ADRDA Work Group. Neurology 34, 939–944, 1984.

McLellan, A.T., Luborsky, L., Woody, G.E., O'Brien, C.P.: An improved diagnostic evaluation instrument for substance abuse patients. The Addiction Severity Index. J. Nerv. Ment. Dis. 168(1), 26–33, 1980.

McNamara, B., Ray, J.L., Arthurs, O.J., Boniface, S.: Transcranial magnetic stimulation for depression and other psychiatric disorders. Psychol. Med. 31, 1141–1146, 2001.

Mellinger, G.D., Balter, M.B., Uhlenhuth, E.H.: Prevalence and correlates of the long-term regular use of anxiolytics. J. Am. Med. Assoc. 251, 375–379, 1984.

Meltzer, H.Y.: Clinical studies on the mechanism of action of clozapine: the dopamine–serotonin hypothesis of schizophrenia. *Psychopharmacology* **99**, 518–527, 1989.

Meltzer, H.Y., Fatemi, S.H.: Treatment of schizophrenia. In: Schatzberg, A.F., Nemeroff, Ch.B. (eds): *Textbook of Psychopharmacology*, 2nd edn. American Psychiatric Press, Washington, DC, 1998, pp. 747–774.

Meltzer, H.Y., Fatemi, S.H.: Treatment of schizophrenia. In: Schatzberg, A.F., Nemeroff, C.B. (eds): *Essentials of Clinical Psychopharmacology*. American Psychiatric Assocation, Washington, DC, 2001, pp. 399–429.

Meltzer, H.Y., Cola, P., Way, L., *et al.*: Cost effectiveness of clozapine in neuroleptic-resistant schizophrenia. *Am. J. Psychiatry* **150**, 1630–1638, 1993.

Meltzer, H.Y., Alphs, L., Green, A.I., *et al.*: Clozapine treatment for suicidality in schizophrenia: International Suicide Prevention Trial (InterSePT). *Arch. Gen. Psychiatry* **60**(1), 82–91, 2003.

Mercier, M.A., Stewart, W., Quitkin, F.M.: A pilot sequential study of cognitive therapy and pharmacotherapy of atypical depression. *J. Clin. Psychiatry* **53**, 166–170, 1992.

Meterissian, G.B., Bradwejn, J.: Comparative studies on the efficacy of psychotherapy, pharmacotherapy, and their combination in depression: Was adequate pharmacotherapy provided? *J. Clin. Psychopharmacol.* **9**, 334–339, 1989.

Meyer, J.H., Wilson, A.A., Ginovart, N., *et al.*: Occupancy of serotonin transporters by paroxetine and citalopram during the treatment of depression: a [(11C)] DASB PET imaging study. *Am. J. Psychiatry* **158**(11), 1843–1849, 2001.

Meyer-Lindenberg, A., Rammsayer, T., Ulferts, J., Gallhofer, B.: The effects of sulpiride on psychomotor performance and subjective tolerance. *Eur. Neuropsychopharmacol.* **7**, 219–223, 1997.

Miller, I.W., Norman, W.H., Keitner, G.I.: Cognitive–behavioral treatment of depressed inpatients: six- and twelve-month follow-up. *Am. J. Psychiatry* **146**, 1274–1279, 1989.

Mintun, M., Raichle, M., Kilbourn, M., *et al.*: A quantitative model for the *in vivo* assessment of drug binding sites with positron emission tomography. *Ann. Neurol.* **15**, 217–227, 1984.

Moghaddam, B., Adams, B.W.: Reversal of phencyclidine effects by group II metabotropic glutamate receptor agonists in rats. *Science* **281**, 1349–1352, 1998.

Mojtabai, R., Nicholson, R.A., Carpenter, B.N.: Role of psychosocial treatments in management of schizophrenia: a meta-analytic review of controlled outcome studies. *Schizophr. Bull.* **24**, 569–587, 1998.

Möller, H.J.: Therapieresistenz auf Antidepressiva: Risikofaktoren und Behandlungsmöglichkeiten. *Nervenarzt* **62**, 658–669, 1991.

Möller, H.J.: Klinische Prüfstudien. In: Riederer, P., Laux, G., Pöldinger, W. (eds): *Neuro-Psychopharmaka*, Bd.1. Springer, Vienna, 1992, pp. 177–199.

Möller, H.J.: Niedrigdosierte Neuroleptika in Tranquilizer-Indikationen. *Sandorama* **1**, 22–25, 1993.

Möller, H.J.: The negative component in schizophrenia. *Acta Psychiatr. Scand.* **91** (Suppl. 388), 11–14, 1995.

Möller, H.J., Müller, W.E.: *Opipramol, Sigmaligand und stimmungsaufhellendes Anxiolytikum*. LinguaMed Verlags-GmbH, Neu-Isenburg, 2001.

Montgomery, S.A.: The need for long term treatment of depression. *Eur. Neuropsychopharmacol.* **7**, S309–S313, 1997.

Montgomery, S.A.: The failure of placebo-controlled studies. ECNP Consensus Meeting, September 13, 1997, Vienna. *Eur. Neuropsychopharmacol.* **9**, 271–276, 1999.

Montgomery, S.A., Asberg, M.: A new depression scale designed to be sensitive to change. *Br. J. Psychiatry* **134**, 382–389, 1979.

Moore, C.M., Demopulos, C.M., Henry, M.E., *et al.*: Brain-to-serum lithium ratio and age: an *in vivo* magnetic resonance spectroscopy study. *Am. J. Psychiatry* **159**(7), 1240–1242, 2002.

Morris, J.B., Beck, A.T.: The efficacy of antidepressant drugs. *Arch. Gen. Psychiatry* **30**, 667–674, 1974.

Moser, D.J., Schultz, S.K., Arndt, S., Benjamin, M.L., Fleming, F.W.: Capacity to provide informed consent for participation in schizophrenia and HIV research. *Am. J. Psychiatry* **159**(7), 1201–1207, 2002.

MTA Cooperative Group: A 14-month randomized clinical trial of treatment strategies for attention-deficit/hyperactivity disorder. *Arch. Gen. Psychiatry* **56**, 1073–1086, 1999.

Müller, Ch.: Psychotherapie und Soziotherapie der endogenen Psychosen. In: Kisker, K.P., Meyer, J.-E., Müller, M., Strömgren, E. (eds): *Psychiatrie der Gegenwart*, Bd. II/1. Springer, Berlin, 1972, pp. 291–342.

Müller, P., Schöneich, D.: Einfluss kombinierter Pharmako- und Psychotherapie in einer Schizophrenie-Ambulanz auf Rehospitalisierungszeiten und Behandlungskosten. *Psychiatr. Prax.* **19**, 91–95, 1992.

Münte, T.F., Heinze, H.F., Künkel, H.: Use of endogenous event-related potentials (ERP) in the evaluation of psychotropic substances: towards an ERP profile of drug effects. *Neuropsychobiology* **16**, 135–145, 1986.

Mural, R.J., Adams, M.D., Myers, E.W., *et al.*: A comparison of whole-genome shotgun-derived mouse chromosome 16 and the human genome. *Science* **296**, 1661–1671, 2002.

Murphy, G.E., Simons, A.D., Wetzel, R.D., Lustman, P.J.: Cognitive therapy and pharmacotherapy: singly and together in the treatment of depression. *Arch. Gen. Psychiatry* **41**, 33–41, 1984.

Naber, D., Lambert, M., Krauz, M., Haasen, C., Pickar, D.: *Atypical Antipsychotics in the Treatment of Schizophrenic Patients*. Uni-Med Verlag, Bremen, 2002.

Nathan, P.J., Baker, A., Carr, E., *et al.*: Cholinergic modulation of cognitive function in healthy subjects: acute effects of donepezil, a cholinesterase inhibitor. *Hum. Psychopharmacol.* **16**, 481–483, 2001.

Neftel, K.A., Adler, R.H., Kaeppeli, L., *et al.*: Stage fright in musicians: a model illustrating the effect of beta blockers. *Psychosom. Med.* **44**, 461–469, 1982.

Nemeroff, Ch.B.: Evolutionary trends in the pharmacotherapeutic management of depression. *J. Clin. Psychiatry* **55**, 3–15, 1994.

Nemeroff, Ch.B., Schatzberg, A.F.: Pharmacological treatments for unipolar depression. In: Nathan, P.E., Gorman, J.M. (eds): *A Guide for Treatments that Work*. Oxford University Press, New York, 2002, pp. 229–243.

Newhouse, P.A., Rama Krishnan, K.R., Doraiswamy, P.M., *et al.*: A double-blind comparison of sertraline and fluoxetine in depressed elderly outpatients. *J. Clin. Psychiatry* **61**, 559–568, 2000.

Niklson, I.A., Reimitz, P.E.: Baseline characteristics of major depressive disorder patients in clinical trials in Europe and United States: is there a transatlantic difference? *J. Psychiatr. Res.* **35**(2), 71–81, 2001.

Ninan, Ph.T., Cole, J.O., Yonkers, K.A.: Nonbenzodiazepine anxiotytics. In: Schatzberg, A.F., Nemeroff, Ch.N. (eds): *Textbook of Psychopharmacology*, 2nd edn. American Psychiatric Press, Washington, DC, 1998, pp. 287–300.

Nishimura, T., Saito, A., Yagyu, T., *et al.*: Psychotropic properties of fluvoxamine maleate: pharmaco-EEG study and pharmacodynamics on healthy subjects. *Jpn. J. Neuropsychopharmacol.* **18**, 319–329, 1996.

Noda, Y., Kamei, H., Nabeshima, T.: Sigma-receptor ligands and anti-stress actions. *Nippon Yakurigaku Zasshi* **114**, 43–49, 1999.

Norman, R.M., Townsend, L., Malla, A.K.: Duration of untreated psychosis and cognitive functioning in first-episode patients. *Br. J. Psychiatry* **179**, 340–345, 2001.

Nuijten, M.J.C., van Iperen, P.O., Palmer, C., van Hilten, B.J., Snyder, E.: Cost-effectiveness analysis of entacapone in Parkinson's disease: a Markov process analysis. *Value Health* **4**(4), 316–327, 2001.

Nyberg, S., Nakashima, Y., Nordström, A.L., *et al.*: Positron emission tomography of *in-vivo* binding characteristics of atypical antipsychotic drugs. Review of D2 and 5-HT2 receptor occupancy studies and clinical response. *Br. J. Psychiatry* **168** (Suppl. 29), 40–44, 1996.

O'Brien, D., Skelton, K.H., Owens, M.J., Nemeroff, C.B.: Are CRF receptor antagonists potential antidepressants? *Hum. Psychopharmacol. Clin. Exp.* **16**, 81–87, 2001.

O'Carroll, R.: Cognitive impairment in schizophrenia. *Adv. Psychiatr. Treat.* **6**, 161–168, 2000.

O'Hara, M.W., Hinrichs, J.V., Kohut, F.J., Wallace, R.B., Lemke, J.H.: Memory complaint and memory performance in the depressed elderly. *Psychol. Aging* **1**, 208–214, 1986.

Odejide, D.A., Aderounmu, A.F.: Double-blind placebo substitution: withdrawal of fluphenazine decanoate in schizophrenic patients. *J. Clin. Psychiatry* **43**, 195–196, 1982.

Ogawa, S., Tank, D.W., Menon, R., *et al.*: Intrinsic signal changes accompanying sensory stimulation: functional brain mapping with magnetic resonance imaging. *Proc. Natl. Acad. Sci. USA* **89**, 5951–5955, 1992.

Olney, J.W.: Exitotoxic amino acids and neuropsychiatric disorders. *Ann. Rev. Pharmacol. Toxicol.* **30**, 47–61, 1990.

Olver, J.S., Burrows, G.D., Norman, T.R.: Third-generation antidepressants. Do they offer advantages over the SSRIs? *CNS Drugs* **15**, 941–954, 2001.

Orgogozo, J.M., Spiegel, R.: Critical review of clinical trials in senile dementia. *Postgrad. Med. J.* **63**, 237–240, 337–343, 1987.

Ornstein, R.E.: *The Psychology of Consciousness*. Freeman, San Francisco, 1972.

Oswald, I.: Drugs and sleep. *Pharmacol. Rev.* **20**, 273–303, 1968.

Overall, J.E., Gorham, D.R.: The brief psychiatric rating scale. *Psychol. Rep.* **10**, 799–812, 1962.

Overstreet, D.H., Pucilowski, O., Rezvani, A.H., Janowsky, D.S.: Administration of antidepressants, diazepam and psychomotor stimulants further confirms the utility of Flinders Sensitive Line rats as an animal model of depression. *Psychopharmacology* **121**, 27–37, 1995.

Owen, R.T., Tyrer, P.: Benzodiazepine dependence: a review of the evidence. *Drugs* **25**, 385–398, 1983.

Owens, M.J., Risch, S.C.: Atypical antipsychotics. In: Schatzberg, A.F., Nemeroff, Ch.B. (eds): *Textbook of Psychopharmacology*, 2nd edn. American Psychiatric Press, Washington, DC, 1998, pp. 323–348.

Pachman, J.S.: The dawn of a revolution in mental health. *Am. Psychol.* **51**, 213–215, 1996.

Pacifici, G.M., Gustaffson, L.L., Sawe, J., Rane, A.: Metabolic interaction between morphine and various benzodiazepines. *Acta Pharmacol. Toxicol. (Copenhagen)* **58**(4), 249–252, 1986.

Palmer, B.W., Heaton, R.K., Paulsen, J.S., *et al.*: Is it possible to be schizophrenic yet neuropsychologically normal? *Neuropsychology* **11**, 437–446, 1997.

Papp, M., Vassout, A., Gentsch, C.: The NK-1 receptor antagonist NKP608 has an antidepressant-like effect in the chronic mild stress model of depression in rats. *Behav. Brain Res.* **115**, 19–23, 2000.

Parascandola, J.: The development of receptor theory in discoveries in pharmacology. In: Parnham, M.J., Bruinvels, J. (eds): *Pharmacological Methods, Receptors and Chemotherapy.* Elsevier, New York, 1986.

Pare, W.P., Redei, E.: Depressive behavior and stress ulcer in Wistar Kyoto rats. *J. Physiol.* **87**, 229–238, 1993.

Parrino, L., Terzano, M.G.: Polysomnographic effects of hypnotic drugs. *Psychopharmacology* **126**, 1–16, 1996.

Patat, A.: Clinical pharmacology of psychotropic drugs. *Hum. Psychopharmacol.* **15**, 361–387, 2000.

Paykel, E.S., Di Mascio, A., Klerman, G.L., Prusoff, B.A., Weissman, M.M.: Maintenance therapy of depression. *Pharmacopsychiatry* **9**, 127–136, 1976.

Pazzaglia, P.J., Post, R.M., Ketter, T.A., *et al.*: Preliminary controlled trial of nimodipine in ultra-rapid cycling affective dysregulation. *Psychiatry Res.* **49**, 257–272, 1993.

Pazzaglia, P.J., Post, R.M., Ketter, T.A., *et al.*: Nimodipine monotherapy and carbamazepine augmentation in patients with refractory recurrent affective illness. *J. Clin. Psychopharmacol.* **18**, 404–413, 1998.

Peck, A.W., Bye, C.E., Clubley, M., Henson, T., Riddington, C.: Comparison of bupropion hydrochloride with dexamphetamine and amitriptyline in healthy subjects. *Br. J. Clin. Pharmacol.* **7**, 469–478, 1979.

Peck, C.C.: The randomized concentration controlled clinical trial: an information rich alternative to the randomized controlled trial. *Clin. Pharmacol. Ther.* **47**, 126, 1990.

Pelham, W.E., Kipp, H.L., Gnagy, E.M., Hoza, B.: Effects of methylphenidate and expectancy on ADHD children's performance, self-evaluations, persistence, and attributions on a cognitive task. *Exp. Clin. Psychopharmacol.* **5**, 3–13, 1997.

Pelham, W.E., Gnagy, E.M., Greiner, A.R., *et al.*: Behavioral versus behavioral and pharmacological treatment in ADHD children attending a summer treatment program. *J. Abnorm. Child Psychol.* **28**, 507–525, 2000.

Perna, G., Bertani, A., Caldirola, D., *et al.*: Anti-panic drug modulation of 35% CO_2 hyperreactivity and short-term treatment outcome. *J. Clin. Psychopharmacol.* **22**, 300–308, 2002.

Perry, E.K., Tomlinson, B.E., Blessed, G., *et al.*: Correlation of cholinergic abnormalities with senile plaques and mental test scores in senile dementia. *Br. Med. J. ii*, 1457–1459, 1978.

Perry, P.J., Alexander, B.: Dosage and serum levels. In: Johnson, F.N. (ed.): *Modern Lithium Therapy.* MTP Press, Lancaster, 1987, pp. 67–73.

Perry, W., Geyer, M.A., Braff, D.L.: Sensorimotor gating and thought disturbance measured in close temporal proximity in schizophrenic patients. *Arch. Gen. Psychiatry* **56**, 277–281, 1999.

Petersen, R.C., Doody, R., Kurz, A., *et al.*: Current concepts in mild cognitive impairment. *Arch. Neurol.* **58**, 1985–1992, 2001a.

Petersen, R.C., Stevens, J.C., Ganguli, M., *et al.*: Practice parameter: early detection of dementia: mild cognitive impairment (an evidence-based review). *Neurology* **56**, 1133–1142, 2001b.

Petroff, O.A., Rothman, D.L., Behar, K.L., Mattson, R.H.: Human brain GABA levels rise after initiation of vigabatrin therapy but fail to rise further with increasing dose. *Neurology* **46**(5), 1459–1463, 1996.

Pfefferbaum, A.: Psychotherapy and psychopharmacology. In: Barchas, J.D., Berger, Ph.A., Ciaranello, R.D., Elliott, G.R. (eds): *Psychopharmacology: from Theory to Practice.* Oxford University Press, New York, 1977, pp. 481–492.

Phelps, M.E., Mazziota, J.C., Schelbert, H.R.: *Positron Emission Tomography and Autoradiography: Principles and Applications for the Brain and Heart.* Raven Press, New York, 1986.

Podewils, L.J., Lyketsos, C.G.: Tricyclic antidepressants and cognitive decline. *Psychosomatics* **43**, 31–35, 2002.

Pöldinger, W.: *Kompendium der Psychopharmakotherapie.* Editiones 'Roche', Basel, 1975.

Pooviboonsuk, P., Dalton, J.A., Curran, H.V., Lader, M.H.: The effects of single doses of lorazepam on event-related potentials and cognitive function. *Hum. Psychopharmacol.* **11**, 241–252, 1996.

Pope, H.G., Keck, P.E., McElroy, S.L.: Frequency and presentation of neuroleptic malignant syndrome in a large psychiatric hospital. *Am. J. Psychiatry* **143**, 1227–1233, 1986.

Pope, H.G., Jr., McElroy, S.L., Keck, P.E., Jr., *et al.*: Valproate in the treatment of acute mania: a placebo-controlled study. *Arch. Gen. Psychiatry* **48**, 62–68, 1991.

Potkin, S.G., Fleming, K., Jin, Y., Gulasekaram, B.: Clozapine enhances neurocognition and clinical symptomatology more than standard neuroleptics. *J. Clin. Psychopharmacol.* **21**, 479–483, 2001.

Potkin, S.G., Anand, R., Hartman, R., *et al.*: Impact of Alzheimer's disease and rivastigmine treatment on activities of daily living over the course of mild to moderately severe disease. *Prog. Neuro-Psychopharmacol. Biol. Psychiatry* **26**, 713–720, 2002.

Potts, N.L., Book, S., Davidson, J.R.: The neurobiology of social phobia. *Int. Clin. Psychopharmacol.* **11** (Suppl. 3), 43–48, 1996.

Preda, L., Alberoni, M., Bressi, S., *et al.*: Effects of acute doses of oxiracetam in the scopolamine model of human amnesia. *Psychopharmacology (Berlin)* **110**(4), 421–426, 1993.

Pretorius, J.L., Phillips, M., Langley, R.W., *et al.*: Comparison of clozapine and haloperidol on some autonomic and psychomotor functions, and on serum prolactin concentration. *Br. J. Clin. Pharmacol.* **52**, 322–326, 2001.

Prien, R.F., Gelenberg, A.J.: Alternatives to lithium for preventive treatment of bipolar disorder. *Am. J. Psychiatry* **146**, 840–848, 1989.

Procyshyn, R.M., Thompson, D., Tse, G., Pharmacoeconomics of clozapine, risperidone and olanzapine. A review of the literature. *CNS Drugs* **13**(1), 47–76, 2000.

Prusoff, B.A., Weissman, M.M., Klerman, G.L., Rounsaville, B.J.: Research diagnostic criteria subtypes of depression: their role as predictors of differential response to psychotherapy and drug treatment. *Arch. Gen. Psychiatry* **37**, 796–801, 1980.

Rabiner, E.A., Gunn, R.N., Castro, M.E., *et al.*: beta-blocker binding to human 5-HT(1A) receptors *in vivo* and *in vitro*: implications for antidepressant therapy. *Neuropsychopharmacology* **23**(3), 285–293, 2000.

Radloff, L.S.: The Centre for Epidemiologic Studies – Depression Scale (CES-D); a self report depression scale for research in the general population. *Appl. Psychol. Meas.* **1**, 385–401, 1977.

Raedler, T.J., Knable, M.B., Lafargue, T., *et al*.: *In vivo* determination of muscarinic cholinergic receptor occupancy in patients treated with olanzapine. *Schizophr. Res.* **36**, 245, 1999.

Raiteri, M., Maura, G., Folghera,'S., *et al*.: Modulation of 5-hydroxytryptamine release by presynaptic inhibitory alpha 2-adrenoceptors in the human cerebral cortex. *Naunyn-Schmiedebergs Arch. Pharmacol.* **342**(5), 508–512, 1990.

Ramaekers, J.G., Louwerens, J.W., Munjewerff, N.D., *et al*.: Psychomotor, cognitive, extrapyramidal, and affective functions of healthy volunteers during treatment with an atypical (amisulpride) and a classic (haloperidol) antipsychotic. *J. Clin. Psychopharmacol.* **19**, 209–221, 1999.

Ramsay, E.R., Pryor, F.M.: Gabapentin – adverse effects. In: Levy, R.H., Mattson, R.H., Meldrum, B.S., Perucca, E. (eds): *Antiepileptic Drugs*, 5th edn. Lippincott Williams & Wilkins, Philadelphia, 2002, pp. 354–362.

Ranstam, J., Merlo, J., Blennow, G., *et al*.: Impaired cognitive function in elderly men exposed to benzodiazepines or other anxiolytics. *Eur. J. Publ. Health* **7**, 149–152, 1997.

Rappaport, G.C., Ornoy, A., Tannenbaum, A.: Is early intervention effective in preventing ADHD? *Isr. J. Psychiatry Relat. Sci.* **35**(4), 271–279, 1998.

Raskin, A., Schulterbrandt, J., Reating, N., *et al*.: Replication of factors of psychopathology in interview, ward behavior, and self-report ratings of hospitalized depressives. *J. Nerv. Ment. Dis.* **148**(1), 87–98, 1969.

Reimherr, F.W., Amsterdam, J.D., Quitkin, F.M., *et al*.: Optimal length of continuation therapy in depression: a prospective assessment during long-term fluoxetine treatment. *Am. J. Psychiatry* **155**, 1247–1253, 1998.

Reisberg, B., Borenstein, J., Salob, S.P., *et al*.: Behavioral symptoms in Alzheimer's disease. Phenomenology and treatment. *J. Clin. Psychiatry* **48** (Suppl.), 9–15, 1987.

Reivich, M., Kuhl, D., Wolf, A., *et al*.: The [18F] fluorodeoxyglucose method for the measurement of local cerebral glucose utilization in man. *Circ. Res.* **44**(1), 127–137, 1979.

Reul, J.M., Holsboer, F.: Corticotropin-releasing factor receptors 1 and 2 in anxiety and depression. *Curr. Opin. Pharmacol.* **2**, 23–33, 2002.

Riccio, C.A., Waldrop, J.J.M., Reynolds, C.R., Lowe, P.: Effects of stimulants on the continuous performance test (CPT): implications for CPT use and interpretation. *J. Neuropsych. Clin. Neurosci.* **13**, 326–335, 2001.

Rickels, K., Schweizer, E.E.: Current pharmacotherapy of anxiety and panic. In: Meltzer, H.Y. (ed.): *Psychopharmacology: the Third Generation of Progress*. Raven, New York, 1987, pp. 1193–1203.

Rickels, K., Schweizer, E.E., Case, W.G., Greenblatt, D.J.: Long-term therapeutic use of benzodiazepines. I. Effects of abrupt discontinuation. *Arch. Gen. Psychiatry* **47**, 899–907, 1990.

Rief, W., Fichter, M.: The Symptom Check List SCL-90-R and its ability to discriminate between dysthymia, anxiety disorders, and anorexia nervosa. *Psychopathology* **25**(3), 128–138, 1992.

Riemann, D., Lis, S., Fritsch-Montero, R., *et al*.: Effects of tetrahydroaminoacridine on sleep in healthy subjects. *Biol. Psychiatry* **39**, 796–802, 1996.

Rifkin, A., Doddi, S., Karajgi, B., Borenstein, M., Wachspress, M.: Dosage of haloperidol for schizophrenia. *Arch. Gen. Psychiatry* **48**, 166–170, 1991.

Rinne, T., Westenberg, H.G., den Boer, J.A., van den Brink, W.: Serotonergic blunting to meta-chlorophenylpiperazine (m-CPP) highly correlates with sustained childhood abuse in impulsive and autoaggressive female borderline patients. *Biol. Psychiatry* **47**(6), 548–556, 2000.

Robbe, H.W.J., O'Hanlon, J.F.: Acute and subchronic effects of paroxetine 20 and 40 mg on actual driving, psychomotor performance and subjective assessments in healthy volunteers. *Eur. Neuropsychopharmacol.* **5**, 35–42, 1995.

Rohloff, A., Ott, H., Fichte, K.: ZNS-Profil von Bromergurid anhand von Pharmako-EEG, psychometrischen Tests und Fragebogen im Vergleich zu Haloperidol und Placebo nach einmaliger Gabe. In: Oldigs-Kerber, L.J., Leonard, J.P. (eds): *Pharmakopsychologie: experimentelle und klinische Aspekte.* G. Fischer, Jena, 1992, pp. 285–304.

Rosen, G.: *Madness in Society.* Harper & Row, New York, 1969.

Rosen, W.G., Mohs, R.C., Davis, K.L.: A new rating scale for Alzheimer's disease. *Am. J. Psychiatry* **11**, 1356–1364, 1984.

Rosenbaum, J.F., Fava, M., Hoog, S.L., *et al.*: Selective serotonin reuptake inhibitor discontinuation syndrome: a randomized clinical trial. *Biol. Psychiatry* **44**, 77–87, 1998.

Rosenheck, R., Cramer, J., Xu, W., *et al.*: A comparison of clozapine and haloperidol in hospitalized patients with refractory schizophrenia: Department of Veterans Affairs Co-operative Study Group on clozapine in refractory schizophrenia. *N. Engl. J. Med.* **337**, 809–815, 1997.

Rosenthal, R., Rubin, D.B.: Interpersonal expectancy effects: the first 345 studies. *Behav. Brain Sci.* **3**, 377–415, 1978.

Rosenzweig, P., Canal, M., Patat, A., *et al.*: A review of the pharmacokinetics, tolerability and pharmacodynamics of amisulpride in healthy volunteers. *Hum. Psychopharmacol.* **17**, 1–13, 2002.

Roth, M.: Senile dementia and its borderlands. In: Cole, J.O., Barrett, J.E. (eds): *Psychopathology in the Aged.* Raven, New York, 1980, pp. 205–232.

Roy-Byrne, P., Cowley, D.S.: Pharmacological treatments for panic disorder, generalized anxiety disorder, specific phobia, and social anxiety disorder. In: Nathan, P.E., Gorman, J.M. (eds): *A Guide to Treatments that Work.* Oxford University Press, Oxford, 2002, pp. 337–365.

Roy-Byrne, P., Fleishaker, J., Arnett, C., *et al.*: Effects of acute and chronic alprazolam treatment on cerebral blood flow, memory, sedation, and plasma catecholamines. *Neuropsychopharmology* **8**(2), 161–169, 1993a.

Roy-Byrne, P., Wingerson, D., Cowley, D., Dager, S.: Psychopharmacologic treatment of panic, generalized anxiety disorder, and social phobia. *Psychiatr. Clin. North Am.* **16**, 719–735, 1993b.

Rudorfer, M.V., Potter, W.Z.: Antidepressants: a comparative review of the clinical pharmacology and therapeutic use of the 'newer' versus the 'older' drugs. *Drugs* **37**, 713–738, 1989.

Rund, B.R., Borg, N.E.: Cognitive deficits and cognitive training in schizophrenic patients: a review. *Acta Psychiatr. Scand.* **100**, 85–95, 1999.

Rupniak, N.M.: Elucidating the antidepressant actions of substance P (NK1 receptor) antagonists. *Curr. Opin. Invest. Drugs* **3**, 257–261, 2002.

Rupniak, N.M., Kramer, M.S.: Discovery of the antidepressant and anti-emetic efficacy of substance P receptor (NK1) antagonists. *Trends Pharmacol. Sci.* **20**, 485–490, 1999.

Rush, A.J., Guillon, C.M., Basco, M.R., Jarrett, R.B., Trivedi, M.H.: The inventory of depressive symptomatology (IDS): psychometric properties. *Psychol. Med.* **26**(3), 477–486, 1996.

Rush, C.R., Griffith, R.R.: Zolpidem, triazolam, and temazepam: behavioral and subject-rated effects in normal volunteers. *J. Clin. Psychopharmacol.* **16**, 146–157, 1996.

Rush, C.R., Higgins, S.T., Bickel, W.K., Hughes, J.R.: Acute behavioral effects of lorazepam and caffeine, alone and in combination, in humans. *Behav. Pharmacol.* **5**, 245–254, 1994.

Rush, C.R., Madakasira, S., Hayes, C.A., *et al.*: Trazodone and triazolam: acute subject-rated and performance-impairing effects in healthy volunteers. *Psychopharmacology* **131**, 9–18, 1997.

Rutten-van Molken, M.P., Bakker, C.H., van Doorslaer, E.K., van der Linden, S.: Methodological issues of patient utility measurement. Experience from two clinical trials. *Med. Care* **33**, 922–937, 1995.

Sachdeo, R.C., Karia, R.M.: Topiramate – adverse effects. In: Levy, R.H., Mattson, R.H., Meldrum, B.S., Perucca, E. (eds): *Antiepileptic Drugs*, 5th edn. Lippincott Williams & Wilkins, Philadelphia, 2002, pp. 760–766.

Sachdev, P.S., McBride, R., Loo, C.: Effects of different frequencies of transcranial magnetic stimulation (TMS) on the forced swim test model of depression in rats. *Biol. Psychiatry* **15**, 474–479, 2002.

Sack, R.L., De Fraites, E.: Lithium and the treatment of mania. In: Barchas, J.D., Berger, Ph.A., Ciaranello, R.D., Elliott, G.R. (eds): *Psychopharmacology: from Theory to Practice*. Oxford University Press, New York, 1977, pp. 208–225.

Sadock, B.J., Sadock, V.A.: *Kaplan & Sadock's Pocket Handbook of Psychiatric Drug Treatment*, 3rd edn. Lippincott, Williams & Wilkins, Philadelphia, 2001.

Sadzot, B., Mayberg, H.S., Frost, J.J.: Detection and quantification of opiate receptors in man by positron emission tomography. Potential applications to the study of pain. *Neurophysiol. Clin.* **20**(5), 323–334, 1990.

Safer, D.J.: Design and reporting modifications in industry-sponsored comparative psychopharmacology trials. *J. Nerv. Ment. Dis.* **190**(9), 583–592, 2002.

Safer, D.J., Allen, R.P.: Absence of tolerance to the behavioral effects of methylphenidate in hyperactive and inattentive children. *J. Pediatr.* **115**, 1003–1008, 1989.

Sajatovic, M., Ramirez, L.F.: *Rating Scales in Mental Health*. Lexi Comp Inc., Ohio, 2002.

Sakulsripong, M., Curran, H.V., Lader, M.: Does tolerance develop to the sedative and amnesic effects of antidepressants? *Eur. J. Clin. Pharmacol.* **40**, 43–48, 1991.

Saletu, B.: *Psychopharmaka, Gehirntätigkeit und Schlaf*. Bibl. Psychiat. No. 155. Karger, Basel, 1976.

Sams-Dodd, F.: Phencyclidine-induced stereotyped behaviour and social isolation in rats: a possible animal model of schizophrenia. *Behav. Pharmacol.* **7**: 3–23, 1996.

Sanchez, C., Papp, M.: The selective sigma2 ligand Lu 28-179 has an antidepressant-like profile in the rat chronic mild stress model of depression. *Behav. Pharmacol.* **11**, 117–124, 2000.

Santarelli, L., Gobbi, G., Debs, P.C., *et al.*: Genetic and pharmacological disruption of neurokinin 1 receptor function decreases anxiety-related behaviors and increases serotonergic function. *Proc. Natl. Acad. Sci. USA* **98**, 1912–1917, 2001.

Sartorius, N., Ban, T.A.: *Assessment of Depression*. Springer Verlag, Berlin, 1986.

Sartory, G., Maurer, J.: Benzodiazepine: Entzugsprobleme und unterstützende Behandlung des Entzugs. *Psychol. Rundsch.* **42**, 187–194, 1991.

Satel, S.L., Nelson, J.C.: Stimulants in the treatment of depression: a critical overview. *J. Clin. Psychiatry* **50**, 241–249, 1989.

Sawa, A., Snyder, H.S.: Schizophrenia: diverse approaches to a complex disease. *Science* **296**, 692–695, 2002.

Schachar, R., Mota, V.L., Logan, G.D., *et al.*: Confirmation of an inhibitory control deficit in attention deficit/hyperactivity disorder. *J. Abnorm. Child Psychol.* **28**, 227–235, 2000.

Schachter, S.C.: Tiagabine – adverse effects. In: Levy, R.H., Mattson, R.H., Meldrum, B.S., Perucca, E. (eds): *Antiepileptic Drugs*, 5th edn. Lippincott Williams & Wilkins, Philadelphia, 2002, pp. 711–715.

Schatzberg, A.F., Kraemer, H.C.: Use of placebo control groups in evaluating efficacy of treatment of unipolar major depression. *Biol. Psychiatry* **47**, 736–744, 2000.

Schatzberg, A.F., Cole, J.O., Blumer, D.P.: Speech blockage: a tricyclic side effect. *Am. J. Psychiatry* **135**, 600–601, 1978.

Schildkraut, J.J.: The catecholamine hypothesis of affective disorders: a review of supporting evidence. *Am. J. Psychiatry* **122**, 509–522, 1965.

Schmidt, M.E.: Neuroimaging and the pharmacological treatment of schizophrenia. In: Breier, A., Tran, P.V., Herrera, J., *et al.* (eds): *Current Issues in the Psychopharmacology of Schizophrenia.* Lippincott Williams and Williams, Philadelphia, 2001, pp. 131–147.

Schmidt, M.E., Ernst, M., Matochik, J.A., *et al.*: Cerebral glucose metabolism during pharmacologic studies: test-retest under placebo conditions. *J. Nucl. Med.* **37**, 1142–1149, 1996.

Schmidt, M.E., Matochik, J.A., Goldstein, D.S., *et al.*: Gender differences in brain metabolic and plasma catecholamine responses to alpha2-adrenoceptor blockade. *Neuropsychopharmacology* **16**(4), 298–310, 1997.

Schmidt, M.E., Oshinsky, R.J., Kim, H.G., *et al.*: Cerebral glucose metabolic and plasma catecholamine responses to the alpha (2) adrenoceptor antagonist ethoxyidazoxan given to healthy volunteers. *Psychopharmacology* **146**(2), 119–127, 1999.

Schmitt, J.A.J., Kruizinga, M.J., Riedel, W.J.: Non-serotoninergic pharmacological profiles and associated cognitive effects of serotonin reuptake inhibitors. *J. Psychopharmacol.* **15**, 173–180, 2001.

Schmitt, J.E.J., Riedel, W.J., Vuurman, E.F.P.M., *et al.*: Modulation of the critical flicker fusion effects of serotonin reuptake inhibitors by concomitant pupillary changes. *Psychopharmacology* **160**, 381–386, 2002.

Schmutz, J., Eichenberger, E.: Clozapine. In: Bindra, J.S., Ledniger, D. (eds): *Chronicles of Drug Discovery.* John Wiley, New York, 1983, pp. 39–59.

Schneider, P.J.: *Entwurf zu einer Heilmittellehre gegen psychische Krankheiten–oder Heilmittel in Beziehung auf psychische Krankheitsformen.* Tübingen, 1824.

Schooler, N.R.: Maintenance medication for schizophrenia: strategies for dose reduction. *Schizophr. Bull.* **17**, 311–324, 1991.

Schooler, N.R., Hogarty, G.E.: Medication and psychological strategies in the treatment of schizophrenia. In: Meltzer, H.Y. (ed.): *Psychopharmacology: the Third Generation of Progress.* Raven, New York, 1987, pp. 1111–1119.

Schooler, N.R., Keith, S.J., Severe, J.B., *et al.*: Relapse and rehospitalization during maintenance treatment of schizophrenia. *Arch. Gen. Psychiatry* **54**, 453–463, 1997.

Schöpf, J.: Psychische Abhängigkeit bei Benzodiazepin-Langzeitbehandlung. *Nervenarzt* **56**, 585–592, 1985.

Schou, M., Juel-Nielson, N., Stromgen, E., *et al.*: The treatment of manic psychoses by administration of lithium salts. *J Neurol. Neurosurg. Psychiatry* **17**, 250–260, 1954.

Schrenk, M.: *Ueber den Umgang mit Geisteskrankheiten.* Springer, Berlin, 1973.

Schultz, S.K., Andreasen, N.C.: Schizophrenia. *Lancet* **353**, 1425–1430, 1999.

Schulz, H., Jobert, M.: Effects of hypericum extract on the sleep EEG in older volunteers. *J. Geriatr. Psychiatry Neurol.* **7** (Suppl. 1): S39–S43, 1994.

Schweizer, E., Rickels, K., Case, W.G., Greenblatt, D.J.: Long-term therapeutic use of benzodiazepines. II. Effects of gradual taper. *Arch. Gen. Psychiatry* **47**, 908–915, 1990.

Scott, J., Teasdale, J.D., Paykal, E.S., *et al.*: Effects of cognitive therapy on psychological symptoms and social functioning in residual depression. *Br. J. Psychiatry* **177**, 440–446, 2000.

Seemann, P.: Brain dopamine receptors. *Pharmacol. Rev.* **32**, 229–313, 1980.

Seifritz, E., Gillin, J.Ch., Rapaport, M.H., *et al.*: Sleep electroencephalographic response to muscarinic and serotonin1A receptor probes in patients with major depression and in normal controls. *Biol. Psychiatry* **44**, 21–33, 1998.

Sellwood, W., Haddock, G., Tarrier, N., Yusupoff, L.: Advances in the psychological management of positive symptoms of schizophrenia. *Int. Rev. Psychiatry* **6**, 201–215, 1994.

Senn, S.: The AB/BA crossover: past, present and future? *Stat. Methods Med. Res.* **3**(4), 303–324, 1994.

Shader, R.I., Greenblatt, D.J.: Use of benzodiazepines in anxiety disorders. *N. Engl. J. Med.* **328**, 1398–1405, 1993.

Shalev, A., Munitz, H.: The neuroleptic malignant syndrome: agent and host interaction. *Acta Psychiatr. Scand.* **73**, 337–347, 1986.

Sharpley, A.L., Williamson, D.J., Attenburow, M.E.J., *et al.*: The effects of paroxetine and nefazodone on sleep: a placebo controlled trial. *Psychopharmacology* **126**, 50–54, 1996.

Sharpley, A.L., McGavin, C.L., Whale, R., *et al.*: Antidepressant-like effect of hypericum perforatum (St John's wort) on the sleep polygram. *Psychopharmacology* **139**, 286–287, 1998.

Shear, C.M., Brown, T.A., Barlow, D.H., *et al.*: Multicenter Collaborative Panic Disorder Severity Scale. *Am. J. Psychiatry* **154**, 1571–1575, 1997.

Sheehan, D.V., Harnett-Sheehan, K., Raj, B.A.: The measurement of disability. *Int. Clin. Psychopharmacol.* **II** (Suppl. 3), 89–95, 1996.

Sheehan, D.V., Lecrubier, Y., Sheehan, K.H., *et al.*: The Mini-International Neuropsychiatric Interview (M.I.N.I.): the development and validation of a structured diagnostic psychiatric interview for DSM-IV and ICD-10. *J. Clin. Psychiatry* **59** (Suppl. 20), 22–33, 1998.

Sheitman, B.B., Lieberman, J.A.: The natural history and pathophysiology of treatment resistant schizophrenia. *J. Psychiatr. Res.* **32**(3/4), 143–150, 1998.

Shinotoh, H., Iyo, M., Yamada, T., *et al.*: Detection of benzodiazepine receptor occupancy in the human brain by positron emission tomography. *Psychopharmacology* **99**, 202–207, 1989.

Shorter, E.: *A History of Psychiatry.* John Wiley, New York, 1997.

Silva, M., Hetem, L.A.B., Guimaraes, F.S., Graeff, F.G.: Opposite effects of nefazodone in two human models of anxiety. *Psychopharmacology* **156**, 454–460, 2001.

Simons, A.D., Murphy, G.E., Levine, J.L., Wetzel, R.D.: Cognitive therapy and pharmacotherapy for depression. *Arch. Gen. Psychiatry* **43**, 43–48, 1986.

Small, G.S., Rabins, P.V., Barry, P.P., *et al.*: Diagnosis and treatment of Alzheimer disease and related disorders. Consensus Statement. *J. Am. Med. Assoc.* **278**, 1363–1371, 1997.

Smith, D., Dempster, C., Glanville, J., *et al.*: Efficacy and tolerability of venlafaxine compared with selective serotonin reuptake inhibitors and other antidepressants: a meta-analysis. *Br. J. Psychiatry* **180**, 396–404, 2002.

Snowden, J.S., Neary, D.: Neuropsychiatric aspects of frontotemporal dementias. *Curr. Psychiatry Rep.* **1**, 93–98, 1999.

Snyder, S.H.: Neurotransmitters and CNF disease. Schizophrenia. *Lancet ii*, 970–974, 1982.

Sokoloff, L.: Cerebral circulation, metabolism, and synthesis. In: Phelps, M.E., Mazziota, J.C., Schelbert, H.R. (eds): *Positron Emission Tomography and Autoradiography: Principles and Applications for the Brain and Heart.* Raven Press, New York, 1986, pp. 1–71.

Sokoloff, L., Reivich, M., Kennedy, C., *et al.*: The [14C] deoxyglucose method for the measurement of local cerebral glucose utilization: theory, procedure, and normal values in the conscious and anesthetized albino rat. *J. Neurochem.* **28**(5), 897–916, 1977.

Solberg, L.C., Losee Olson, S., Turek, F.W., Redei, E.: Altered hormone levels and circadian rhythm of activity in the WKY rat, a putative animal model of depression. *Am. J. Physiol. Regul. Integr. Comp. Physiol.* **281**, R786–R794, 2001.

Sommerville, K.W.: Tiagabine – clinical efficacy and use in nonepileptic disorders. In: Levy, R.H., Mattson, R.H., Meldrum, B.S., Perucca, E. (eds): *Antiepileptic Drugs*, 5th edn. Lippincott Williams & Wilkins, Philadelphia, 2002, pp. 705–710.

Song, F., Freemantle, N., Sheldon, T.A., *et al.*: Selective serotonin reuptake inhibitors: meta-analysis of efficacy and acceptability. *Br. Med. J.* **306**, 683–687, 1993.

Song, H., Stevens, C., Gage, F.H.: Astroglia induce neurogenesis from adult neural stem cells. *Nature* **417**, 39–44, 2002.

Southwick, S.M., Morgan, C.A., 3rd, Charney, D.S., *et al.*: Yohimbine use in a natural setting: effects on posttraumatic stress disorder. *Biol. Psychiatry* **46**(3), 442–444, 1999.

Sperling, R., Greve, D., Dale, A., *et al.*: Functional MRI detection of pharmacologically induced memory impairment. *Proc. Natl. Acad. Sci. USA* **99**(1), 455–460, 2002.

Spiegel, R.: *Sleep and Sleeplessness in Advanced Age, Advances in Sleep Research*, Vol. 5. Spectrum, Kluwer Academic Publishers, New York, 1981.

Spiegel, R.: Aspects of sleep, daytime vigilance, mental performance and psychotropic drug treatment in the elderly. *Gerontology* **28** (Suppl. 1), 68–82, 1982.

Spiegel, R.: Zur Voraussage des Therapieerfolgs mit Antidepressiva: Sind kurze REM-Latenzen diagnostisch und prognostisch zuverlässige Merkmale? *Fortschr. Neurol. Psychiatr.* **52**, 302–311, 1984.

Spiegel, R.: *Psychopharmacology – an Introduction*, 2nd edn. John Wiley, Chichester, 1989.

Spiegel, R.: Zur prädiktiven Validität von Phase-I-Studien mit Anti-Demenz-Substanzen (Nootropika). In: Oldigs-Kerber, J., Leonard, J.P. (eds): *Pharmakopsychologie – experimentelle und klinische Aspekte.* G. Fischer, Jena, 1992, pp. 445–458.

Spiegel, R.: *Psychopharmacology – an Introduction*, 3rd edn. John Wiley, Chichester, 1996.

Spiegel, R., Aebi, H.J.: *Psychopharmacology: an Introduction.* John Wiley, Chichester, 1983.

Spiegel, R., Dixon, K.: Psychotropic drug experiments in normal subjects: their relation to animal studies and clinical trials. In: Spiegelstein, M.Y., Levy, A. (eds): *Behavioral Models and the Analysis of Drug Action*. Proc. 27th OHOLO Conf. Elsevier, Amsterdam, 1982, pp. 39–55.

Spielberger, C.D.: *State–Trait Anxiety Inventory: a Comprehensive Bibliography*. Consult Psychologists Press, Palo Alto, 1984.

Spitzer, R.L.: Discussion of paper by Weissman *et al*. In: Spitzer, R.L., Klein, D.F. (eds): *Evaluation of Psychological Therapies*. Johns Hopkins University Press, Baltimore, 1976, p. 178.

Spitzer, R.L., Robins, E., Endicott, J.: Research diagnostic criteria: rationale and reliability. *Arch. Gen. Psychiatry* **35**, 773–782, 1978.

Spooren, W.P.J.M., Schoeffter, P., Gasparini, F., *et al*.: Pharmacological and endocrinological charaterisation of stress-induced hyperthermia in singly housed mice using classical candidate anxiolytics (LY314582, MPEP and NKP608). *Eur. J. Pharmacol.* **435**, 161–170, 2002.

Sramek, J.J., Hurley, D.J., Wardle, T.S., *et al*.: The safety and tolerance of xanomeline tartrate in patients with Alzheimer's disease. *J. Clin. Pharmacol.* **35**, 800–806, 1995.

Staehelin, J.E., Kielholz, P.: Largactil, ein neues vegetatives Dämpfungsmittel bei psychischen Störungen. *Schweiz. Med. Wochenschr.* **83**, 581–586, 1953.

Stain-Malmgren, R., Khoury, A.E., Aberg-Wistedt, A., Tham, A.: Serotonergic function in major depression and effect of sertraline and paroxetine treatment. *Int. Clin. Psychopharmacol.* **16**(2), 93–101, 2001.

Starr, J.M., Whalley, L.J.: Drug-induced dementia. *Drug Safety* **11**, 310–317, 1994.

Stein, E.A., Pankiewicz, J., Harsch, H.H., *et al*.: Nicotine induced limbic cortical activation in the human brain: a functional MRI study. *Am. J. Psychiatry* **155**(8), 1009–1015, 1998.

Stein, M.B., Uhde, T.W.: Biology of anxiety disorders. In: Schatzberg, A.F., Nemeroff, Ch.B. (eds): *Textbook of Psychopharmacology*, 2nd edn. American Psychiatric Press, Washington, DC, 1998, pp. 609–628.

Steiner, M., Steinberg, S., Stewart, D., *et al*.: Fluoxetine in the treatment of premenstrual dysphoria. *N. Engl. J. Med.* **332**, 1529–1534, 1995.

Stenzel-Poore, M.P., Cameron, V.A., Vaughan, J., *et al*.: Development of Cushing's syndrome in corticotropin-releasing factor transgenic mice. *Endocrinology* **130**, 3378–3386, 1992.

Stenzel-Poore, M.P., Heinrichs, S.C., Rivest, S., Koob, G.F., Vale, W.W.: Overproduction of corticotropin-releasing factor in transgenic mice: a genetic model of anxiogenic behavior. *J. Neurosci.* **14**, 2579–2584, 1994.

Stephen, L.J., Brodie, M.J.: Lamotrigine – clinical efficacy and use in epilepsy. In: Levy, R.H., Mattson, R.H., Meldrum, B.S., Perucca, E. (eds): *Antiepileptic Drugs*, 5th edn. Lippincott Williams & Wilkins, Philadelphia, 2002, pp. 389–402.

Sternbach, L.: The benzodiazepine story. In: Jucker, E. (ed.): *Progress in Drug Research*, Vol. 22. Birkhäuser, Basel, 1978, pp. 229–266.

Sternberg, D.E., Jarvik, M.: Memory functions in depression. *Arch. Gen. Psychiatry* **33**, 219–224, 1976.

Steru, L., Chermat, R., Thierry, B., Simon, P.: The tail suspension test: a new method for screening antidepressants in mice. *Psychopharmacology* **85**, 367–370, 1985.

Stille, G., Fischer-Cornelssen, K.: Die Entwicklung von Clozapin (Leponex) – ein Mysterium? [The development of clozapine (Leponex) – a mystery?]. In: Linde, O.K. (ed.): *Pharmakopsychiatrie im Wandel der Zeit*. Tilia-Verlag, Klingenmünster, Germany, 1988, pp. 333–348.

Stoll, W.A.: Lysergsäure-Diäthylamid, ein Phantasticum aus der Mutterkorn-Gruppe. *Schweiz. Arch. Neurol. Psychiatry* **60**, 279–323, 1947.

Stout, S.C., Owens, M.J., Nemeroff, C.B.: Neurokinin-1 receptor antagonists as potential antidepressants. *Annu. Rev. Pharmacol. Toxicol.* **41**, 877–906, 2001.

Strohle, A., Kellner, M., Yassouridis, A., *et al.*: Effect of flumazenil in lactate-sensitive patients with panic disorder. *Am. J. Psychiatry* **155**(5), 610–612, 1998.

Stubbe, D.E.: Attention-deficit/hyperactivity disorder overview. Historical perspective, current controversies, and future directions. *Child Adolesc. Psychiatr. Clin. North Am.* **9**, 469–479, 2000.

Stuppaeck, C.H., Barnas, C., Schwitzer, J., Fleischhacker, W.W.: Carbamazepine in the prophylaxis of major depression: a 5-year follow-up. *J. Clin. Psychiatry* **55**, 146–150, 1994.

Sullivan, J.T., Sykora, K., Schneiderman, J., *et al.*: Assessment of alcohol withdrawal: the revised clinical institute withdrawal assessment for alcohol scale (CIWA-Ar). *Br. J. Addict.* **84**(11), 1353–1357, 1989.

Summers, W.K., Majovski, L.V., Marsh, G.M., Tachiki, K., Kling, A.: Oral tetrahydroaminoacridine in long-term treatment of senile dementia, Alzheimer type. *N. Engl. J. Med.* **315**, 1241–1245, 1986.

Suzman, M.M.: Use of β-adrenergic receptor blocking agents in psychiatry. In: Palmer, G.C. (ed.): *Neuropharmacology of Central Nervous System and Behavioral Disorders.* Academic Press, New York, 1981, pp. 339–391.

Swazey, J.P.: *Chlorpromazine in Psychiatry.* MIT Press. Cambridge, MA, 1974.

Szasz, I.: Some observations on the use of tranquilizing drugs. *Arch. Neurol. Psychiatry* **77**, 86–92, 1957.

Szelies, B.: Brain mapping zur Darstellung altersabhängiger Veränderungen in Abgrenzung von Demenz. *Nervenarzt* **63**, 609–618, 1992.

Talairach, J., Tournoux, P.: *Co-planar Stereotaxic Atlas of the Human Brain: Three-dimensional Proportional System, an Approach to Cerebral Imaging.* Thieme Medical, New York, 1988.

Talamini, L.M., Ellenbroek, B., Koch, T., Korf, J.: Impaired sensory gating and attention in rats with developmental abnormalities of the mesocortex. Implications for schizophrenia. *Ann. NY Acad. Sci.* **911**, 486–494, 2000.

Tancer, M.E., Mailman, R.B., Stein, M.B., Mason, G.A., Carson, S.W., Golden, R.N., *et al.*: Neuroendocrine responsivity to monoaminergic system probes in generalized social phobia. *Anxiety* **1**(5), 216–223, 1994.

Targum, S.D.: Differential responses to anxiogenic challenge studies in patients with major depressive disorder and panic disorder. *Biol. Psychiatry* **28**, 21–34, 1990.

Taylor, J.L., Tinklenberg, J.R.: Cognitive impairment and benzodiazepines. In: Meltzer, H.Y. (ed.): *Psychopharmacology: the Third Generation of Progress.* Raven, New York, 1987, pp. 1449–1454.

Tecce, J.J., Savignano-Bowman, J., Cole, J.O.: Drug effects on contingent negative variation and eyeblinks: the distraction–arousal hypothesis. In: Lipton, M.A., DiMascio, A., Killam, K.F. (eds): *Psychopharmacology: a Generation of Progress.* Raven, New York, 1978, pp. 745–758.

Temple, R.: Are surrogate markers adequate to assess cardiovascular disease drugs? *J. Am. Med. Assoc.* **282**, 790–795, 1999.

Thase, M.E.: How should efficacy be evaluated in randomized clinical trials of treatment for depression. *J. Clin. Psychiatry* **60** (Suppl. 4), 23–31, 1999.

Thase, M.E., Entsuah, A.R., Rudolph, R.I.: Remission rates during treatment with venlafaxine or selective serotonin reuptake inhibitors. *Br. J. Psychiatry* **178**, 234–241, 2001.

Thompson, C.: The use of high-dose antipsychotic medication. *Br. J. Psychiatry* **164**, 448–458, 1994.

Thompson, J.M., Neave, N., Moss, M.C., et al.: Cognitive properties of sedation agents: comparison of the effects of nitrous oxide and midazolam on memory and mood. *Br. Dent. J.* **187**, 557–562, 1999.

Thompson, P.J.: Antidepressants and memory: a review. *Hum. Psychopharmacol.* **6**, 79–90, 1991.

Timoshanko, A., Stough, C., Vitetta, L., Nathan, P.J.: A preliminary investigation on the acute pharmacodynamic effects of hypericum on cognitive and psychomotor performance. *Behav. Pharmacol.* **12**, 635–640, 2001.

Tohen, M., Sanger, T.M., McElroy, S.L., et al.: Olanzapine versus placebo in the treatment of acute mania. *Am. J. Psychiatry* **156**, 702–709, 1999.

Tohen, M., Jacobs, T.C., Grondy, S.L., et al.: A double-blind, placebo-controlled study of olanzapine in patients with acute bipolar mania. *Arch. Gen. Psychiatry* **57**, 841–849, 2000.

Tohen, M., Baker, R.W., Milton, D.R., et al.: Olanzapine versus divalproex sodium for the treatment of acute mania. *Bipolar Disorders* **3**, 60–61, 2001.

Tölle, R.: *Psychiatrie*. Springer, Berlin, 1985.

Tollefson, G.D., Rampey, A.H., Potvin, J.H., et al.: A multicenter investigation of fixed-dose fluoxetine in the treatment of obsessive compulsive disorder. *Arch. Gen. Psychiatry* **51**, 559–567, 1994.

Tomotake, M., Hanano, M., Matsuoka, K., et al.: The acute effects of antidepressants on the human aep (auditory evoked potential) and EEG. *Shikoku Acta Med.* **53**: 75–82, 1997.

Torrance, G.W., Feeny, D.: Utilities and quality-adjusted life years. *Int. J. Technol. Assess. Health Care* **5**, 559–575, 1989.

Tsai, G., Coyle, J.T.: Glutamatergic mechanisms in schizophrenia. *Annu. Rev. Pharmacol. Toxicol.* **42**, 165–179, 2002.

Tsai, G., Yang, P., Chung, L., et al.: D-Serine added to antipsychotic for the treatment of schizophrenia. *Biol. Psychiatry* **44**, 1081–1089, 1998.

Tupper, D., Hotten, T., Moore, N.: Presentation on olanzapine, given at the *Society for Medicines Research Millennial Case Histories of Drug Discovery and Design Meeting*, London, 2 December 1999.

Turner, P.: Drugs and the special senses. *Semin. Drug Treat.* **1**, 335–353, 1971.

Uhlenhuth, E.H.: Depressives, doctors, and antidepressants. *J. Am. Med. Assoc.* **248**, 1879–1880, 1982.

Uhlenhuth, E.H., DeWitt, H., Balter, M.B., Johanson, Ch.E., Mellinger, G.D.: Risks and benefits of long-term benzodiazepine use. *J. Clin. Psychopharmacol.* **8**, 161–167, 1988.

Uhr, L., Miller, J.C.: *Drugs and Behavior*. John Wiley, New York, 1964.

Urata, J., Uchiyama, M., Iyo, M., et al.: Effects of a small dose of triazolam on P300 and resting EEG. *Psychopharmacology* **125**, 179–184, 1996.

Van Eijk, M.E.C., Avorn, J., Porsius, A.J., de Boer, A.: Reducing prescribing of highly anticholinergic antidepressants for elderly people: randomised trial of group versus individual academic detailing. *Br. Med. J.* **322**, 1–6, 2001.

Van Laar, M.W., Volkerts, E.R., Verbaten, M.N., et al.: Differential effects of amitriptyline, nefazodone and paroxetine on performance and brain indices of visual selective attention and working memory. *Psychopharmacology* **162**, 351–363, 2002.

Van Leeuwen, T.H., Verbaten, M.N., Koelega, H.S., et al.: Effects of oxazepam on event-related brain potentials, EEG frequency bands, and vigilance performance. *Psychopharmacology* **122**, 244–262, 1995.

Van Putten, T., May, P.R.A., Marder, S.R.: Response to antipsychotic medication, the doctor's and the consumer's view. *Am. J. Psychiatry* **141**, 16–19, 1984.

Van Vliet, I.M., Westenberg, H.G., Slaap, B.R., *et al.*: Anxiogenic effects of pentagastrin in patients with social phobia and healthy controls. *Biol. Psychiatry* **42**(1), 76–78, 1997.

Varga, E., Sugerman, A.A., Varga, V., *et al.*: Prevalence of spontaneous oral dyskinesia in the elderly. *Am. J. Psychiatry* **139**, 329–331, 1982.

Vassout, A., Veenstra, S., Hauser, K., *et al.*: NKP608: a selective NK1 receptor antagonist with anxiolytic-like effects in the social interaction and social exploration test in rats. *Regul. Pept.* **96**, 7–16, 2000.

Vogel, G.W., Buffenstein, A., Minter, K., Hennessey, A.: Drug effects on REM sleep and on endogenous depression. *Neurosci. Biobehav. Rev.* **14**, 49–63, 1990.

Volavka, J., Czobor, P., Sheitman, B., *et al.*: Clozapine, olanzapine, risperidone, and haloperidol in the treatment of patients with chronic schizophrenia and schizoaffective disorder. *Am. J. Psychiatry* **159**, 255–262, 2002.

Volkow, N.D., Mullani, N., Gould, L., *et al.*: Effects of acute alcohol intoxication on cerebral blood flow measured by PET. *Psychiatry Res.* **24**(2), 201–209, 1988.

Volkow, N.D., Wang, G.J., Fowler, J.S., *et al.*: Relationship between blockade of dopamine transporters by oral methylphenidate and the increases in extracellular dopamine: therapeutic implications. *Synapse* **43**(3): 181–187, 2002.

Wahlstrom, A., Lenhammar, L., Ask, B., Rane, A.: Tricyclic antidepressants inhibit opioid receptor binding in human brain and hepatic morphine glucuronidation. *Pharmacol. Toxicol.* **75**(1), 23–27, 1994.

Walsh, B.T., Seidman, S.N., Sysko, R., Gould, M.: Placebo response in studies of major depression. *J. Am. Med. Assoc.* **287**, 1840–1847, 2002.

Wang, D., Chalk, J.B., Rose, S.E., *et al.*: MR image-based measurement of rates of change in volumes of brain structures. Part II: Application to a study of Alzheimer's disease and normal aging. *Magn. Res. Imag.* **20**, 41–48, 2002.

Wang, G.J., Volkow, N.D., Franceschi, D., *et al.*: Regional brain metabolism during alcohol intoxication. *Alcohol. Clin. Exp. Res.* **24**(6), 822–829, 2000.

Wardle, J.: Behaviour therapy and benzodiazepines: Allies or antagonists? *Br. J. Psychiatry* **156**, 163–168, 1990.

Ware, J.E. Jr.: SF-36 *Health Survey: Manual and Interpretation Guide.* The Health Institute, New England Medical Center, Boston, MA, 1993.

Ware, J.E. Jr., Kosisnski, M., Keller, S.D.: *SF-36: Physical and Mental Health Summary Scores: a User's Manual.* The Health Institute, New England Medical Center, Boston, MA, 1994.

Wechsler, D.: *Wechsler Intelligence Scale for Children, Third Edition – Revised.* Psychological Corporation, New York, 1992.

Weingartner, H.: Human state dependent learning. In: Ho, B.T., Richards, D.N., Chute, D.L. (eds): *Drug Discrimination and State Dependent Learning.* Academic Press, New York, 1978, pp. 361–382.

Weingartner, H., Silberman, E.: Models of cognitive impairment: cognitive changes in depression. *Psychopharmacol. Bull.* **18**, 27–42, 1982.

Weisbrod, B.A., Test, M.A., Stein, L.I.: Alternatives to mental hospital treatment: economic cost–benefit analysis. *Arch. Gen. Psychiatry* **37**, 400–405, 1980.

Weiss, B., Laties, V.C.: Enhancement of human performance by caffeine and the amphetamines. *Pharmacol. Rev.* **14**, 1–36, 1962.

Weiss, E.M., Bilder, R.M., Fleischhacker, W.W.: The effects of second-generation antipsychotics on cognitive functioning and psychosocial outcome in schizophrenia. *Psychopharmacology* **162**, 11–17, 2002.

Weiss, G., Hechtman, L.T.: *Hyperactive Children Grown Up: Empirical Findings and Theoretical Considerations.* Guilford Press, New York, 1986.

Weissman, M.M.: Psychotherapy and its relevance to the pharmacotherapy of affective disorders: from ideology to evidence. In: Lipton, M.A., DiMascio, A., Killam, K.F. (eds): *Psychopharmacology: a Generation of Progress.* Raven, New York, 1978, pp. 1313–1321.

Weissman, M.M., Klerman, G.L., Paykel, E.S., Prusoff, B., Hanson, B.: Treatment effects on the social adjustment of depressed patients. *Arch. Gen. Psychiatry* **30**, 771–778, 1974.

Weissman, M.M., Prusoff, B.A., Di Mascio, A., *et al.*: The efficacy of drugs and psychotherapy in the treatment of acute depressive episodes. *Am. J. Psychiatry* **136**, 555–558, 1979.

Weissman, M.M., Jarrett, R.B., Rush, J.A.: Psychotherapy and its relevance to the pharmacotherapy of major depression: a decade later (1976–1985). In: Meltzer, H.Y. (ed.): *Psychopharmacology: the Third Generation of Progress.* Raven, New York, 1987, pp. 1059–1069.

Welkowitz, L.A., Papp, L.A., Cloitre, M., *et al.*: Cognitive–behavior therapy for panic disorder delivered by psychopharmacologically oriented clinicians. *J. Nerv. Ment. Dis.* **179**, 473–477, 1991.

Welner, A., Welner, Z., Robins, E.: Effect of tricyclic antidepressants on individual symptoms. *J. Clin. Psychiatry* **41**, 306–309, 1980.

Wennberg, J.E.: Dealing with medical practice variations: a proposal for action. *Health Affairs (Millwood)* **3**(2), 6–32, 1984.

Westra, H.A., Stewart, S.H.: Cognitive behavioral therapy and pharmacotherapy: complementary or contradictory approaches to the treatment of anxiety? *Clin. Psychol. Rev.* **18**, 307–340, 1998.

Wettstein, A., Spiegel, R.: Clinical trials with the cholinergic drug RS 86 in Alzheimer's disease (AD) and senile dementia of the Alzheimer type (SDAT). *Psychopharmacology* **84**, 572–573, 1984.

Whalen, C.K., Henker, B., Collins, B.E., Finck, D., Dotemoto, S.: A social ecology of hyperactive boys: medication effects in structured classroom environments. *J. Appl. Behav. Anal.* **12**, 65–81, 1979.

Wiggins, J.G.: Would you want your child to be a psychologist? *Am. Psychol.* **49**, 485–492, 1994.

Wilcox, C.S., Cohn, J.B., Linden, R.D., *et al.*: Predictors of placebo response: a retrospective analysis. *Psychopharmacol. Bull.* **28**(2), 157–162, 1992.

Wilens, T.E., Biederman, J.: The stimulants. *Psychiatr. Clin. North Am.* **15**, 191–222, 1992.

Wilens, T.E., Biederman, J., Spencer, T.J.: Pharmacotherapy of attention deficit hyperactivity disorder in adults. *CNS Drugs* **9**, 347–356, 1998.

Willam, A.R., Pater, J.L.: Carryover and the two-period crossover clinical trial. *Biometrics* **42**(3), 593–599, 1986.

Williams, J.B.W.: A structured interview guide for the Hamilton Depression Rating Scale. *Arch. Gen. Psychiatry* **45**, 742–747, 1988.

Wilson, S.J., Bailey, J.E., Alford, C., Nutt, D.J.: Sleep and daytime sleepiness the next day following single night-time dose of fluvoxamine, dothiepin and placebo in normal volunteers. *J. Psychopharmacol.* **14**, 378–386, 2000.

Wistedt, B., Jorgensen, A., Wiles, D.: A depot neuroleptic withdrawal study. *Psychopharmacology* **78**, 301–304, 1982.

Wittern, R.: Die Geschichte psychotroper Drogen vor der Aera der modernen Psychopharmaka. In: Langer, G., Heimann, H. (eds): *Psychopharmaka: Grundlagen und Therapie.* Springer, Vienna, 1983, pp. 3–19.

Woggon, B.: Neuroleptika-Absetzversuche bei chronisch schizophrenen Patienten. *Int. Pharmacopsychiatry* **14**, 34–56, 1979.

Wolfson, C., Oremus, M., Shukla, V., *et al.*: Donepezil and rivastigmine in the treatment of Alzheimer's disease: a best-evidence synthesis of the published data on their efficacy and cost-effectiveness. *Clin. Ther.* **24**, 862–886, 2002.

Wolozin, B.: Cholesterol and Alzheimer's disease. *Biochem. Soc. Trans.* **30**, 525–529, 2002.

Wooley, D.W., Shaw, E.: A biochemical and pharmacological suggestion about certain mental disorders. *Proc. Natl. Acad. Sci. USA* **40**, 228–231, 1954.

World Health Organization: *The World Health Report 2001. Mental Health, New Understanding, New Hope.* World Health Organization, Geneva, 2001.

Wyatt, R.J.: Early intervention with neuroleptics may decrease the long-term morbidity of schizophrenia. *Schizophr. Res.* **5**(3), 201–202, 1991..

Wyatt, R.J., Henter, I. Rationale for the study of early intervention. *Schizophr. Res.* **51**, 69–76, 2001.

Yoshii, F., Barker, W.W., Chang, J.Y., Loewenstein, D., Apicella, A., Smith, D., *et al.*: Sensitivity of cerebral glucose metabolism to age, gender, brain volume, brain atrophy, and cerebrovascular risk factors. *J. Cerebr. Blood Flow Metab.* **8**(5), 654–661, 1988.

Young, R.C., Biggs, J.T., Ziegler, V.E., *et al.*: A rating scale for mania: reliability, validity and sensitivity. *Br. J. Psychiatry* **133**, 420–435, 1978.

Zethof, T.J.J, van der Heyden, J.A.M., Tolboom, J.B.M., Olivier, B.: Stress-induced hyperthermia in mice: a methodological study. *Physiol. Behav.* **55**, 109–115, 1994.

Zigmond, A.S., Snaith, R.P.: The hospital anxiety and depression scale. *Acta Psychiatr. Scand.* **67**, 361–370, 1983.

Zipursky, R.B., Schulz, S.C.: *The Early Stages of Schizophrenia.* American Psychiatric Press, Washington, DC, 2002.

Zobel, A.W., Nickel, T., Künzel, H.E., *et al.*: Effects of the high-affinity corticotropin-releasing hormone receptor 1 antagonist R121919 in major depression: the first 20 patients treated. *J. Psychiatr. Res.* **34**, 171–181, 2000.

Zomberg, G.L., Pope, M.C., Jr.: Treatment of depression in bipolar disorder: new directions for research. *J. Clin. Psychopharmacol.* **13**, 397–408, 1993.

Zung, W.W.: The depression status inventory: an adjunct to the Self-Rating Depression Scale. *J. Clin. Psychol.* **28**(4), 539–543, 1972.

Zwanzger, P., Baghai, T.C., Schuele, C., *et al.*: Vigabatrin decreases cholecystokinin-tetrapeptide (CCK-4) induced panic in healthy volunteers. *Neuropsychopharmacology* **25**(5), 699–703, 2001.

Index

Note: page numbers in *italics* refer to figures; page numbers in **bold** refer to tables.

Psychopharmacology, Fourth Edition. By R. Spiegel
© 2003 John Wiley & Sons, Ltd: ISBN 0 471 56039 1: 0 470 84691 7 (PB)

Index compiled by L. N. Derrick